Scientific and Philosophical Perspectives in Neuroethics

While neuroscience has provided insights in to the structure and function of nervous systems, hard questions remain about the nature of consciousness, mind, and self. Perhaps the most difficult questions involve the meaning of neuroscientific information, and how to pursue and utilize neuroscientific knowledge in ways that are consistent with some construal of social ``good.''

Written for researchers and graduate students in neuroscience and bioethics, *Scientific and Philosophical Perspectives in Neuroethics* explores important developments in neuroscience and neurotechnology, and addresses the philosophical, ethical, and social issues and problems that such advancements generate. It examines three core questions. First, what is the scope and direction of neuroscientific inquiry? Second, how has progress to date affected scientific and philosophical ideas, and finally, what ethical issues and problems do this progress and knowledge incur, both now and in the future?

JAMES J. GIORDANO is a Fellow of the Centre for Philosophical Psychology, Blackfriars Hall, University of Oxford, and Director of the Center for Neurotechnology Studies, Potomac Institute for Policy Studies, Arlington, VA (USA). His interests center around the neuroscience and neurophilosophy of pain, and the neuroethical issues arising from the development and uses of neurotechnologies in pain care, psychiatry, and public life.

BERT GORDIJN is Professor of Ethics and Director of the Institute of Ethics at Dublin City University. He is also Secretary of the European Society for Philosophy of Medicine and Health Care and the Irish Chapter of the European Business Ethics Network. His current research interests focus on ethical issues in nanotechnology, geoengineering, and neurotechnology.

Scientific and Philosophical Perspectives in Neuroethics

Edited by

JAMES J. GIORDANO, PH.D.
IPS Centre for Philosophical Psychology
University of Oxford, UK

BERT GORDIJN, PH.D.
Dublin City University
Dublin, Ireland

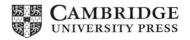
CAMBRIDGE
UNIVERSITY PRESS

CAMBRIDGE UNIVERSITY PRESS
Cambridge, New York, Melbourne, Madrid, Cape Town, Singapore,
São Paulo, Delhi, Dubai, Tokyo

Cambridge University Press
The Edinburgh Building, Cambridge CB2 8RU, UK

Published in the United States of America by
Cambridge University Press, New York

www.cambridge.org
Information on this title: www.cambridge.org/9780521878555

First published 2010

Printed in the United Kingdom at the University Press, Cambridge

A catalogue record for this publication is available from the British Library

Library of Congress Cataloguing in Publication data
Scientific and philosophical perspectives in neuroethics /
   [edited by] James J. Giordano, Bert Gordijn.
      p. ; cm.
   Includes bibliographical references and index.
   ISBN 978-0-521-87855-5 (hardback) – ISBN 978-0-521-70303-1 (Pbk.)
   1. Neurology–Moral and ethical aspects.   2. Neurosciences–Moral
   and ethical aspects.   I. Giordano, James J.   II. Gordijn, Bert, 1965–
   III. Title.
   [DNLM: 1. Neurology–ethics.   2. Neurosciences–ethics.   3. Bioethical
   Issues. WL 21 S416 2010]
   RC343.S35 2010
   174.2′968–dc22   2009037854

ISBN 978-0-521-87855-5 Hardback
ISBN 978-0-521-70303-1 Paperback

To Edmund Pellegrino,
physician, scholar, teacher, mentor, friend, and inspiration
``. . . *recta ratio agibilium*´´

Contents

List of contributors	*page* ix
Preface	xiii
N. LEVY	
Acknowledgments	xxiii
Introduction	xxv
J. J. GIORDANO	
1	Developments in neuroscience	1
	D. F. SWAAB	
2	The origins of the modern concept of ``neuroscience´´	37
	N. KOHLS & R. BENEDIKTER	
3	On the cusp	66
	R. D. ELLIS	
4	The mind–body issue	95
	D. BIRNBACHER	
5	Personal identity and the nature of the self	117
	P. COSTA	
6	Religious issues and the question of moral autonomy	134
	A. AUTIERO & L. GALVAGNI	
7	Toward a cognitive neurobiology of the moral virtues	146
	P. M. CHURCHLAND	
8	From a neurophilosophy of pain to a neuroethics of pain care	172
	J. J. GIORDANO	
9	Transplantation and xenotransplantation	190
	G. J. BOER	
10	Neurogenetics and ethics	216
	K. FITZGERALD & R. WURZMAN	

11   Neuroimaging   230
     J. VANMETER
12   Can we read minds?   244
     E. RACINE, E. BELL & J. ILLES
13   Possibilities, limits, and implications of
     brain–computer interfacing technologies   271
     T. HINTERBERGER
14   Neural engineering   283
     B. GORDIJN & A. M. BUYX
15   Neurotechnology as a public good   302
     A. M. JEANNOTTE, K. N. SCHILLER,
     L. M. REEVES, E. G. DERENZO & D. K. MCBRIDE
16   Globalization: pluralist concerns and contexts   321
     R. H. BLANK
17   The human condition and strivings to flourish   343
     A. GINI & J. J. GIORDANO
18   The limits of neuro-talk   355
     M. B. CRAWFORD

     Afterword   370
     W. GLANNON
     Index   375

Contributors

Antonio Autiero
Seminar für Moraltheologie, Westfälische Wilhelms-Universität Münster, Zimmer 17, Johannisstrasse 8–10, D-48143 Münster, Germany

Emily Bell
Neuroethics Research Unit, Institut de recherches cliniques de Montréal (IRCM), 110, avenue des Pins Quest, Montréal, Québec, Canada H2W 1R7

Roland Benedikter
Orfalea Center for Global and International Studies, University of California at Santa Barbara, Humanities and Social Sciences Building, Room 3044, Mail Code 7065, Santa Barbara, CA 93106–7065, USA

Dieter Birnbacher
Philosophisches Institut, Heinrich-Heine-Universität, Universitäts-strasse 1, 40225 Düsseldorf, Germany

Robert H. Blank
Political Science and Communication, University of Canterbury, Private Bag 4800, Christchurch, New Zealand

Gerard J. Boer
Department of Neuroregeneration, Netherlands Institute for Neuro-science, Meibergdreef 47, 1105 BA Amsterdam, The Netherlands

Alena M. Buyx
Institut für Ethik, Geschichte und Theorie der Medizin, Universitäts-klinikum Münster, Von-Esmarch-Strasse 62, D-48149 Münster, Germany

Paul M. Churchland
Cognitive Science Faculty, University of California, San Diego, 9500 Gilman Drive, La Jolla, CA 92093–0119, USA

Paolo Costa
Instituto Trentino di Cultura, Via Santa Croce 77, 38100 Trento, Italy

Matthew B. Crawford
Institute for Advanced Studies in Culture, University of Virginia, P. O.
Box 400816, University of Virginia, Charlottesville, VA 22904–4816, USA

Evan G. DeRenzo
Center for Ethics, Washington Hospital Center, 110 Irving Street, NW,
Washington, DC 20010, USA

Ralph D. Ellis
Department of Religion and Philosophy, Clark Atlanta University, 223
James P. Brawley Drive, SW Atlanta, GA 30314, USA

Kevin FitzGerald
Center for Clinical Bioethics, Georgetown University, 4000 Reservoir
Rd, Washington, DC 20057, USA

Lucia Galvagni
Instituto Trentino di Cultura, Via Santa Croce 77, 38100 Trento, Italy

Adriana Gini
Faculty of Bioethics, Regina Apostolorum Pontifical Athenaeum, Via
degli Aldobrandeschi 190, 00163 Rome, Italy

James Giordano
IPS Centre for Philosophical Psychology, University of Oxford, OX1, UK,
and Potomac Institute for Policy Studies, 901 N. Stuart St. Suite 900,
Arlington, VA 22203, USA

Walter Glannon
Department of Philosophy, University of Calgary, Calgary, Alberta,
Canada T2N 1N4

Bert Gordijn
Ethics Institute, Dublin City University, Dublin 9, Ireland

Thilo Hinterberger
Institut für Umweltmedizin und Krankenhaushygiene (Department of
Environmental Health Sciences), Universitätsklinikum Freiburg, Breisa-
cher Strasse 115 b, 79106 Freiburg, Germany

Judy Illes
2211 Wesbrook Mall, National Core for Neuroethics, Koerner S124,
Vancouver, BC, Canada V6T 2B5

Alexis M. Jeannotte
Center for Neurotechnology Studies, Potomac Institute for Policy Studies, 901 N. Stuart St. Suite 900, Arlington, VA 22203, USA

Niko Kohls
Humanwissenschaftlichen Zentrum, Ludwig-Maximilians-Universität München, Prof.-Max-Lange-Platz 11, 83646 Bad Tölz, Germany

Neil Levy
Faculty of Philosophy, University of Oxford, 10 Merton Street, Oxford OX1 4JJ, UK

Dennis K. McBride
Potomac Institute for Policy Studies, 901 N. Stuart St. Suite 900, Arlington, VA 22203, USA

Eric Racine
Neuroethics Research Unit, Institut de Recherches Cliniques de Montréal (IRCM), 110, avenue des Pins Ouest, Montréal, Québec H2W 1R7, Canada

Leah M. Reeves
Center for Neurotechnology Studies, Potomac Institute for Policy Studies, 901 N. Stuart St. Suite 900, Arlington, VA 22203, USA

Kathryn N. Schiller
Center for Neurotechnology Studies, Potomac Institute for Policy Studies, 901 N. Stuart St. Suite 900, Arlington, VA 22203, USA

D. F. Swaab
Netherlands Institute for Neuroscience, Meibergdreef 47, 1105 BA Amsterdam, The Netherlands

John VanMeter
Department of Neuroimaging, Georgetown University Medical Center, 4000 Reservoir Road NW, Suite 120, Washington, DC 20007, USA

Rachel Wurzman
Interdisciplinary Program in Neurosciences, Georgetown University Medical Center, 4000 Reservoir Road NW, Suite 120, Washington, DC 20007, USA

Preface

NEIL LEVY

Neuroethics is a truly exciting endeavor. For a very long time, human beings have puzzled over questions concerning the fundamental nature of the world in which we live and of ourselves. Why be moral? Do we have free will? How should we behave towards one another? Can we know anything? These are the questions of the discipline that has come to be called philosophy. For most of human history, these questions were pursued using the full range of tools available, but sometime in the recent past – perhaps as late as the nineteenth century – the philosophical questions became separated from scientific questions. Each was seen to have its own distinctive methodology, its own tools and conceptual resources; philosophers thought it was a mistake to think that science could shed much light on their research.

Neuroethics, along with a number of related developments (experimental philosophy; philosophy of biology; cognitive science) is part of a backlash against this separation. Science is the crowning achievement of human epistemology; its distinctive methods help to compensate for our cognitive limitations and to build a cumulative and reliable body of knowledge to an extent unprecedented in human history. For philosophers to cut themselves off from this body of knowledge would be madness. But philosophers have skills, in conceptual analysis and logic, that prove invaluable in understanding the human significance of science. Moreover, philosophers have a tradition of their own to draw upon, the fruits of which are, in some ways, no less impressive than the fruits of science. Drawing together science and philosophy promises to contribute to our understanding of human life, of our philosophical questions, to a degree unmatched by either alone.

But neuroethics is also important for another reason. The ethical issues with which it is concerned are truly pressing. It is illuminating, in this regard, to compare neuroethics to the applied ethics discipline that preceded it: bioethics. Bioethics grew out of concerns over the potential for abuse of the dizzying array of new technologies stemming from the life sciences over the past three or four decades. These technologies were concerned with central aspects of human existence: with nothing less than the power of bringing life into the world and of extending it or ending it. Thus, the relevant technologies (from IVF through to stem cells and the genomic revolution) were properly the focus of moral concern. Yet, significant though these technologies undoubtedly are, there is a case for saying that techniques and technologies stemming from the sciences of the mind raise yet more profound questions about what it means to be human, and pose greater challenges to moral thought.

What could be more significant than life? There is a traditional answer to this question: the soul. Now the soul, if there is any such thing, is the province of theologians. But the closest secular equivalent of the soul is surely the mind. It is our minds that make us the individuals we are, at least on one plausible conception of personal identity; indisputably it is our minds that make us matter, morally, and which make our relationships meaningful. But the sciences of the mind seem to promise, or threaten, nothing less than the power to take control of the human mind, altering it, enhancing it, and remaking it as we wish. Given that the mind is the closest secular equivalent to the soul, there is no surprise that many wonder if this is a power that we ought to have.

Consider some of the potential applications envisaged – some of them arguably already available, in a crude form – as stemming from the sciences of the mind. Already there are technologies that their advocates hold allow us to determine, with some degree of certitude, whether someone is lying or telling the truth. But this is only the first step toward the development of mind-reading technologies, some think. We have made huge steps in the direction of directly reading thoughts from the brain: judging how subjects have chosen to resolve an ambiguous figure, thinking of a particular person or building; we can even predict, with 60% accuracy, which of two buttons a subject will choose to push a full ten seconds before they press! Some fear that this is a technology with frightening implications, putting Orwellian paranoia in the shade. In the wrong hands, reliable thought-reading machines would be the ultimate invaders of our privacy. Moreover, with a technology this powerful, are any hands right? We should recall the adage: power corrupts; absolute power corrupts absolutely.

Some philosophers suspect that we have little to worry about, at least for the near future, and perhaps always; that genuine mind-reading machines will be forever out of reach. But if mind-reading is frightening, how much more worrying is mind *control*? This, unfortunately, is not a technology likely to prove impossible: in some form it is already here.

We can use techniques from the sciences of the mind covertly to modulate thought in a variety of ways. We can use oxytocin, a neurotransmitter that is potentially deliverable in a gas, to increase the propensity of people to trust. Trust, we might think, is generally a good thing – but think of how this power might be used by demagogic politicians, or used car salespeople. We can structure the environment that subjects encounter in ways known to run down their resources of self-control: we might do this, too, to increase sales. We can administer a beta-blocker, Propranolol, to dim people's memories. In the future, we might be able to intervene more dramatically, perhaps erasing precisely targeted memories or inserting new beliefs (though once again some philosophers think that this will prove impossible, given the holistic nature of belief).

These are obviously frightening possibilities. But perhaps we ought to worry less about what might be done, sometime in the future, and instead be concerned with what is happening right now. We need not wait to see technologies stemming from the sciences of the mind widely applied. It is happening right now, on a truly vast scale. In 2004, twelve million prescriptions for anti-depressants were dispensed through the Pharmaceutical Benefits Scheme in Australia alone (Bell 2005); this is a state of affairs that is replicated across the developed world (and increasingly common in the developing world too). More worrying for many people is the use of methylphenidate for the treatment of attention deficit hyperactivity disorder (ADHD), since this is a drug that is overwhelmingly dispensed to children and adolescents. Are we medicating away childhood, some ask?

Concerns about the widespread use of psychopharmaceuticals center on issues concerned with authenticity (Elliott 1998), the mechanization of mind (Freedman 1998), and the proper attitude we ought to have toward them (Sandel 2007), as well as on the potential for injustice they seem to carry when they enhance cognitive ability (e.g. Sahakian & Morein-Zamir 2007). All these questions are urgent and intrinsically fascinating; on their resolution rests the shape of the society we shall shape for ourselves.

So neuroethics has two branches: ethical reflection on new technologies and techniques produced by neuroscience (and other sciences of the mind), closely analogous to – sometimes overlapping with – the kinds of issues that are the traditional territory of bioethics, and a second branch, which resembles more closely traditional philosophy of mind and moral psychology than it does bioethics. Roskies (2002) calls these two enterprises the ethics of neuroscience and the neuroscience of ethics. A central reason for the fascination of neuroethics is that these two branches are not separate; instead, the results we obtain from reflecting on the mind in ways that are informed by the sciences of the mind inform our understanding of the ethical issues we consider under the heading of the ethics of neuroscience. In the rest of this foreword, I consider how this comes about.

RATIONALITY

When we reflect upon moral problems, we hope thereby to come to rational solutions. We aim to assess whether, say, cognitive enhancement will really have the effects that some fear on the texture of our society, or whether it is really innocuous; if it is likely to have negative effects we need to discover what are the best ways to avoid or mitigate these effects and how effective social policy is best implemented to this end. All of this requires rational enquiry. One way in which the sciences of the mind could dramatically affect our ethical enquiries is by demonstrating that we cannot engage in this kind of rational thought, at all, or to anything like the extent to which we hitherto believed.

The sciences of the mind threaten our conception of ourselves as able to engage in rational reflection in many ways. First, they apparently show that far fewer of our actions are guided by reasons than we might have thought. The evidence here comes largely from work in social psychology, on the *automaticity* of actions. Automatic actions are effortless, ballistic (uninterruptible once initiated), and typically unconsciously initiated; that is, they are not made in response to conscious reasons of ours but are instead more like reflexes, triggered by features of the situation in which we find ourselves. In the influential terminology introduced by Stanovich (1999), automatic actions are system 1 processes, not slow, effortful, conscious, and deliberative system 2 processes. System 1 processes are evolutionarily more ancient; they are the kind of cognitive process we share with many other animals, whereas system 2 processes are the kind distinctive of us. If we are rational animals, and that is what distinguishes us, it is only inasmuch as we deploy system 2 processes that this is true. The threatening finding from social psychology is not that we often deploy system 1 processes; it is that these are *by far* the more common. The overwhelming majority of human actions are guided by automatic mental processes (Bargh & Chartrand 1999). In the light of the sciences of the mind, our claim to be rational animals suddenly looks somewhat shaky.

Worse is to come. Even when we do deploy system 2 processes, the rationality of our thought is less than we might have hoped. The evidence for this claim comes largely from cognitive psychology, especially work in the heuristics and biases traditions. *Heuristics* are mental short cuts and rules of thumb that we deploy, usually without realizing we are doing so; *biases* are the ways in which we weight the significance of information in making judgments. There is a huge mass of evidence showing that when we assess arguments or make decisions, we deploy such heuristics and biases, often in ways that mislead us. I shall mention only a few of the ways in which we assess information badly.

Human beings are pervasively subject to the *confirmation bias*, a systematic tendency to search for evidence that supports a hypothesis we are entertaining, rather than evidence that refutes it, and to interpret ambiguous evidence so that it supports our hypothesis (Nickerson 1998). The confirmation bias (along with a substantial dose of wishful thinking) helps to explain many people´s belief in supernatural events. Suppose your hypothesis is that dreams foretell the future. The confirmation bias makes it likely that you will pay attention to confirming evidence (that time you dreamt that your aunt was unwell, only to learn that around that time she had a bad fall) and disregard disconfirming evidence (all the times when you dreamt about good or bad things happening to people you know when no such event occurred). The confirmation bias works in conjunction with the *availability heuristic*, our tendency to base assessments of the probability of an event on the ease with which instances can be brought to mind (Tversky & Kahneman 1973). Because confirming instances are more easily recalled, memory searches, carried out in good faith, lead us to conclude that our hypothesis is true.

You may think that the tendency to believe in the supernatural is harmless and trivial. This may or may not be right (think of the occasional cases of parents preferring to have their seriously ill children treated by new-age healers rather than qualified physicians), but there is no doubt that the kind of biases at issue here do real world harm. One instance is the recent rash of claims involving ``recovered memories´´ of sexual assault. There is no evidence that *any* such recovered memories were true, but we do know that many of them were false. There is therefore no reason to regard such memories as reliable. Yet on the basis of this evidence, many people were imprisoned, and many more families ruptured irrevocably. Why was there this sudden rash of recovered memories? Part of the explanation lies in the techniques used by some therapists to elicit possible repressed memories. Since they believed that these memories were deeply repressed, they encouraged their patients to visualize events they could not recall, or to pretend that they happened. But these techniques are known to be effective in producing false memories, or in otherwise bringing people to mistake imaginings for reality (Loftus 1993). Why did they do this? Confirmation bias helps to explain their behavior: they noticed that patients sometimes appeared to improve when they used these techniques, and ignored alternative explanations of these improvements (was the mere fact that someone was listening to them helping their mental state? Might the passing of time by itself be playing a role?) and ignored cases in which the techniques failed to help (Tavris & Aronson 2007). Ignorance of our systematic biases and cognitive limitations – for instance, on the part of patients who take the vividness of a ``memory´´ as evidence of its veracity, of therapists who are unaware of the need to test hypotheses systematically, and courts who take sincere memory and eyewitness testimony as irrefutable evidence – can cause great harm.

The example of repressed memory has two morals for us. First, it helps to suggest how the issues dealt with by neuroethics are practically important. Applying the knowledge gained from the sciences of the mind, in court rooms and in clinical practices, would lead to less harm and more good. Second, however, we should appreciate how disturbing is the evidence of the limitations of our rationality, the fallibility of our memory, and the unreliability of our experience as a guide to reality. We think we are rational beings; we think that our memories are transcriptions of past events, we think that we have a good grasp of what the world immediately around us is like, but we may be wrong.

MORALITY

Threats to rationality are perfectly general; they threaten our ability to engage in rational deliberation across all domains. In addition to these general threats, there are threats more particularly to *moral* deliberation. In the eyes of some, the sciences of the mind demonstrate that we are not capable of deliberating about moral questions. The threats to moral deliberation are of two kinds: those that threaten moral deliberation across the board, and those that focus on a particular account of moral judgment or a particular (purportedly) moral principle.

Much of this work purports to show that moral deliberation is too emotional to be truly rational, thereby placing pressure on particular moral theories. One of the most influential theories, the theory that (arguably at least) underlies the notion of human rights, is *deontology*, the theory, most closely associated with Immanuel Kant, that morality is essentially about rights and duties. One way to understand deontology and its associated rights and duties is as follows: these rights and duties place constraints on what we might do to improve general welfare. That is, we ought always to improve welfare, *except when* doing so would infringe a right; then we have a duty to refrain from acting to improve general welfare. Consider a well-known illustration, the famous trolley problem (Foot 1978). The problem is designed to demonstrate how rights constrain welfare maximization. In the problem, we are presented with two variants of a scenario in which we might act to maximize welfare, by saving the greater number of people:

(1)   Imagine you find yourselves by the tracks when you see an oncoming trolley heading for a group of five people. The people cannot escape from their predicament and will certainly be killed if you do nothing. In front of you is a lever; if you pull it, you will divert the trolley to a side-track, where it will certainly hit and kill one person. Should you pull the lever?

Most philosophers have the intuition that we ought to pull the lever; moreover, most ordinary people, tested by the growing number of psychologists interested in morality, agree (Cushman *et al.* 2006). But now consider this variation on the problem:

(2)   Imagine you find yourself on a bridge over the tracks when you see an oncoming trolley heading for a group of five people. The people cannot escape from their predicament and will certainly be killed if you do nothing. Next to you is a very large man. You realize that if you push the large man onto the tracks, his great bulk will stop the trolley (whereas your slight frame will not); he will certainly die, but the five people on the tracks will be safe. Should you push the large man?

Most philosophers have the intuition that you should *not* push the large man; once again, most ordinary people agree (in fact, the split is about the same in both cases, with around 90% of people in the same camp (Hauser 2006)). At first glance, this is puzzling: the cases seem to be relevantly similar. In both, you are faced with the choice of acting to save five people at the cost of one. Why should it be right to save the five in case (1), but not (2)?

The standard answer is that people have rights, including a right to life, and that pushing the large man would infringe his rights. But redirecting the trolley is not infringing anyone's rights (perhaps because we use the large man as a means to an end – were it not for his bulk, we could not stop the trolley – but since the presence of the man on the side-track is not necessary for stopping the trolley, we do not use him as a means). Recent research by neuroscientists has thrown doubt on this explanation.

Greene *et al.* (2001) scanned the brains of subjects considering the trolley problem and similarly structured dilemmas. They found that when subjects consider *impersonal* dilemmas – in which harms caused are not up close and personal – regions of the brain associated with working memory showed a significant degree of activation, while regions associated with emotion showed little activation. But when subjects considered *personal* moral dilemmas, regions associated with emotion showed a significant degree of activity, whereas regions associated with working memory showed a degree of activity *below* the resting baseline. The authors plausibly suggest that the thought of directly killing someone is much more personally engaging than is the thought of failing to help someone, or using indirect means to harm them. But the real significance of this result lies in the apparent threat it poses to some of our moral judgments. What it apparently shows is that only some of our judgments – those concerned with maximizing welfare – are the product of rational thought, whereas others are the product of our rational processes being swamped by raw emotion. This result has been taken as evidence for discounting deontological intuition, in favor of a thoroughgoing consequentialism (Singer 2005).

If Greene's results seem to challenge one important class of moral judgments, revealing them to be irrational, other work seems to threaten the entire edifice of morality, conceived of as a rational enterprise. In a series of studies, Jonathan Haidt has apparently shown that ordinary people's moral judgments are driven by their emotional responses, and that the theories they offer to justify their judgments are *post hoc* confabulations, designed to protect their judgments (Haidt 2001). We assume that we reason our way to our moral judgments, but in fact our reasons are just rationalizations, Haidt suggests. Together with Wheatley,

Haidt has shown that inducing emotional responses by using post-hypnotic suggestion influences people´s moral judgments (Wheatley & Haidt 2005). These results seem to suggest that the idea, beloved of philosophers, that morality is responsive to reasons is false. They also threaten the notion that moral argument can lead to moral progress.

Once again, the implications of this work for our self-conception are potentially dramatic. When we proudly proclaim that we are moral animals, we do not mean that our behavior is driven by affective responses, in the kinds of ways which characterize the reciprocal altruism and sense of fairness possessed by chimps, monkeys, and even much simpler animals (see Trivers 1985; de Waal 1996). Instead, we pride ourselves on a rational morality, which transcends our merely animal inheritance. This flattering image of ourselves may need heavy qualification. More immediately and practically, there may be policy implications of some of these findings. If, for instance, it can be shown that some (and only some) of our moral responses are irrational, because driven by raw emotion, then we have a powerful reason for rewriting policy to discount these responses.

These are just some of the topics covered by the incipient discipline of neuroethics. You will find many covered in these pages. Here you will find introductions to, as well thoughtful reflections on, much of the work in contemporary neuroscience that is challenging our conception of ourselves as a rational and moral animal, as well as important contributions to both branches of neuroethics: the ethics of neuroscience and the neuroscience of ethics. These will not be the last words on these topics, but they will serve as indispensable guides to this rapidly growing and fascinating field.

REFERENCES

Bargh, J. A. & Chartrand, T. L. 1999. The unbearable automaticity of being. *American Psychologist* **54**: 462–79.
Bell, G. 2005. The worried well. *Quarterly Essay* **18**: 1–74.
Cushman, F. A., Young, L. & Hauser, M. D. 2006. The role of conscious reasoning and intuitions in moral judgment: testing three principles of harm. *Psychological Science* **17**: 1082–9.
de Waal, F. 1996. *Good Natured: The Origins of Right and Wrong in Humans and Other Animals*. Cambridge, MA: Harvard University Press.
Elliott, C. 1998. The tyranny of happiness: ethics and cosmetic psychopharmacology. In Parens, E. (ed.) *Enhancing Human Traits: Ethical and Social Implications*. Washington, D.C.: Georgetown University Press, pp. 177–88.
Foot, P. 1978. The problem of abortion and the doctrine of the double effect. In Foot, P. (ed.) *Virtues and Vices*. Oxford: Basil Blackwell, pp. 19–32.

Freedman, C. 1998. Aspirin for the mind? Some ethical worries about psychopharmacology. In Parens, E. (ed.) *Enhancing Human Traits: Ethical and Social Implications*. Washington, D.C.: Georgetown University Press, pp. 135–50.

Greene, J. Sommerville, R. B., Nystrom, L. E., Darley, J. M. & Cohen, J. D. 2001. An FMRI investigation of emotional engagement in moral judgment. *Science* **293**: 2105–8.

Haidt, J. 2001. The emotional dog and its rational tail: a social intuitionist approach to moral judgment. *Psychological Review* **108**: 814–34.

Hauser, M. 2006. *Moral Minds*. New York: Ecco/HarperCollins Publishers.

Loftus, E. D. 1993. The reality of repressed memories. *American Psychologist* **48**: 518–37.

Nickerson, R. S. 1998. Confirmation bias: a ubiquitous phenomenon in many guises. *Review of General Psychology* **2**: 175–220.

Roskies, A. 2002. Neuroethics for the new millennium. *Neuron* **35**: 21–3.

Sahakian, B. & Morein-Zamir, S. 2007. Professor's little helper. *Nature* **450**: 1157–9.

Sandel, M. 2007. *The Case against Perfection: Ethics in the Age of Genetic Engineering*. Cambridge, MA: Belknap Press.

Singer, P. 2005. Ethics and intuitions. *Journal of Ethics* **9**: 331–52.

Stanovich, K. E. 1999. *Who is Rational? Studies of Individual Differences in Reasoning*. Mahwah, NJ: Lawrence Erlbaum.

Tavris, C. & Aronson, A. 2007. *Mistakes Were Made (but Not by Me)*. Orlando, FL: Harcourt.

Trivers, R. 1985. *Social Evolution*. Menlo Park, CA: Benjamin/Cummings Publishing.

Tversky, A. & Kahneman, D. 1973. Availability: a heuristic for judging frequency and probability. *Cognitive Psychology* **5**: 207–32.

Wheatley, T. & Haidt, J. 2005. Hypnotic disgust makes moral judgments more severe. *Psychological Science* **16**: 780–4.

Acknowledgments

Of course, a book such as this is indubitably a group effort, and thus, we thank all of the scholars who have taken the time to reflect upon the issues of this somewhat new and developing field, and comment about the state of maturation of both the science and ethics. Martin Griffiths at Cambridge University Press was the ideal publications' editor: patient, helpful, encouraging, and of a fine sense of humor, and we appreciate his ongoing support and enthusiasm for this project since its inception. A special thanks to Sherry Loveless, who served as coordinator and project manager, for her sometimes herculean efforts to bring authors together, coordinate conversations, serve as liaison between the editors, authors, and publisher, and essentially both make the process workable, and ultimately make this book a reality. In no uncertain terms, this could not have been achieved without her tireless labor, eagerness to help, and boundless optimism and amiability.

The idea for this book arose from conversations while the editors were both at Georgetown University Medical Center, Washington, DC; JG as Samueli–Rockefeller Professor, BG as a visiting scholar; the visiting scholar program has been, and continues to be, a wonderful forum for creating just the type of collaboration and energy that has given rise to this - and several other - projects. JG's work at Georgetown University was funded by The Laurance S. Rockefeller Trust, and much gratitude is extended for the Trust's ongoing support of the Brain–Mind and Healing Research Program. Thanks also to the Samueli Institute of Alexandria Virginia for support of related projects within this Program.

Much appreciation for the ongoing support of the Centre for Philosophical Psychology, Oxford, UK and the Center for Neurotechnology Studies of the Potomac Institute for Policy Studies, Arlington,

VA, USA, that have provided (JG) excellent forums to address how neuroethical issues impact psychosocial dimensions of the human condition; in this regard JG is particularly grateful to the warm collegiality and friendship of Drs. Gladys Sweeney, Richard Finn, and Roger Scruton. Parts of the project were engaged while JG was an American Academy of Pain Medicine National Visiting Professor at the Texas Tech University Health Sciences Center, TX, and thanks go to Dr. Mark Boswell for his insights, perspectives, great brainstorming sessions – and humor – about the ``shape of things to come´´. Long and enjoyable conversations with Dr. Dennis McBride at the Center for Neurotechnology Studies of the Potomac Institute for Policy Studies, were important to ``. . . turning over stones, looking over horizons and considering possibilities´´, and colleagues engaged in the Decade of the Mind Project were wholly instrumental in shaping this project toward meeting the ethical issues, questions, possibilities, and fears that studies and applications of brain–mind sciences might incur. In this regard, thanks to Drs. James Olds, Michael Schwartz, James Albus, Christof Koch, Michael Schulman, and Chris Forsythe, among many others.

As with any book, this project involved a fair number of long days and (very) late nights, and we most humbly thank our wives, Sherry (Giordano) and Ellis (Gordijn) for their support, motivation, good cheer, patience, and love.

Introduction

Neuroethics: coming of age and facing the future

J. J. GIORDANO

The field of neuroscience has ``evolved´´ as an inter-disciplinarity of neurobiology, anatomy, physiology, pharmacology, and psychology, to focus upon the structure and function of nervous systems (in both human and non-human organisms). Growing from older iterations of experimental and physiological psychology, neuroscience initially addressed mechanisms of neural function as related to sensory and motor systems, learning and memory, cognition, and ultimately consciousness. These basic approaches fostered subsequent studies that were specifically relevant to medicine (e.g. neurology, psychiatry, and pain care), and, more recently, social practices (such as consumer behavior, and spiritual and religious practices and experiences).

In the United States, the congressionally dedicated Decade of the Brain (1990–2000) provided political incentive to support neuroscientific research with renewed intensity. As a result, significant discoveries were achieved in a variety of areas including neurogenetics, neuro- and psychopharmacology, and neuroimaging. This progress was not limited to the United States; rather, the Decade of the Brain served to provide a funding base that catalyzed international cooperation. We feel that this was the beginning of a ``culture of neuroscience´´ that was created from, and continues to engage a world-wide ``think tank´´ atmosphere that facilitates academic, medical, and technological collaboration, rapid scientific developments, and widely distributed effects in research, health care, and public life.

In addition, neuroscience has become a venue for the employment of cutting edge biotechnology that is extending the capabilities and boundaries of both investigation and intervention. Still, what

David Chalmers refers to as the "hard problems" of neuroscience remain, about the nature of consciousness, viability of the concept of "mind" and "self", notions of free will, and validity of moral beliefs and action. While these questions might be seen as philosophical, they are nonetheless practical and vital to consider, as neuroscientific findings are increasingly used and applied in social contexts – despite the rapidly changing nature of what we hold to be (neuroscientifically relevant) "facts". Thus, perhaps the most difficult questions involve the "meaning" of neuroscientific information, and how to pursue and utilize neuroscientific knowledge in ways that are consistent with some construal of social "good". This is the work of neuroethics.

The term "neuroethics" was first used in the United States by *NY Times* journalist William Safire at a 2002 Dana Foundation conference, and has subsequently become part of the academic and public lexicon. The term actually reflects two interactive traditions; the first entails study of the neural basis of moral thought, while the second describes the ethical (legal and social) issues arising in and from neuroscientific research and its applications. These definitions (1) necessitate appreciation for a grounding natural philosophy, and (2) axiomatically link neuroscience (inclusive of its constituent disciplines and scientific interdisciplinarity) to the humanities, and in this way sustain a transdisciplinary approach. We argue that for such an approach to be valid, it must be based upon an understanding of facts (and acknowledgment of the relative contingency of these facts), philosophical constructs, doctrines, biases, and practical contexts of science (as an institution and practice), and the realities and values of society and culture. This allows recognition of (1) the issues and exigencies that are inherent to neuroscience; (2) moral dimensions, obligations, and responsibilities that such issues involve; and (3) how various ethical systems and approaches might be used to address and resolve these issues, questions, and problems.

The structure and functions of neuroethics might be envisioned as depicted in Figure A.1. We think of this as being analogous to an egg: the "living", developing, content is on the inside, while the "shell" that provides shape, structure, and support is on the outside. But these are not mutually exclusive; without the "living content" of epistemic capital, focus, and goals of neurophilosophy and neuroscience, etc. that give rise to moral obligation and ethical enactment of tasks and responsibilities, the "shell" (i.e. guidelines and policies for research, clinical and social applications, etc.) would be "hollow", and easily crumble. Likewise, without the structure and support provided by the

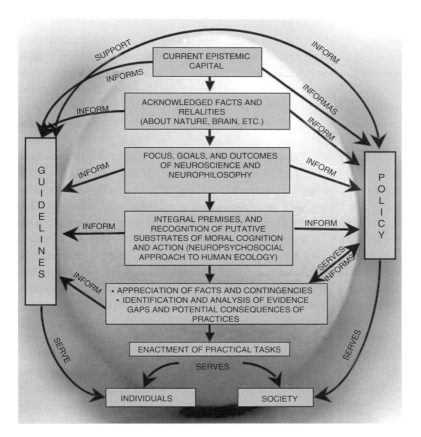

Figure A.1

``shell'' of well-conceived, realistic, and prudent guidelines and polices, the ``living content'' (i.e. the epistemic capital, and philosophic and ethical claims) of neuroscience could not develop, would be shapeless and vulnerable, and could not be practically applied. The points of contact are the dimensions in which neuroscience and neuroethics serve individuals and society. But these are also the points of maximum pressure, incurred by the forces of an ever-changing knowledge base, newly generated moral issues, diverse ethical systems, and polyglot politico-cultural values. If neuroethics is to serve a public good, it must accommodate, withstand, and apportion these forces; we believe that to do so will require ongoing sharing and reciprocity of information, ideas, and incentives between the participatory and involved stakeholders from science, humanities, funding agencies, law makers, and society.

In many ways, this may bespeak a new worldview that recognizes what Thomas Kuhn has called ``an epistemic crisis´´ – a time of social change based upon mass-effect of new knowledge. Previously accepted ideas about the nervous system, brain, and concept of mind are being revised (if not abandoned) in favor of new notions and novel ways of thinking about the human condition.

But what of lessons learned? The questions of neuroscience are those that address how we know, what we are, and thus the very nature of being and understanding. The technological advances that have allowed much of this inquiry have progressed with tremendous speed, yet, as so frequently, the philosophy and ethics that should guide the use of such technology and knowledge, and foster prudent application(s) in medicine and society tend to occur after the fact. In recognition and response, neuroethics – although somewhat nascent as a field – is steadily developing a canon that seeks to (1) identify the humanistic importance of neuroscience, both epistemologically and in application, and (2) provide reflective direction to the pace and trajectory of technological progress.

In this light, this volume provides information about important developments in neuroscience and neurotechnology, and addresses the philosophical, ethical, and social questions, issues, and problems that such advancements generate. To re-iterate, the field is young, but many of the issues have rapidly matured, and have been the focus of considerable debate and discussion. Throughout, we have tried to base the discourse upon three core questions: First, what is the scope and direction of neuroscientific inquiry? Second, how has progress to date affected scientific and philosophical ideas, and what potential for epistemic revision lies ahead; and third, what ethical issues and problems does (and could) this progress and knowledge incur, both now and in the future?

To address these questions, the book is organized into four major ``domains´´ that we feel sustain a contemporary and forward-looking neuroethics. The first presents a history of neuroscience, as relevant to the current state of neuroethics (chapters 1–3). The second identifies how the ``hard problems´´ of neuroscience have created philosophical and social issues of ethical importance (chapters 4–8). The third discusses developments in neurotechnology, and how such devices, techniques, and the information and outcomes they provide have spawned ethical, legal, and social dilemmas (and what might – or should – be done to resolve these questions and problems before they become irretrievable, intractable or unforgiveable; chapters 9–15). The final section frames neuroethics in the contexts of a pluralized world-stage, poses thoughts on what international policy could achieve given the need for any ethics of brain-science to consider the neural basis of what it may mean ``to be human´´, and urges equal consideration of the tentative nature of this information, and the limits and limitations of such ``frontier knowledge´´ (Chapters 16–18). Overall, our goal was to provide the reader with a view to how neuroethics has come of age. The inertia of the United States´ Decade of the Brain, and Decade of Pain Control and Research (2000–2010) – together with international efforts – have done much to advance the pace and progress of brain science. However, this has also revealed the work that remains to be done. We do not know how ``mind´´ and consciousness occur in the brain. And while this may, in fact represent ``merely´´ an evidence gap, such uncertainty engenders considerable philosophic, theological, social, legal, and political insecurity and debate. Revealing the mechanisms of the brain to understand consciousness, the ``self´´, and the ethical, legal, and social implications and impact of such studies are the intended goals of the proposed Decade of the Mind. Clearly, the Decade of the Mind project and neuroethics as a profession and practice necessitate a consilient, international effort. Our hope is that this volume will be useful to students, scholars, scientists, and all those involved with both this endeavor and the field at large.

1

Developments in neuroscience

Where have we been; where are we going?

D. F. SWAAB

INTRODUCTION

My introduction to this book on neuroethics, a volume with a large diversity of topics, is based upon a very personal selection of some of the numerous highlights that form the contributory history of the field of neuroscience. This volume shows how the way in which we look upon the brain has changed – in a relatively short period of time – from being just one of the organs that housed a soul to being the focus of a huge multidisciplinary endeavor to study the source of the mind. The focus of brain research has moved through that endeavor from the study of macroscopically visible pathologies of the brain to the subtle structural and functional differences that form the basis of psychiatric disorders and of our character. The sexual differentiation of our brain in utero – the programming of our gender identity and sexual orientation for the rest of our life – is discussed as an example of one of the many aspects of our character that become hardwired in our brain during early development. The concept of a critical window during which a developmental process can take place in order to structure brain systems and their function for the rest of our life is also why it is so difficult to repair lesions in the adult brain. In spite of this difficulty, it is now possible to sketch a series of new technical developments in neuroscience that bear the promise of leading to new, effective therapeutic strategies to tackle brain disorders in the near future.

Scientific and Philosophical Perspectives in Neuroethics, ed. J. J. Giordano & B. Gordijn. Published by Cambridge University Press. © Cambridge University Press 2010.

WE ARE OUR BRAINS

Everything we think, believe, and do is determined and carried out by our brains. The unprecedented evolutionary success of humankind – as well as the many limitations of individual people – are determined by this fabulous organ, our brain, which determines our possibilities, our limitations, and our character, as was already recognized by Hippocrates and Descartes[1]; *we are our brains.* The rest of our body only serves to feed our brain, to move it around, and to make new brains through procreation. Brain research therefore not only deals with disorders, but is increasingly becoming a search for the answer to the question why we are the way we are, a search for the self.

Nerve cells, also called neurons, are the building blocks of our brains. These cells are specialized in (1) gathering information from the rest of our body via other nerve cells and from hormones and, through our senses, from the environment; (2) the integration and processing of information and the decision-making on the basis of this information; and (3) the carrying out of these decisions in the form of movements, changes in hormone levels, the regulation of physical processes, and the production of a never-ending stream of thoughts. Faults in this efficient, information-processing machine may be genetically based, may occur in a developmental stage or later in life, and may lead to psychiatric or neurological disorders, or

---

[1] It should be generally known that the source of our pleasure, merriment, laughter, and amusement, as of our grief, pain, anxiety, and tears, is none other than the brain. It is this organ in particular that enables us to think, see and hear, and to distinguish the ugly from the fair, the bad from the good, and the pleasant from the unpleasant. It is the brain, too, that is the seat of madness and insanity, of terrors and fears that crowd in upon us, usually at night, but sometimes even during the day; this is the cause of insomnia and somnambulism, of thoughts that will not come, of forgotten duties and strange phenomena.

Hippocrates, fifth century BC

I want you to look upon all the functions I attribute to this machine (the brain), such as digestion, nutrition, respiration, waking and sleeping, taking in light, sound, smell, the impression of images in the organ of observation and imagination, the retaining of these ideas in the memory, the lower movements of lusts and passions, and lastly the moving of all outer limbs, I want you to look upon all these functions as taking place naturally in this machine exclusively as a result of the nature of its organs, no less than the movements of a clock.

Descartes, 1596–1650.

to a great variety of behavioral disorders, including aggression and criminal behavior.

The computer metaphor

When we look at the building blocks of our brains and see how they are linked, the computer metaphor appears obvious. The brain weighs 1500 g, contains 100 billion (10×10^{10}) neurons (16 times the number of people in the world), twice as many glial cells (the cells that support the neurons in their functions) and at least 1000 times as many places where nerve cells make contact or, as Santiago Ramón y Cajal (1852–1934) put it, ``hold hands´´: the synapses. The nerve cells are connected by more than 100,000 km of nerve fibers. A possibly even better metaphor for the brain, a central control room, was proposed by Tolman in 1948. He wrote:

> We assert that the central office itself is far more like a map control room than it is like an old- fashioned telephone exchange. The stimuli which are allowed in are not connected by just simple one-to-one switches to the outgoing responses. Rather, the incoming impulses are usually worked over and elaborated in the central control room into a tentative, cognitive-like map of the environment. And it is this tentative map, indicating routes and paths and environmental relationships, which finally determines what responses, if any, the animal will finally release.
>
> Cited in Repovš & Bresjanac 2006.

The staggering numbers of cells and synapses work so efficiently that our brains do not consume the energy of more than a mere 15 W bulb. Michel Hofman has calculated that this means that the total energy costs of the brain of one individual are only 1200 euro per life time at the current price level. You cannot even buy a decent computer with that kind of money. But what this means is that one can make one billion neurons work for 80 years at a cost of 1200 euro! A fantastically efficient machine, then, with parallel circuits, better equipped for image processing and association than any computer. The volume of the biological clock of the brain, the suprachiasmatic nucleus (see Figure 1.1A), is only $0.5 \, \text{mm}^3$, and this is sufficient to regulate all our day/night rhythms (waking, sleeping, eating, drinking, procreation, hormone levels, etc.). Try imagining what $1500 \, \text{cm}^3$ (3 million times more) can do!

The product of the functions and interactions of all those billions of nerve cells is our ``mind´´. ``The brain secretes thoughts, as the kidney secretes urine´´ (Jakob Moleschott, 1822–93). One can actually see a human being think during a functional scanning session: which

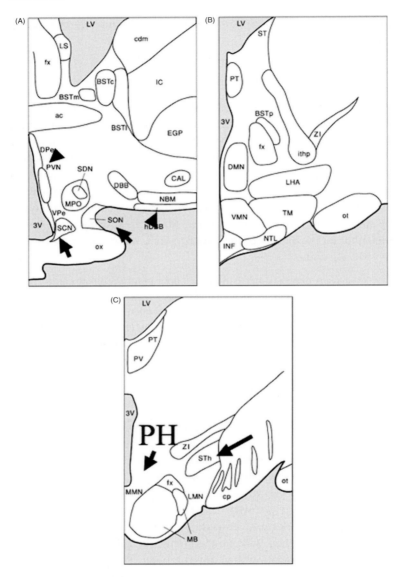

Figure 1.1 Scheme of the hypothalamic area. Arrows indicate the structures mentioned in the text. NBM, nucleus basalis of Meynert; PH, posterior hypothalamus; PVN, paraventricular nucleus; SCN, suprachiasmatic nucleus; SON, supraoptic nucleus; STh, subthalamic nucleus.

brain areas are activated when we read, calculate, listen to music, hallucinate, are in love, or are sexually aroused. Using real-time functional MRI as a biofeedback system, it is even possible to train brain areas to function in a different way. Patients thus trained to control the frontal part of the anterior cingulate gyrus (see Figures 1.2, 1.3) were able to diminish their chronic pain (DeCharms *et al.* 2005).

There are still people who credit the heart with special, mystical properties, in relation to our feelings, our emotions, our character, our love, and even our soul. Of course, our heart rate increases when we experience emotions, but only because the autonomic nervous system commands it. Yet there are anecdotes about heart transplant recipients who underwent a change of character reminiscent of the donor. The *Telegraaf*, a big Dutch newspaper, printed the headline: ``Is the soul localized in the heart? Claire Sylvia (47) got the heart transplant from a boy. She now whistles to girls and is drinking beer´´. Sylvia, in 1997, wrote in her book that she was convinced that the character of her donor, a young motor cyclist, was transplanted along with his heart and lungs. There are also anecdotes of heart transplant patients whose taste in music, favorite color, or preference for art, food, recreation, or career changed into that of the donor. Someone who had received a

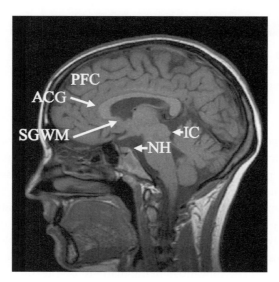

Figure 1.2 Frontal MRI scan. ACG, anterior cingulate gyrus; IC, inferior colliculus; NH, neurohypophysis; PFC, prefrontal cortex; SGWM, subgenual cingulate white matter.

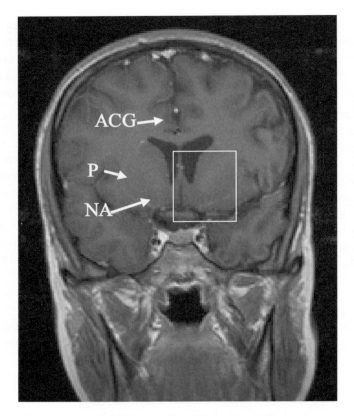

Figure 1.3 Frontal MRI scan. The white square indicates the hypothalamic area that is shown in more detail in Figure 1.1. ACG, anterior cingulate gyrus; NA, nucleus accumbens; P, putamen.

donor heart reported to have seen the face of the murderer of his donor in a dream (Pearsall *et al.* 2002). A woman reported that she could suddenly play chess after receiving the heart of a professional chess player. One may wonder how the presumed information from the heart is transported to the brain after a transplantation during which all nerve connections are cut, so before we can take these reports seriously we need a well-controlled study that completely excludes any possibility that the recipient receives information about the donor, that makes unwanted manipulations of the interviews impossible, and that takes into consideration the effects of the immunosuppressive medication that is taken after a transplant and that might affect behavior.

BRAIN DEVELOPMENT

During development we make our own brains into a unique machine

The computer metaphor only partially applies to the brain. The ``hardware´´ of our brain is soft, and some systems are very malleable. Our brain is a living machine that changes continuously with use, especially during development. Everything we do or observe during development may result in lasting changes in the numbers of cells, circuits, and cell contacts. Our environment and the use of our brain strongly and permanently influence its structure, and therefore its function, which makes it unique. Each of the brains of identical twins has already become unique in this way at the moment of birth (Steinmetz et al. 1994). The brain thus only partly develops on the basis of hereditary information. A child´s brain development is influenced in the womb, by hormones and its mother´s stress, and by the random silencing of genes, and it is threatened there, too, by any medication, alcohol, and nicotine taken by the mother during pregnancy. If the mother smokes during pregnancy the chances of the child´s later showing Attention Deficit Hyperactivity Disorder (ADHD), becoming aggressive, or displaying criminal behavior, increase (Brennan et al. 1999; Neuman et al. 2007).

During development the brain makes an excess of cells and connections. The brain systems´ functioning determines which of these cells and connections are effective and will ultimately survive. This competition among brain cells to survive is called ``neuronal Darwinism´´. It is thus not just a child´s practicing its movements that determines the construction of its brain and any ensuing functions; the child´s learning, experiencing, seeing, and thinking also organize the structure, and therefore the function, of its brain. A multitude of factors that influence the structure of the brain during early development determine our character. Whether we will feel like a man or like a woman (gender identity) and our sexual orientation are determined in utero. Although it has often been postulated that postnatal development is also important for the direction of our sexual differentiation, any solid proof of this possibility is lacking (Swaab 2007).

During our first couple of years our environment also determines the structure of the brain systems that are involved in language, and this gives us our mother tongue. This system is not plastic, as is apparent from our accent when we learn another language later on.

Moreover, we are exposed to the religious convictions of our environment at an age when whatever our parents say is considered to be the truth, and our religious convictions are thus imprinted in our brains and not easily changed. However, the synapses are a brain system that does remain plastic throughout life. They undergo small alterations in brain areas where, for example, memories are stored.

The brain is thus only partly created on the basis of genetic information and for a major part built under the influence of its functioning during early development. As no one's experiences and thoughts are exactly the same, every brain becomes unique in the process of development. This is how our character is determined. The environment is also involved, especially in early development, through such influences as language and religion. Our brain makes our culture and our culture shapes our brain development.

In the course of our development we make our own brain into a unique feature, a person, and sometimes a personality.

Development causes restrictions

During our development our options become ever more limited by the growing organization of our brain. This process has already started in the womb. We are not born a *tabula rasa*, as Locke and Rousseau thought. At the moment the ovum is fertilized the risk of many of our future deviations (e.g. dementia) are already genetically determined. The choice of mother tongue, sexual orientation and gender identity, and level of aggression is made for us during our development. It is impossible to dissuade transsexuals from their idea that they are living in a body of the wrong sex and that the body should be changed. There is no other option; once the brain is organized it is virtually impossible to change anything. Our last bit of elbow room is taken from us once we are born, by the only efficient manipulation of the brain in existence: a thorough upbringing. Commercials and television finish the job. That is why all over the world teenagers are listening to exactly the same music in exactly the same designer clothes. Neuronal Darwinism seems to underlie the neurobiological processes for these continuous limitations, which cause our brains to function more and more efficiently, but at the same time to lose increasingly more degrees of freedom, leaving us with the paradox that the only person with any real freedom is the fetus, who is unable to enjoy this freedom owing to its immature nervous system. Once we have reached adulthood, our ability to modify our brains, and therefore our behavior, has met with too many structural restrictions of our brain. We have then acquired our ``character''.

We are indeed limited in our choices not only by the conventions of society but also by the way our brain has developed. Child abusers were abused when they themselves were children. How ``free'' is the abuser not to go down the road of abuse himself? How ``free'' is an adolescent, whose brain must learn to deal, in a very short time, with sex hormones, which change the function of nearly every brain structure during puberty? In adulthood brain disorders can change a person completely. The brain of RAF terrorist Ulrike Meinhof turned out to be damaged when it was examined after her suicide in prison in 1976. She had had an aneurysm, a widening of a blood vessel, that was pressing on the amygdala (Figures 1.4 and 1.5) earlier and her prefrontal cortex was damaged during surgery. The pressure on the amygdala can give aggression while the damage done to the prefrontal cortex during surgery may cause impulsive behavior. So both lesions could explain the change in behavior from discerning journalist to terrorist. How free was her will?

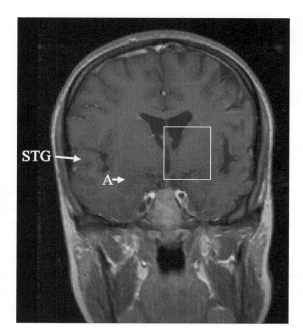

Figure 1.4 Frontal MRI scan. The white square indicates the hypothalamic area that is shown in more detail in Figure 1.1. A, amygdala; STG, superior temporal gyrus.

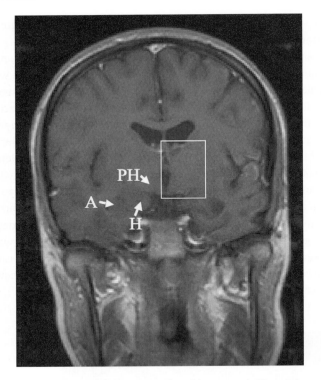

Figure 1.5 Frontal MRI scan. The white square indicates the
hypothalamic area that is shown in more detail in Figure 1.1. A,
amygdala; H, hippocampus; PH, posterior hypothalamus.

Sexual differentiation of the brain as an example of early imprinting

Sexual differentiation of our brain starts in the womb and brings about
permanent changes in brain structures and functions, mainly through
the interaction of the developing neurons with the sex hormones of
the child.

The testicles and ovaries develop in the sixth week of pregnancy.
This happens under the influence of a cascade of genes, for which the
sex-determining gene on the Y chromosome of boys, SRY, is a trigger.
The production of testosterone by a boy´s testes is necessary for the
sexual differentiation of his sexual organs between the sixth and
twelfth week of pregnancy. The development of the female sexual
organs in the womb is primarily based on the absence of testosterone.
The brain of a boy is permanently organized by two peaks in

testosterone. The first peak occurs during mid-pregnancy, and the second peak takes place in the first 3 months after birth. These two peaks of testosterone in boys cause a programming of structures in the brain for the rest of their lives. The rising hormone levels during puberty ``activate´´ circuits that were built during early development. In humans, the *direct* effects of testosterone on the developing brain appear to be the main mechanism involved in gender identity and sexual orientation, as appears from the androgen insensitivity syndrome (see Glossary). This is a genetic disorder by which the entire body is not sensitive for the male sex hormone testosterone. The genetic (XY) males develop into heterosexual females, showing that testosterone in development is crucial for the male appearance, gender identity, and sexual orientation towards females. The sex differences in brain structures and functions that result from the interaction of hormones and developing brain cells are thought to be the basis of the sex differences in our later behavior, such as our feeling of being a man or a woman (gender identity), the way in which we behave as men or women in society (gender role), our sexual orientation (hetero-, homo-, and bisexuality), and sex differences regarding cognition and aggressive behavior. Factors that interfere with the interaction between hormones and the developing brain in the womb may permanently influence our later behavior (Swaab 2007).

Sexual differentiation of the brain: little or no effect of the social environment

In the period between the 1950s and 1970s it was postulated that a child was born as a *tabula rasa* and was forced into the male or female direction by society´s conventions. John Money put this as follows (Money 1975):

> Gender identity is sufficiently incompletely differentiated at birth as to permit successful assignment of a genetic male as a girl. Gender identity then differentiates in keeping with the experiences of rearing.

This concept has had devastating results, as shown by the well-known story of John–Joan–John (or John–Joan as Money, a well-known psychologist and sexologist, used to refer to the case). John is a pseudonym of David Reimer (see Colapinto 2001), the little boy that had to go to surgery for a small operation, i.e. the removal of the foreskin of the penis at the age of 8 months. The boy lost his penis due to a mistake during this minor surgery. According to Money, gender imprinting did not start until the age of 1 year and its development would be far advanced by the ages of 3–4 (Money & Erhardt 1972). This was the basis for the decision to make a girl (Brenda) out of this 8-month-old boy (Bruce). The testicles of this child were removed before the age of 17 months in order to facilitate feminization. The child was dressed in girls´ clothes, received psychological counselling, and was given estrogens in puberty. Money described the development of this child as ``normal female´´. However, at age 13, Brenda decided to assume a male gender identity, calling himself David. Later Milton Diamond described how Brenda changed back to male, married, and adopted children (Diamond & Sigmundson 1997). Unfortunately, David lost money on the stock exchange, was divorced, and eventually committed suicide in May 2004. This story illustrates the strong influence of programming of the intrauterine period on our gender identity. Even removal of the penis, cross dressing and educating him as a girl, giving psychological guidance, and administering female sex hormones during puberty did not change his gender identity.

The apparent impossibility of forcing someone to change sexual orientation is also a major argument against the importance of the social environment in the emergence of homosexuality, as well as against the idea that homosexuality is a lifestyle choice. The mind boggles at what has been tried to achieve this: hormonal treatments, such as castration, administering testosterone or estrogens, treatments that appeared to affect libido but not sexual orientation; psychoanalysis; apomorphine, a compound that causes vomiting, given in combination with homo-erotic pictures without changing the person´s feelings about these pictures; psychosurgery (i.e. lesions in the hypothalamus); electroshock treatment; chemical induction of epileptic insults; and imprisonment. As none of these interventions has led to a well-documented change in sexual orientation, and since children who were born after artificial insemination with donor sperm and were raised by a lesbian couple tend to be heterosexually oriented (Swaab 2007; LeVay 1996), there can be little doubt that our sexual orientation has become fixed by the time we reach adulthood and is beyond influencing later on. It is sad that even nowadays some children are forbidden to play with homosexual friends, an unimaginable relic from the idea that homosexuality would be contagious.

Transsexuality

Transsexuality is characterized by a conviction of having have been born in the wrong body. Gender problems often crop up early in development.

Mothers report that, from the moment their sons learned to talk, they insisted on wearing their mother's clothes and shoes, only showed an interest in girls' toys, and mostly played with girls.

There is a vast array of factors that may lead to gender problems. Twin and family research have shown that genetic factors play a part (Coolidge *et al.* 2002), and it was recently found that polymorphisms (i.e. small alterations in the DNA of certain genes) (see Glossary) of the genes for the estrogen receptors α and β and for aromatase also produced an increased risk (Henningsson *et al.* 2005). The chance that a girl becomes transsexual after exposure to high levels of testosterone in utero is also greater. This occurs in the case of congenital adrenal hyperplasia (CAH) (see Glossary). Epileptic women who were given phenobarbital or diphantoin during pregnancy also have an increased risk of giving birth to a transsexual child. Both these substances change the metabolism of the sex hormones and may act on the sexual differentiation of the brain of the child (Dessens *et al.* 1999). There are no indications that postnatal social factors could be responsible for the occurrence of transsexuality. Whether endocrine disrupters, i.e. chemicals in the environment, for instance from industry, influence sexual differentiation of the brain is an important question for the future (Swaab 2007).

Transsexuality and the brain

The theory of the origin of transsexuality is based on the fact that the sexual differentiation of our sexual organs takes place during the first couple of months of pregnancy, well before the sexual differentiation of the brain. As these two processes have different timetables it is possible, in principle, that they take different routes. If that is the case, one would expect, in transsexuals, female structures in a male brain and vice versa. And indeed, we did find such a reversal of sex in the central nucleus of the bed nucleus of the stria terminalis (BSTc), a brain structure that, as we know from experiments in rodents, is involved in many aspects of sexual behavior.

A clear sex difference is present in the human BSTc. In men this area is twice as large as that of females and contains 70% more somatostatin neurons (this is a major population of neurons in the BSTc, containing somatostatin as a neurotransmitter). No difference was found regarding size or number of neurons in this area in relation to sexual orientation. In male-to-female transsexuals we found a completely female BSTc (Figure 1.6). Until now we have only been able

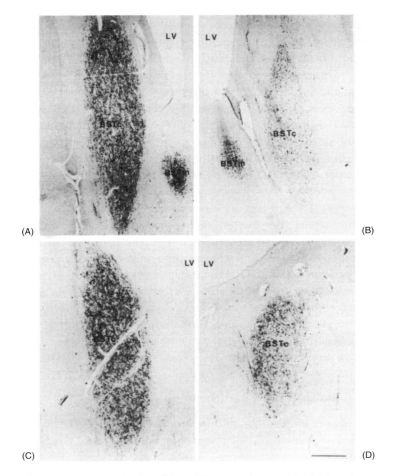

Figure 1.6 Representative slides of the central part of the bed nucleus of the stria terminalis (BSTc) innervated by fibers stained for vasoactive intestinal polypeptide (VIP). (A) Heterosexual man; (B) heterosexual woman; (C) homosexual man; (D) male-to-female transsexual. Scale bar, 0.5 mm. LV, lateral ventricle. Please note the sex difference (the males in A and C vs. the female in B) and that the male-to-female transsexual (D) has a female BSTc as far as size and innervation are concerned (from Zhou *et al.* 1995, with permission).

to obtain material from one female-to-male transsexual, and his BSTc indeed turned out to have all the male characteristics. We were able to exclude that the reversal of sex differences in the BSTc was caused by changing hormone levels in adulthood (Zhou *et al.* 1995; Kruijver *et al.*

2000), and it therefore seems that we are dealing with a developmental effect. Our observations thus support the above-mentioned neurobiological theory about the origin of transsexuality. The size of the BSTc and the number of neurons match the gender that transsexuals feel they belong to and not the sex of their sexual organs, birth certificate or passport.

In conclusion, during our intrauterine period the brain develops in the male direction through a direct action of a boy's testosterone on the developing nerve cells, and in the female direction through absence of this hormone in a girl. In this way not only our gender identity (the feeling of being a man or a woman) but also our sexual orientation is programmed into our brain structures when we are still in the womb (Swaab 2007). The possibility that pedophilia may also be explained as an early developmental disorder of sexual differentiation of the brain should be investigated.

MIND VERSUS SOUL

Are we "just" the unique, fantastically complex, neuronal machine that produces the mind and that is programmed largely in early development as far as its structure and function are concerned? Is there more than the brain as a neuronal machine? Freud had already recognized that all cultures, all religions, carry within them the concept that after we die there is the continued existence of "something" immaterial of our personality. That "something" is called the soul, which is generally thought to stay near the body for a short while after death before moving on for ever to an afterlife. In 1906, MacDougall (USA) weighed dying patients with bed and all. When these patients had breathed their last breath they were weighed again. They turned out to be 21 grams lighter and MacDougall said he had weighed "the soul". He did not find this difference in animals and concluded that they did not have a soul. However, Professor Twining (Los Angeles) claimed that animals lost several (milli) grams when they died and therefore had to have some soul (Heindel 1913).

Some give brain-related arguments in favor of the existence of a soul and an afterlife, such as the direct contact with God that some temporal lobe epilepsy patients have, and the occurrence of near-death experiences. Some patients suffering from temporal lobe epilepsy have indeed very deeply religious experiences. While the attack rages the patients are generally in a dreamlike state and experience auditory and visual hallucinations, often with strong religious overtones. Sometimes these patients have out-of-body experiences as well. The attacks and the "visitations from God" tend to last only seconds but may change one's personality for ever. In addition, such patients undergo emotional changes and may become hyperreligious. These patients often have a personality disorder known as the "Geschwind syndrome" that consists of hypergraphy (they write an enormous amount of works), hyposexuality and hyperreligiosity (Wuerfel *et al.* 2004; Saver & Robin 1997). Some founders of large religious movements and some prophets and religious leaders, among them the apostle Paul and Joan of Arc, suffered from epilepsy. The same goes for Van Gogh and Dostoevsky. As the latter wrote in "The Idiot":

> The air was filled with a big noise, and I thought it had engulfed me. I have really touched God. He came into me myself; yes, God exists, I cried, and I don't remember anything else. You all, healthy people, he said, can't imagine the happiness we epileptics feel during the second before our attack. I don't know if this felicity lasts for seconds, hours, or months, but believe me, for all the joys that life may bring, I would not exchange this one.

A patient with ecstatic epileptic attacks, who sometimes saw a figure resembling Jesus, turned out to have a brain tumor in the temporal lobe. The attacks disappeared after temporal lobectomy, which supports the neurological explanation for this ecstatic phenomenon. Apparently stimulation in the temporal region by a tumor or other lesions releases the religious experiences that are imprinted during early development. Patients in the Far East with a temporal lobe epilepsy never reported contact with a Western God, but see local religious figures instead.

Near-death experiences are also often used as "proof" that there is a hereafter, and as proof that we do not need brain function for consciousness (Parnia & Fenwick 2002; Van Lommel *et al.* 2001). Near-death experiences tend to feature a tunnel, bright light, deceased relatives, and mysterious figures. One sees one's life flashing before one, feels as if one is leaving one's body and is able to look down upon it while hovering above it (autoscopy). These images are usually considered pleasant rather than frightening, and very often people who have experienced near-death take a greater interest in spiritual things and begin to believe in a hereafter, while their fear of death lessens. Near-death experiences may occur when the brain does not obtain sufficient oxygen, e.g. due to heart failure. It may also occur when a fighter pilot loses consciousness when he accelerates too quickly, or may be due to hyperventilation due to extreme stress, e.g. in a car accident. The sense of leaving one´s body apparently occurs once in the lifetime of some 10%–20% of the population, without ever finding a cause for it.

Patients who had a near-death experience in a clinic were actually diagnosed to be clinically dead, i.e. unconscious due to cessation of circulation and respiration. Sometimes clinical death was objectified by the absence of ECG or EEG and sometimes wide, unresponsive pupils are reported. It is generally believed that irreversible damage to the brain cells will occur within 5-10 minutes after cessation of circulation and respiration. This is a ``truth´´ that will have to be revised, however, as it turns out that we are able to culture human neurons and keep them alive for months when they are obtained within 10 h after the death of a patient (Verwer *et al.* 2002).

Because only a small percentage (6%–18%) of clinically dead patients report a near-death experience it has been proposed that this cannot be explained purely by the hypoxia. This is, of course, not a valid argument because this form of hallucination requires stimulation of the brain in a certain way by a certain degree of hypoxia. Besides, memory must have remained at least sufficiently intact for the patient to remember this experience. Fewer near-death experiences are reported when memory has been damaged after lengthy resuscitation (Blanke *et al.* 2002). When the gyrus angularis (at the parieto-temporal junction, see Figure 1.7) was electrically stimulated, one patient felt as if her legs were getting shorter and that she was floating above the bed. In 6 neurological patients (5 epileptics and 1 with migraine and a small brain infarct) who had repeated out-of-body experiences, abnormal activity was located in that particular brain area as well (Blanke *et al.* 2002, 2004). These experiences are accompanied by impulses from the sense of equilibrium, such as hovering, flying, elevation, and rotation. These ``experiences´´ thus seem to be based on a disturbance of the brain mechanisms involved in processing of information coming from the muscles, the sense of equilibrium, and the visual system. Visual information is not required for near-death experiences: they have also been reported by blind people. It is not clear whether near-death experiences are induced at the very start of the period of unconsciousness or in the recovery phase. It is true that there are also anecdotes about detailed memories about the surroundings of the unconscious patient, but this does not mean that those observations did not need a brain, merely that it is possible to observe and remember even when your brain is not functioning properly. Sometimes patients even recall conversations held between surgeons while they were under anesthesia. All in all, near-death experiences are not proof of consciousness beyond the brain, nor are they proof of a life after death.

Moreover, are we so important that something of us should remain when we die? Rather, the idea of a soul seems to be based on a universal fear of death, inflated ego, and, of course, the hope of seeing loved ones again. At the moment a much simpler hypothesis explains just as much: the mind is the result of the functioning of the brain. I think that the "soul" is a misconception. And indeed, with this fabulous machine – our brain – we do not need extra immaterial explanations; there is no such thing as a "psychon", there are only neurons.

When we die, our brain stops functioning and nothing remains of the mind. At the present moment we can keep brain cells of a deceased person in culture for months (Verwer *et al.* 2002). In that sense there is life after death, at least for a while. The only other ways of living on seem to be to pass on hereditary information to our children. But that does not mean that *our* mind lives on. Our children develop their own unique brains and will become unique personalities, who tend to have surprisingly little in common with us. Nothing or almost nothing of us remains. Brought forth by evolution and from DNA, environment, and functioning we, or rather, our brains, have become unique. Of course we will become dust (Genesis 3.19), because even during our lives we were nothing but a physical being.

NEUROTHERAPY: TREATMENT OF BRAIN DISORDERS
AND RESTORATIVE NEUROSCIENCE

Where are we going to?

Although the brain may be considered as a neuronal machine, it is so complex that brain diseases still remain difficult to treat. However, the era of defeatism has been replaced by one of excitement about recent technological progress and new insights coming from the different disciplines in neuroscience. A great international effort creates new optimism in clinics, where better diagnostic and therapeutic opportunities are expected in the near future.

Both neurology and psychiatry use the great diagnostic potentials of molecular and imaging techniques. Alterations in the DNA of genes that have a function in the chemical transfer of information in the brain have been discovered that increase the risk of excessive aggression (Manuck *et al.* 1999, 2000). MRI scans have changed the diagnostics in neurology fundamentally. Scanning has to be applied more routinely in psychiatry as well, since surprises have been reported. A small hypothalamic tumor might mimic all the signs and symptoms of the eating disorder anorexia nervosa, and even of schizophrenia (Swaab 2004). Lesions in the prefrontal cortex may lead to disturbed social and moral behavior (Anderson *et al.* 1999) and to criminal behavior (Popma & Raine 2006). Lesions in or near the amygdala (Figures 1.4, 1.5) may lead to aggression or murder (Blair 2003). Brain scanning may thus also have legal consequences. The diagnostic and therapeutic potentials of functional scans have only recently become apparent. For instance, this approach makes it possible to predict which depressive patient will respond to anti-depressives and which to psychotherapy (Osuch & Williamson 2006).

For more and more brain disorders we are beginning to understand the pathogenesis and the molecular networks involved, using new powerful techniques such as microarrays that allow the determination of the expression levels of all genes and proteomics, determining the amount of all proteins in a brain sample. This leads to new therapeutic strategies. For a long time Parkinson´s disease has been treated with L-dopa, but now fetal brain grafts are also implanted in the brain. AIDS dementia has disappeared, owing to an effective combination therapy. Psychiatric syndromes can now be treated by influencing the chemical messengers in the brain with anti-psychotics, anti-depressants, and anxiolytics. Under the microscope one can see that brain development of a schizophrenic patient is disturbed in early pregnancy. Schizophrenia can now be treated with medication, while transcranial magnetic stimulation can reduce hallucinations. In cases of tinnitus in deaf patients, such stimulation of the auditory cortex may put an end to the irritating songs they hear continuously.

FUNCTIONAL IMPROVEMENTS BY PSYCHOPHARMACA, REACTIVATION OF NEURONS, DEEP BRAIN STIMULATION, AND PLACEBOS

I believe that the great diseases of the brain ... will be shown to be connected with specific chemical changes in neuroplasm ... It is probable that by the aid of chemistry, many derangements of the brain and mind, which are at present obscure, will become accurately definable and amenable to precise treatment, and what is now an object of anxious empiricism will become one for the proud exercise of exact science.

J. L.W. Thudicum *A Treatise on the Chemical Constitution of the Brain – Based Throughout upon Original Researches* (1884)

The treatment of depression: the future ``analytical psychiatrist´´ for patient-tailored therapy

The hypothalamo-pituitary–adrenal (HPA) axis, the stress axis (see Glossary), is considered to be the ``final common pathway´´ for a major part of the depressive symptomatology. Genetic risk factors for depression, small size at birth, smoking of the pregnant mother, child abuse and early maternal separation all cause an increased HPA-axis activity and risk of depression in adulthood. Following treatment with antidepressants, electroconvulsive therapy, or when patients show spontaneous remission, the HPA axis function returns to normal. Activity of the corticotropin-releasing hormone (CRH) neurons in the hypothalamic paraventricular nucleus (Figure 1.1A) (PVN) forms the basis of the hyperactivity of the HPA axis. The CRH neurons co-express vasopressin, which potentiates the CRH effects. CRH neurons project not only to the median eminence but also into brain areas where they affect mood. Both centrally released CRH and increased levels of cortisol contribute to the signs and symptoms of depression. The hypothalamo-neurohypophysial system is also involved in the stress response. It releases AVP from the PVN and the supraoptic nucleus (Figure 1.1A) (SON) via the neurohypophysis (Figure 1.2) into the bloodstream. Increased levels of circulating AVP are also associated with the risk of suicide. A decreased activity in the suprachiasmatic nucleus (SCN), the hypothalamic clock, in depression is the basis for the disturbances of circadian and circannual fluctuations in mood, sleep, and hormonal rhythms. Alterations in the systems from the brainstem that use amines as chemical messenger (noradrenergic, serotonergic, and histaminergic systems) or the prefrontal cortex (Figures 1.2, 1.7) may also be causally involved in depression. Genetic polymorphisms and developmental effects on each of these brain systems may be the major reason for depression in a particular patient (for review see Bao *et al.* 2008). On the basis of these findings in a large number of brain systems I foresee that a new kind of ``analytical psychiatry´´ will develop in the near future. After the anamnesis, blood from the depressed patient will be taken in order to determine hormone levels and metabolites of the chemical messengers that are transported from the brain to the blood, and the relevant genetic polymorphisms will be analyzed in the cellular fraction. On the basis of these data an ``analytical psychiatrist´´ will be able to establish which of the neurobiological systems plays a major part in the depressive symptoms of that particular patient (i.e. hyperactivity of CRH or vasopressin, decreased biological clock function, increased adrenal corticosteroids or alterations in the aminergic systems) and a patient-tailored therapy will then be given. This therapy may consist of a combination of chemicals specifically acting on one of the chemical messengers in the brain agonists or antagonists, electrical stimulation of particular brain structures or of the vagal nerve, or transcranial magnetic stimulation of the prefrontal cortex.

Deep brain stimulation in neurology and psychiatry: reversible psychosurgery

Stimulation by means of a microelectrode that is implanted deep into the brain, exactly in the right structure, while the patient is in the awake state, has a great future, not only in neurology but also in psychiatry. This approach started in 1987, when Benabid et al. (1987) reported on the first successful use of thalamic deep brain stimulation (DBS) as a chronic treatment for Parkinson's disease. DBS of the subthalamic nucleus can substantially reduce the slow movements, rigidity, tremor, and gait difficulties in Parkinson's disease. The benefit of DBS is often dramatic and durable and it is very impressive to see how extremely strong tremors suddenly disappear when the patient himself is putting the pulse generator on. DBS in the thalamus can also suppress a post-traumatic tremor or a multiple sclerosis tremor that is refractory to medication (Foote et al. 2006). Pain in terminal cancer, or intractable head or facial pains, can be relieved by DBS in the central grey of the brain, in the cortex or in the sensory thalamus (Owen et al. 2006; Perlmutter & Mink 2006; Green et al. 2005). When stimulated, an electrode in the central grey induces a release of opium-like substances in the brain. Cluster headache is one of the most severe primary headaches, and also known as ``suicide headache´´ because of the unbearably painful attacks that always occur at the same time of the day or night. Depth electrodes in the posterior part of the hypothalamus are effective against cluster headache. This brain area was shown to be activated during cluster headache attacks (Leone et al. 2004). Dystonia, a disorder of the tonicity of muscles, responds poorly to medical treatment but can now be effectively treated with DBS in the internal globus pallidus (Diamond et al. 2006; Kupsch et al. 2006; Vidailhet et al. 2005). DBS in the internal globus pallidus or in the medial thalamus substantially reduces tics and compulsions in Tourette syndrome (Ackermans et al. 2006). The same structure is the target in the case of tardive dyskinesia, a motoric side effect of schizophrenia therapy (Damier et al. 2007).

Interestingly, DBS also has a future in psychiatry. Obsessive compulsive disorder (OCD) patients, who do not have a normal social life anymore because of their disorder, can be treated by DBS of the nucleus accumbens (Figure 1.3). DBS in the subgenual cingulate white matter (Figure 1.2) may improve mood in major depression (Perlmutter & Mink 2006), and DBS of the posterior hypothalamus (Figures 1.1C, 1.5) was reported to have improved disruptive behavior in two mentally retarded patients who were medically intractably impulsive and violent (Franzini *et al.* 2005). In the near future, depth electrodes are expected to be implanted also in case of untreatable obesity.

Now that some 35,000 patients have been treated with DBS, the side effects of this new therapy are beginning to become apparent. Brain hemorrhage during implantation of the electrode, infection, and seizures do occur but are rare. However, psychiatric symptoms may also occur, such as disorders in thinking and memory, changes in character, depressive or manic states, and suicide or gambling. Selection of the right patients for the DBS therapy is thus a challenge for the period to come.

The placebo effect

The placebo effect of medicines can be very strong. Anti-depressants are even thought to have a placebo effect of between 45% and 75%. Placebo effects are real effects based upon our brain´s expectation of the treatment, and caused by unconscious specific alterations in the function of brain systems. If a patient takes a placebo tablet against pain, the brain ``knows´´ it has to release morphine-like peptides. This placebo effect can be blocked by naloxone, an opiate antagonist. In addition, placebo analgesia is accompanied by a decreased activity in pain-sensitive areas, as was shown by fMRI, suggesting that placebos also alter the experience of pain (Wagner *et al.* 2004). A placebo treatment of depressed patients induces an increased activity in the prefrontal cortex and a decreased activity in the hypothalamus, thus counteracting the typical functional alterations of the brain in depression. In Parkinson patients a placebo causes a release of dopamine in the striatum. A mechanism of action of the placebo effect in Parkinson patients has been revealed during the placement of depth electrodes. In the operating room a placebo treatment was causing reduced activity in single neurons in the target of that operation in the subthalamic nucleus (Figure 1.1C). These changes were tightly correlated with a clinical improvement. The rigidity of the arm diminished when ``the new medicine´´ (which was in fact physiological saline) was injected and caused a decrease in neuronal firing rate. Such a positively reacting patient said ``I can feel the new L-dopa´´ or ``I feel much better´´. When there was no decrease in subthalamic firing rate, the rigidity did not diminish and the patient said ``I do not feel anything´´ or ``It does not work´´ (Benedetti *et al.* 2004). Apparently the brain was doing exactly what the depth electrode should do after the operation, i.e. blocking the firing in the subthalamic nucleus when the stimulator is put on. It seems that the brain ``knows´´ what specific circuit should be functionally altered in order to achieve a positive effect. It is conceivable that a better insight into the neurobiological mechanisms of such placebo effects may lead to entirely new therapeutic strategies.

Reactivation of atrophic neurons

The strong atrophy, or diminution of the size of the brain of Alzheimer disease (AD) patients has generally been explained by massive cell death, which was presumed to be the basis of dementia. However, cell death in Alzheimer´s disease appeared not to be a generally occurring major phenomenon. Although the cortex may be strongly atrophic, the total number of neurons was not found to be diminished in AD. Cell death in AD is restricted to a few brain areas, e.g. the CA1 area in the hippocampus (Figure 1.5) and the superior temporal gyrus (Figures 1.6, 1.7). Reduced neuronal activity, resulting in atrophy, is probably one of the major characteristics of AD. It occurs early in the disease process and may underlie the clinical symptoms of dementia. Indeed, a 50%–70% decline of glucose metabolism is found in the brain of Alzheimer patients, causing energy metabolism to be critically lowered (Swaab *et al.* 2002).

A decrease in cerebral glucose metabolism is an early event in AD that may even precede cognitive impairment. Small *et al.* (1995) and Reiman *et al.* (1996) found that late middle-aged, cognitively normal subjects who were homozygous for the APOE-ε4 allele, and thus at risk for AD, already have reduced glucose metabolism in the same region of the brain that is later affected in patients with AD.

Of course, for the demented patient it does not make any difference whether the cells have died, or whether they are still there but no longer function. However, this does make a big difference for the development of therapeutic strategies. The primary focus for therapeutic strategies should thus not be prevention of cell death but rather reactivation of neuronal activity in order to improve neuronal metabolism and thus alleviate the cognitive and behavioral symptoms of AD.

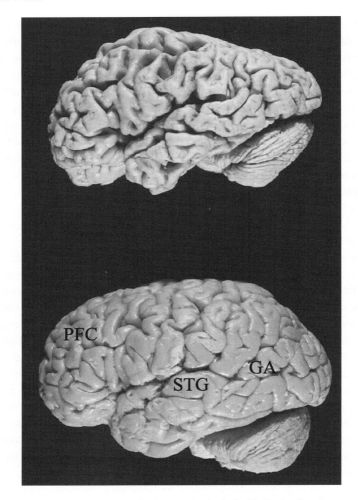

Figure 1.7 Side view of a human brain (left side is the front).
GA, gyrus angularis; PFC, prefrontal cortex; STG, superior temporal
gyrus. Upper panel, the atrophic brain of an Alzheimer patient; lower
panel, an age-matched control.

Activation of neurons may indeed have a beneficial effect on
neuronal function and survival during aging and Alzheimer's disease, a
mechanism we paraphrased as ``use it or lose it´´ (Swaab 1991; Swaab
et al. 2002). Several studies have indicated that education may protect
against dementia. Occupation was shown to be an even stronger
indication of risk for dementia than education (Bonaiuto *et al.* 1995;
Mortel *et al.* 1995). The decrease in time spent on intellectual activities

from early to middle adulthood was associated with a significant risk for AD (Fiedland *et al.* 2001). The observations that glucose administration or increasing glucose availability due to insulin enhances memory in patients with probable AD (Manning *et al.* 1993; Craft *et al.* 1996) not only support the view that AD is basically characterized by a lower brain metabolism, but also indicate that the focus on metabolic stimulation of neurons may be a fruitful strategy.

In order to show the proof of principle that a system affected by AD could still be activated we chose the circadian system. In AD, the suprachiasmatic nucleus (SCN), which is the biological clock of the brain, shows a marked functional deficit that causes sleep–wake pattern fragmentation and nightly restlessness. Increased input by additional bright light improved the rhythms in AD patients (Van Someren *et al.* 1997). In a recent randomized placebo-controlled clinical trial with a 3.5 year follow-up of 189 subjects in 12 homes for the elderly, using increased environmental light during the day and/or melatonin at night, we found a decrease in nightly restlessness by 22%, a decrease in depressive symptoms by 12%, an attenuated decline of 3 MMSE points in 3.5 years, and enhanced rhythms overall (Riemersma-van der Lek 2007). Research of the coming period should be centered around finding effective stimuli for other atrophic brain systems in neurodegenerative disorders.

In order to test for compounds that potentially may reactivate neurons in AD patients, we developed a postmortem brain tissue culture procedure from adult neurological patients and controls. Up to 10 h after death, it appears to be possible to maintain human brain slices in vitro that can be manipulated experimentally for extended periods. Neurons in these cultures (motor cortex, hippocampus, and cerebellum) could be transduced with adeno-associated viral vectors and expressed the reporter genes for as long as 44 days, proving that there is life after the death of the patient. These slice cultures offer new opportunities to study the cellular and molecular mechanisms of aging and neurodegenerative diseases (Verwer *et al.* 2002).

RESTORATIVE NEUROSCIENCE: THE GARAGE CALLED, YOUR BRAIN IS READY

Restoration of function in case of brain disorders can, in principle, be accomplished in very different ways, e.g. by brain–machine interfaces, brain grafts, mechanical or chemical interventions, or by gene, cell or molecular therapies.

Brain–machine interfaces to bypass nervous system damage

Neuroprosthetics aim to bypass the damage in the nervous system that prevents sensory information from going to the brain, or that affects the control of muscular output. Cochlear implants are very successful in cases of cochlear sensory neural hearing loss. Electrodes are positioned within the cochlea to stimulate the neurons that are connected to dysfunctional hearing cells. More than 100,000 people now have a cochlear implant and are often surprisingly successful at understanding speech (Scott 2006). When both auditory nerves are lesioned, an array of 12 electrodes can be placed on the inferior colliculus (Figure 1.3) as an auditory prosthesis. Electrical stimulation of the electrode array produced a significant speech perception and provided a clear improvement in communication ability when paired with lip-reading (Hochberg *et al.* 2006). An individual's cortical motor intentions can, in principle, be recorded and used to control a robotic manipulator or to control a computer mouse, as has been shown by Hochberg *et al.* (2006) in a man with a completely severed spinal cord. They implanted a 96-microelectrode array in his motor cortex that allowed this patient with a paralysis of all four extremities, to control a computer cursor and to close and open a prosthetic hand. This is new and very promising neurotechnology aimed at restoring function in humans with paralysis, although it will take quite some time to develop a fully implantable recording system that can record from thousands of neurons. Successful experiments are performed to restore limited but useful sight in profound blindness, using a miniature video camera built into the nosepiece of a pair of glasses, signal processing electronics carried in the pocket, and an array of microelectrodes implanted in the primary visual cortex (Normann 2007).

Neural transplantation: repair of local lesions

In 1987 the *New England Journal of Medicine* published a paper by Madrazo *et al.* (1987) that reported the amazing recovery of Parkinson patients following transplantation of a piece of their own adrenal medulla into the nucleus caudatus. This was immediately followed up by 200 transplantations in two years' time all over the world. The operation appeared to have produced some improvement after 6 months, but there were no sustained effects of the transplant, while the mortality was 10%–20% in 2 years. Autopsies revealed that the adrenal medulla graft did not survive.

Since 1988, grafts of the fetal substantia nigra, that are indeed able to survive, have been used for transplantation in Parkinson patients. The fetal tissue must be obtained from 6–8 weeks post-conception stages, and the equivalent of four embryos must be used for one transplant. In about 85% of the patients an active transplant may be retrieved by PET scanning. Following transplantation the patients need less L-dopa, while the slowness and rigidity of movements diminish. However, full recovery of these Parkinson patients has never been seen, and the results are highly variable. In some 15% of the patients, dyskinesias (i.e. difficulties in moving) occur, but these are the same patients that also suffer L-dopa dyskinesias. Long-term improvements resulting from fetal substantia nigra transplantations have been reported in Parkinson patients. However, the two double blind studies that were performed did not show an improvement of the primary outcome variables, although some scores were improved and both studies showed long-term survival of the transplant.

A monkey MPTP model is used to improve the efficacy of neural transplantation by trying to answer some general crucial questions for transplantation research. How do we prevent the death of the majority of the cells in a graft? Could neurotrophic factors (i.e. growth factors for the brain) be useful in this respect? How crucial is immuno-suppression, and is there a more suitable, standardized source for dopamine cells than fetal tissue, such as immortalized cell lines that do not generate tumors and do not have to be screened for infectious agents? Xeno-transplants with fetal pig material were tried but do not seem to survive and in addition carry the risk of animal virus transmission to humans (Freed *et al.* 2007).

In a pilot study in Huntington patients the first successful transplants of human fetal grafts implanted bilaterally into multiple caudate and putamen sites were performed. This will be followed by a French multicenter trial (Dunnett & Rosser 2007).

Intervention neurology

Until recently, neurologists could exactly localize the site of the damage but had hardly any therapeutic instruments. Now the work of an intervention neurologist deals with the intravenous administration of an enzyme (i.e. tissue plasminogen activator) that is the most beneficial proven intervention for emergency treatment of stroke. Several interventions, including intra-arterial administration of thrombolytic agents and the placement of stents, show promise. Researchers also investigated the advantages of the various treatments of bleeding from a dilatation of a blood vessel in the brain, and found that there were minimal differences in the long-term cognitive outcome between their method where they brought metallic coils into the dilatation via blood vessels and the classic approach of putting a clip on the dilatation, which demands major surgery. Such developments may make neuro-surgical intervention superfluous, as well as preventing serious brain damage (Martinez-Perez *et al.* 2007; Frazer *et al.* 2007).

Gene, molecular, and cell therapies: repairing neurodegeneration and reconnecting damaged neuronal pathways

Growth factors stimulate cell function and prevent neuronal death and thus offer the potential to prevent neuronal degeneration. Nerve growth factor (NGF) potentially stimulates the survival and functions of basal forebrain cholinergic neurons and may therefore reduce the cholinergic deficit in Alzheimer's disease. Gene therapy can achieve adequate concentrations of growth factors in the brain regions con-taining degenerating neurons and prevent growth factor from spreading to non-targeted regions to avoid side effects. Ongoing clinical programs are testing the hypotheses that NGF will protect cholinergic neurons in the AD brain, and that targeting of the cholinergic system will be sufficient to meaningfully benefit AD patients. Connective tis-sue cells from the skin from these patients were genetically modified to express NGF and injected under general anesthesia in the basal nuclei of AD patients (see Figure 1.1A, NBM). Initial clinical findings from these small, uncontrolled trials suggest that this procedure does indeed yield some positive effects. Now larger-scale, controlled studies of NGF gene delivery in AD are warranted. In addition, studies of NGF delivery by an AAV viral vector that is directly injected into the basal nuclei are in progress (Tuszynski 2007).

In Parkinson's disease, two other open-label clinical trials were started where glial celline-derived neurotrophic factor (GDNF), which has strong neuroprotective effects, was chronically infused using pumps into the putamen. Both of these trials showed functional improvement with a long-term (1 year) increase in dopamine storage in the putamen (Figure 1.3) and a corresponding improvement in the processing of motor output. Additionally, dyskinesia scores were sig-nificantly reduced in both studies. No side effects were noted, showing that site-specific direct GDNF treatment may be safe and beneficial.

However, a randomized controlled trial did not give a positive outcome. Gene therapy with the aim of delivering neurotrophic factors to the affected brain areas of Parkinson patients is currently in preparation (Korecka *et al*. 2007; Yasuhara *et al*. 2007.).

Early initiation of treatment of multiple sclerosis (MS) with interferon beta-1b prevents the development of disability, supporting its use after the first manifestation of relapsing-remitting MS (Kappos *et al*. 2007). In addition, vaccination through intramuscular injection of a DNA plasmid containing a protein from myelin (i.e. myelin basic protein), induced favorable trends on brain MRI and beneficial antigen-specific immune changes (Bar-Or *et al*. 2007). This is an entirely new principle for treatment.

Adult spinal cord injuries may lead to severe damage to both ascending sensory pathways and descending motor nerve pathways without any prospect of complete functional recovery. The paucity of regeneration in the spinal cord is thought to depend on a critical molecular balance between growth-promoting and growth-inhibiting factors. Experimental spinal cord repair strategies focus on the modulation of trophic and inhibitory influences to promote and guide axonal regrowth. Viral vector-mediated transfer of neurotrophin genes to the injured spinal cord is emerging as a novel and effective strategy to express neurotrophins in the injured nervous system. Ex vivo transfer of neurotrophic factor genes as a way for axonal regeneration to bridge lesion cavities is also explored. The genetic modification of different types of cells prior to implantation to the injured spinal cord has resulted in improved cellular nerve guides. Neurotrophic factor gene transfer to the injured spinal cord of animal experimental models, in combination with a range of cellular platforms for ex vivo gene transfer, is currently showing the first significant functional improvements, which offers new perspectives for repair of the injured human nervous system in the near future (Hendriks *et al*. 2004). After very successful animal experimental work, Martin Schwab, in Zürich, now leads a clinical trial to repair spinal cord lesions in freshly paraplegic patients, using antibodies to Nogo, in order to neutralize this protein, which prevents the outgrowth of nerve fibers in the adult nervous system.

The possibility of replacing lost nerve cells by pluripotent stem cells is receiving a great deal of attention. These stem cells can be isolated from autologous bone marrow, from fetal brain, or from the mucous membrane of the nose of the patient. A neuronal cell replacement strategy with embryonic stem (ES) cells is still in a very early stage of development and problems of immune-rejection, tumor formation, and stem cell differentiation must still be overcome. However, adult neural progenitor cells from the human brain survive when transplanted into the rat brain. They show targeted migration and proliferate and differentiate after grafting in the adult rat brain (Olstorn *et al.* 2007), which makes it clear that such cells bear great promise for the future.

CONCLUSIONS

We are our brains. Faults in this information-processing machine may lead to psychiatric, neurological, or neuroendocrine disorders, or to a wide variety of behavioral disorders, including aggression and criminal behavior. The product of the functions and interactions of the 100 billion nerve cells is our ``mind´´, but no argument seems to hold for the concept of the continued existence of a soul, i.e. ``something´´ immaterial that remains of our personality after we die. Some give brain-related arguments in favor of the existence of a soul and an afterlife, i.e. the direct contact with God that some temporal lobe epilepsy patients report and the occurrence of near-death experiences, but for both phenomena there are good neurobiological explanations available.

The extremely complex neuronal machine is programmed for a major part in early development as far as its structure and function are concerned. An example is the sexual differentiation of the brain, which develops in the male direction through the direct action of a boy´s testosterone on the developing nerve cells, and in the female direction through absence of this hormone in a girl. In this way not only our gender identity (the feeling of being a man or a woman) but also our sexual orientation is programmed into our brain structures when we are still in the womb.

Although brain diseases are still difficult to treat, there is now excitement about recent technological progress and new insights that bear great promise for treatment in the near future. For more and more brain disorders we are beginning to understand the pathogenesis and the molecular networks that are involved that lead to new therapeutic strategies.

Functional improvements may be obtained by psychopharmaca, deep brain stimulation (DBS), placebos, or reactivation of neurons. A patient-tailored therapy will become possible for depressed patients on the basis of their genetic background in combination with chemical assays in blood, showing which system is primarily affected, as well as a battery of new pharmacological and non-pharmacological therapeutic possibilities. DBS with microelectrodes that are implanted into exactly the right brain structure has a great future, not only in neurology, but also in psychiatry. A better insight into the neurobiological mechanisms of placebo effects may lead to entirely new therapeutic strategies. Reactivation of atrophic systems in Alzheimer's disease is possible, and active compounds are searched for in slice cultures of postmortem human brain tissue in which neurons survive.

Restorative neuroscience ranges from brain–machine interfacing to molecular techniques. An individual's cortical motor intentions can be recorded and used to reanimate paralyzed muscles or to control a computer mouse by neuroprosthetics. Fetal brain transplantation can be used to repair local lesions in the brain. Intervention neurologists deal with the emergency treatment of stroke. Gene and cell therapies are developed to treat Alzheimer and Parkinson patients and to repair spinal cord lesions.

The chances of growing very old with a healthy brain are constantly being increased by all these new developments in basic and clinical neurosciences.

ACKNOWLEDGMENT

I thank Mrs Wilma Verweij for her secretarial help.

GLOSSARY

Androgen insensitivity syndrome. A syndrome caused by mutations in the receptor gene for the male sex hormone testosterone. People with the syndrome are genetic males (XY) but they develop into women and experience their sexual orientation, fantasies, and experiences as ``heterosexual´´ i.e. towards men, without a gender identity problem.

Congenital adrenal hyperplasia. (CAH). A genetic disorder based on a failure of the adrenal gland to produce cortisol. Since the cortisol feedback on the pituitary and hypothalamus is lacking, the fetal adrenal gland is strongly activated and produces high amounts of male hormones such as testosterone. This masculinizes the female fetus, as is apparent from, for example, an enlarged clitoris at birth and more masculine behavior later.

Hypothalamo-pituitary–adrenal (HPA) axis. Often called the stress axis, this is considered to be the ``final common pathway´´ for a major part of the depressive symptomatology. The adrenal hormone involved is cortisol. The corticotrophin-releasing hormone (CRH) neurons in the paraventricular nucleus of the hypothalamus (see Figure 1.1) co-express vasopressin (AVP), which potentiates the CRH effects. CRH neurons project not only to the median eminence but also into brain areas, where they affect mood. Both centrally released CRH and increased levels of cortisol contribute to the signs and symptoms of depression.

Polymorphisms. Small alterations in the DNA of genes that occur in more that 1% of the population and increase the risk of certain disorders.

REFERENCES

Ackermans, L., Temel, Y., Cath, D. *et al.* 2006. Deep brain stimulation in Tourette´s syndrome: two targets? *Movement Disorders* **21**: 709–13.

Anderson, S. W., Bechara, A., Damasio, H., Tranel, D. & Damasio, A. R. 1999. Impairment of social and moral behavior related to early damage in human prefrontal cortex. *Nature Neuroscience* **2**(11): 1032–7.

Bao, A. –M., Meynen, G. & Swaab, D. F. 2008. The stress system in depression and neurodegeneration: focus on the human hypothalamus. *Brain Research Reviews* **57**: 531–53.

Bar-Or, A., Vollmer, T., Antel, J. *et al.* 2007. Induction of antigen-specific tolerance in multiple sclerosis after immunization with DNA encoding myelin basic protein in a randomized, placebo-controlled phase 1/2 trial. *Archives of Neurology* **64**: 1407–15.

Benabid, A. L., Pollak, P., Louveau, A., Henry, S. & de Rougemont, J. 1987. Combined (thalamotomy and stimulation) stereotactic surgery of the VIM thalamic nucleus for bilateral Parkinson disease. *Applied Neurophysiology* **50**: 344–6.

Benedetti, F., Colloca, L., Torre, E. *et al.* 2004. Placebo-responsive Parkinson patients show decreased activity in single neurons of subthalamic nucleus. *Nature Neuroscience* **7**: 587–8.

Blair, R. J. 2003. Neurobiological basis of psychopathy. *British Journal of Psychiatry* **182**: 5–7.

Blanke, O., Landis, T., Spinelli, L. & Seeck, M. 2004. Out-of-body experience and autoscopy of neurological origin. *Brain* **127**: 243–58.

Blanke, O., Ortigue, S., Landis, T . & Seeck, M. 2002. Stimulating illusory own-body perceptions. *Nature* **419**: 269–70.

Bonaiuto, S., Rocca, W. A., Lippi, A. *et al.* 1995. Education and occupation as risk factors for dementia: a population-based case-control study. *Neuroepidemiology* **14**: 101–9.

Brennan, P. A., Grekin, E. R. & Mednick, S. A. 1999. Maternal smoking during pregnancy and adult male criminal outcomes. *Archives of General Psychiatry* **56**: 215–19.

Colapinto, J. 2001. *As Nature Made Him. The Boy who was Raised as a Girl.* New York: Harper Collins.

Colletti, V., Shannon, R., Carner, M. *et al.* 2007. The first successful case of hearing produced by electrical stimulation of the human midbrain. *Otology and Neurotology* **28**: 39–43.

Coolidge, F. L., Thede, L. L. & Young, S. E. 2002. The heritability of gender identity disorder in a child and adolescent twin sample. *Behavior Genetics* **32**: 251–7.

Craft, S., Newcomer, J., Kanne, S. *et al.* 1996. Memory improvement following induced hyperinsulinemia in Alzheimer's disease. *Neurobiology of Aging* **17**: 123–30.

Damier, P., Thobois, S., Witjas, T. *et al.* 2007. Bilateral deep brain stimulation of the globus pallidus to treat tardive dyskinesia. *Archives of General Psychiatry* **64**: 170–6.

DeCharms, R. C., Maeda, F., Glover, G. H. *et al.* 2005. Control over brain activation and pain learned by using real-time functional MRI. *Proceedings of the National Academy of Sciences, USA* **102**: 18, 626–31.

Dessens, A. B., Cohen-Kettenis, P. T., Mellenbergh, G.-J. *et al.* 1999. Prenatal exposure to anticonvulsants and psychosexual development. *Archives of Sexual Behavior* **28**: 31–44.

Diamond, A., Shahed, J., Azher, S., Dat-Vuong, K. & Jankovic, J. 2006. Globus pallidus deep brain stimulation in dystonia. *Movement Disorder* **21**: 692–5.

Diamond, M. & Sigmundson, K. 1997. Sex reassignment at birth. Long-term review and clinical implications. *Archives of Pediatric and Adolescent Medicine* **151**: 298–304.

Dunnett, S. & Rosser, A. E. 2007. Cell transplantation for Huntington's disease. Should we continue? *Brain Research Bulletin* **72**: 132–47.

Foote, K. D., Seignourel, P., Fernandez, H. H. *et al.* 2006. Dual electrode thalamic deep brain stimulation for the treatment of posttraumatic and multiple sclerosis tremor. *Neurosurgery* **58**: 280–6.

Franzini, A., Marras, C., Ferroli, P., Bugiani, O. & Broggi, G. 2005. Stimulation of the posterior hypothalamus for medically intractable impulsive and violent behavior. *Stereotactic and Functional Neurosurgery* **83**: 63–6.

Frazer, D., Ahuja, A., Watkins, L. & Cipolotti, L. 2007. Coiling versus clipping for the treatment of aneurysmal subarachnoid hemorrhage: a longitudinal investigation into cognitive outcome. *Neurosurgery* **60**: 434–41.

Freed, C. R., Zawada, M., Leehey, M., Zhou, W. & Breeze, R. E. 2007. Transplantation. In Koller, W. C. & Melamed, E. (eds.). *Handbook of Clinical Neurology 84*, Edinburgh: Elsevier, pp. 289–90.

Friedland, R. P., Fritsch, T., Smyth, K.-A. *et al.* 2001. Patients with Alzheimer's disease have reduced activities in midlife compared with healthy control-group members. *Proceedings of the National Academy of Sciences, USA* **98**: 3440–5.

Green, A. L., Owen, S. L. F., Davies, P., Moir, L. & Aziz, T. Z. 2005. Deep brain stimulation for neuropathic cephalalgia. *Cephalalgia* **26**: 561–7.

Heindel, M. 1913. *Rozenkruizers Cosmologie*. Amsterdam: NV Theosofische Uitgeversmaatschappij.

Hendriks, W. T. J., Ruitenberg, M. J., Blits, B., Boer, G. J. & Verhaagen, J. 2004. Viral vector-mediated gene transfer of neurotrophins to promote regeneration of the injured spinal cord. *Progress in Brain Research* **146**: 451–76.

Henningsson, S., Westberg, L., Nilsson, S. *et al.* 2005. Sex steroid-related genes and male-to-female transsexualism. *Psychoneuroendocrinology* **30**: 657–64.

Hochberg, L. R., Serruya, M. D., Friehs, G. M. *et al.* 2006. Neuronal ensemble control of prosthetic devices by a human with tetraplegia. *Nature* **442**: 164–71.

Kappos, L., Freedman, M. S., Polman, C. H. *et al.* 2007. BENEFIT Study Group. Effect of early versus delayed interferon beta-1b treatment on disability after a first clinical event suggestive of multiple sclerosis: a 3-year follow-up analysis of the BENEFIT study. *Lancet* **370**: 389–97.

Korecka, J. A., Verhaagen, J. & Hol, E. M. 2007. Cell replacement and gene therapy strategies for Parkinson's and Alzheimer's disease. *Regenerative Medicine* **2**: 425–46.

Kruijver, F. P. M., Zhou, J. N., Pool, C. W. *et al.* 2000. Male-to-female transsexuals have female neuron numbers in a limbic nucleus. *Journal of Clinical Endocrinology and Metabolism* **85**: 2034–41.

Kupsch, A., Benecke, R., Müller, J. *et al.* 2006. Pallidal deep-brain stimulation in primary generalized or segmental dystonia. *New England Journal of Medicine* **355**: 1978–90.

Leone, M., May, A., Franzini, A. *et al.* 2004. Deep brain stimulation for intractable chronic cluster headache: proposals for patient selection. *Cephalalgia* **24**: 934–7.

LeVay, S. 1996. *Queer Science. The Use and Abuse of Research into Homosexuality.* Cambridge, MA: MIT Press.

Madrazo, I., Drucker-Colín, R., Díaz, V. *et al.* 1987. Open microsurgical autograft of adrenal medulla to the right caudate nucleus in two patients with intractable Parkinson's disease. *New England Journal of Medicine* **316**: 831–4.

Manning, C. A., Ragozzino, M. E., & Gold, P. E. 1993. Glucose enhancement of memory in patients with probable senile dementia of the Alzheimer's type. *Neurobiology of Aging* **14**: 523–8.

Manuck, S. B., Flory, J. D., Ferrell, R. E., Dent, K. M., Mann, J. J. & Muldoon, M. F. 1999. Aggression and anger-related traits associated with a polymorphism of the tryptophan hydroxylase gene. *Biological Psychiatry* **45**: 603–14.

Manuck, S. B., Flory, J. D., Ferrell, R. E., Mann, J. J. & Muldoon, M. F. 2000. A regulatory polymorphism of the monoamine oxidase-A gene may be associated with variability in aggression, impulsivity, and central nervous system serotonergic responsivity. *Psychiatry Research* **95**: 9–23.

Martinez-Perez, M., Canovas-Verge, D. & Carvajal-Diaz, A. 2007. Fibrinolytic treatment with tissue plasminogen activator. Outcomes in clinical practice with a multidisciplinary model of intervention. (In Spanish.) *Revista de Neurologia* **45**: 129–33.

Money J. 1975. Ablatio penis: normal male infant sex-reassigned as a girl. *Archives of Sexual Behavior* **4**: 65–71.

Money, J. & Erhardt, A. A. 1972. *Man and Woman, Boy and Girl: the Differentiation and Dimorphism of Gender Identity from Conception to Maturity.* Baltimore, MD: Johns Hopkins University Press.

Mortel, K. F., Meyer, J. S., Herod, B. & Momby, J. 1995. Education and occupation as risk factors for dementias of the Alzheimer' and ischemic vascular types. *Dementia* **6**: 55–62.

Neuman, R. J., Lobos, E., Reich, W . *et al.* 2007. Prenatal smoking exposure and dopaminergic genotypes interact to cause a severe ADHD subtype. *Biological Psychiatry* **61**: 1320–8.

Normann, R. A. 2007. Technology insight: future neuroprosthetic therapies for disorders of the nervous system. *Nature Neurology* **3**: 444–52.

Olstorn, H., Moe, M. C., Rste, G. K., Bueters, T. & Langmoen, I. A. 2007. Transplantation of stem cells from the adult human brain to the adult rat brain. *Neurosurgery* **60**: 1089–99.

Osuch, E. & Williamson, P. 2006. Brain imaging in psychiatry: from a technique of exclusion to a technique for diagnosis. *Acta Psychiatrica Scandinavica* **114**: 73–4.

Owen, S. L. F., Green, A. L., Stein, J. F. & Aziz, T. Z. 2006. Deep brain stimulation for the alleviation of post-stroke neuropathic pain. *Pain* **120**: 202–6.

Parnia, S. & Fenwick, P. 2002. Near death experiences in cardiac arrest: visions of a dying brain or visions of a new science of consciousness. *Resuscitation* **52**: 5–11.

Pearsall, P., Schwartz, G. E. R. & Russek, L. G. S. 2002. Changes in heart transplant recipients that parallel the personalities of their donors. *Journal of Near-Death Studies* **20**: 191–206.

Perlmutter, J. S. & Mink, J. W. 2006. Deep brain stimulation. *Annual Review of Neuroscience* **29**: 229–57.

Popma, A. & Raine, A. 2006. Will future forensic assessment be neurobiologic? *Child and Adolescent Psychiatric clinics of North America* **15**: 429–44.

Reiman, E. M., Caselli, R. J., Yun, L. S. *et al.* 1996. Preclinical evidence of Alzheimer's disease in persons homozygous for the ε4 allele for apolipoprotein E. *New England Journal of Medicine* **334**: 752–8.

Repovš, G. & Bresjanac, M. 2006. Cognitive neuroscience of working memory: a prologue. *Neuroscience* **139**: 1–3.

Riemersma-van der Lek, R. T. 2007. Keep it bright. Deterioration and reactivation of the biological clock in dementia. Thesis, University of Amsterdam. ISBN 978 90219783.

Saver, J. L. & Rabin, J. 1997. The neural substrates of religious experience. *American Psychiatric Press,* **9** (3): 498–510.

Scott, S. H. 2006. Neuroscience: converting thoughts into action. *Nature* **442**: 141–2.

Small, G. W., Mazziotta, J. C., Collins, M. T. *et al.* 1995. Apolipoprotein E type 4 allele and cerebral glucose metabolism in relatives at risk for familial Alzheimer disease. *Journal of the American Medical Association* **273**: 942–7.

Steinmetz, H., Herzog, A., Huang, Y. & Hackländer T. 1994. Discordant brain-surface anatomy in monozygotic twins. *New England Journal of Medicine* **331**: 952–3.

Swaab, D. F. 1991. Brain aging and Alzheimer's disease: ``wear and tear'' versus ``use it or lose it''. *Neurobiology of Aging* **12**: 317–24.

Swaab, D. F. 2004. *The Human Hypothalamus. Basic and Clinical Aspects. Part II Neuropathology of the Hypothalamus and Adjacent Brain Structures. (Handbook of Clinical Neurology.)* Amsterdam: Elsevier.

Swaab, D. F. 2007. Sexual differentiation of the brain and behavior. *Best Practice & Research in Clinical Endocrinology and Metabolism* **21**: 431–4.

Swaab, D. F., Dubelaar, E. J. G., Hofman, M. A. *et al.* 2002. Brain aging and Alzheimer's disease; use it or lose it. *Progress in Brain Research* **138**: 343–73.

Tuszynski, M. H. 2007. Nerve growth factor gene therapy in Alzheimer disease. *Alzheimer Disease and Associated Disorders* **21**: 179–89.

Van Lommel, P., Van Wees, R., Meyers, V. & Elfferich, I. 2001. Near-death experience in survivors of cardiac arrest: a prospective study in the Netherlands. *Lancet* **358**: 2039–45.

Van Someren, E. J. W., Kessler, A., Mirmiran, M. & Swaab, D. F. 1997. Indirect bright light improves circadian rest-activity rhythm disturbances in demented patients. *Biological Psychiatry* **41**: 955–63.

Verwer, R. W. H., Hermens, W. T. J. M. C., Dijkhuizen, P. A. *et al.* 2002. Cells in human postmortem brain tissue slices remain alive for several weeks in culture. *FASEB Journal* **16**: 54–60.

Vidailhet, M., Vercueil, L., Houeto, J.- L. *et al.* 2005. Bilateral deep-brain stimulation of the globus pallidus in primary generalized dystonia. *New England Journal of Medicine* **352**: 459–67.

Wagner, T. D., Rilling, J. K., Smith, E. E. *et al.* 2004. Placebo-induced changes in fMRI in the anticipation and experience of pain. *Science* **303**: 1162–7.

Wuerfel, J., Krishnamoorthy, E. S., Brown, R. J. *et al.* 2004. Religiosity is associated with hippocampal but not amygdala volumes in patients with refractory epilepsy. *Journal of Neurology, Neurosurgens and Psychiatry* **75**: 640–2.

Yasuhara, T., Shingo, T. & Date, I. 2007. Glial cell line-derived neurotrophic factor (GDNF) therapy for Parkinson´s disease. *Acta Medica Okyama* **61**: 51–6.

Zhou, J. N., Hofman, M. A., Gooren, L. J. G. & Swaab, D. F. 1995. A sex difference in the human brain and its relation to transsexuality. *Nature* **378**: 68–70.

2

The origins of the modern concept of ``neuroscience´´

Wilhelm Wundt between empiricism, and idealism: implications for contemporary neuroethics

N. KOHLS & R. BENEDIKTER

INTRODUCTION

With the Age of Enlightenment, a sociocultural transformation process began on a large scale. This process can defined concisely by the triple trends of individualization, secularization, and scientification (Kohls 2004; Benedikter 2001; 2005). As a consequence, rational and scientific concepts replaced those of religion and spirituality in social life. This was especially true for the role of institutionalized religion as a genuine compass for social values and an epistemological framework as well as for morally and socially acceptable behavior. In the main, religious adherence was gradually substituted by a pluralism of scientific concepts and by philosophical systems. With the rise of academic psychology in the 1880s as a new, independent scientific field of inquiry, the explaining of consciousness and its underlying mechanisms became the focus of science in accordance with the aforementioned *Zeitgeist* as predicted by French thinker Auguste Comte. Psychology as a secular, rational, and ``measuring´´ science overtook religion and philosophy as the new center of intellectual and perhaps social gravity. It was within this new paradigm that the ``essence of the human being´´ was now to be studied.

These developments had enormous impact on the explicit and implicit interpretational frameworks for explaining consciousness and

Scientific and Philosophical Perspectives in Neuroethics, ed. J. J. Giordano & B. Gordijn. Published by Cambridge University Press. © Cambridge University Press 2010.

the scientific theories of mind that emerged of the time. Of note is that, in the first half of the nineteenth century, a paradigm shift also occurred in biology and medicine. The focus of studies about the nature of mind moved from anatomy to physiology. From then on, it became possible and, most importantly, culturally and paradigmatically acceptable, to define terms such as ``life´´ and ``energy´´ mainly in physiological, and not only in philosophical or aesthetic, terms. When physiological research was increasingly applied to scrutinizing perception on the basis of underlying physiological mechanisms, the groundwork for a physiological psychology was formed. Seen from a viewpoint fostered within a history of ideas, the Cartesian ontology that differentiated between body (``res extensa´´) and mind (``res cogitans´´), and the corresponding idea of the ``homunculus´´ as ``primum movens´´ was gradually displaced by a psychophysiological theory of sensation and mentation. This paved the way for the historical separation of philosophy and psychology. However, as enlightened philosophy had engaged a meta-narrative of rationality, psychology (as an upcoming academic endeavor) had to offer stark contrast to mystical and folk beliefs of mental (and behavioral) activity. Psychology was increasingly encouraged to devise a theory of mind that was free of metaphysical concepts such as ``soul´´ or ``spirit.´´

Interestingly, the inception of academic psychology as an independent scientific endeavor, separated from philosophy on the one hand and from the natural sciences on the other, coincided with the rise and eventual clash of two contradicting world views: experimental spiritism and rational empiricism (Kohls 2004; Kohls & Sommer 2006; Stromberg 1989), both of which were exploiting experimental methods in order to substantiate their fundamental hypotheses and premises. Experimental psychology was initiated – at least as an institutionalized academic endeavor independent from philosophy – in 1879, when Wilhelm Wundt established the first genuine psychological laboratory harnessing experimental methods at the University of Leipzig. This is well known as the birth of experimental psychology, the forerunner of cognitive neuroscience, yet it is worthwhile to examine more closely the circumstances surrounding this event, as relevant to the current status and possible trajectories that cognitive neuroscience, neurophilosophy, and neuroethics might assume. Less well known, although well documented, is the fact that from 1877 onwards Wundt – at this time a rather junior figure at the University of Leipzig – had to struggle to establish psychology as an independent academic field (Bringmann & Tweney 1980).

Looking more closely at this historic situation, we argue that it is a basis for the origin of the modern inquiry into consciousness and the human mind. Our hypothesis is that the clash between psychology and spiritism had a major impact on Wundt's later views, which can be seen as explicitly contributory to current cognitive neurosciences.

To build a valid basis for this hypothesis, we present an overview of relevant events from 1877 to 1879. It is useful to start with some background information about Wundt's scientific and philosophical development. We next outline the status of the epistemological debate in the second half of the nineteenth century. We examine the hypothesis that Wundt might have banned altered states of consciousness from the research agenda of experimental psychology, not only because he was traumatized by his encounter with spiritism as a young professor, but mainly because he regarded spiritism as a materialistically distorted form of spirituality. In a final step, we discuss some of the arguments against spiritism originally brought forward by Wundt some 130 years ago in light of the present debates in cognitive neurosciences and the theory of mind, particularly paying attention to ethical considerations of determinism, free will, and moral responsibility.

We pose several core questions. First, can Wundt's rejection of spiritism be interpreted, from a contemporary point of view, as a ``negative'' defense of a dimension of transcendence, that has to be re-integrated adequately – i.e. strictly empirically – in the contemporary quest for an inclusive, holistic concept of consciousness? And if so, does this ``negative defense'' show some similarities to the more recent developments within the leading ``postmodern'' philosophies and world views? Some of them seem to have gone through a late ``ethical and theological turn of deconstruction'' (Caputo 2005; Benedikter 2008a), and, as a consequence, tended to re-integrate both the achievements of radical (secular) rationality and empirically oriented spirituality into a ``spiritual'' concept of the human self, although in negative language. Put bluntly, might there be a convergence in the history of ideas that conjoins developments of the late nineteenth and the early twenty-first century regarding the search for an empirically grounded, inclusive epistemological concept of the human mind? In this case, what can be learned from past developments for the current and future debate on the role of Neuroethics in our progressively plural cultural and intellectual climate?

WILHELM WUNDT: THE FOUNDING FATHER OF EXPERIMENTAL PSYCHOLOGY

Wilhelm Wundt (1832–1920) is well known as the founder of experimental psychology, establishing the first experimental psychology laboratory at the University of Leipzig and training several generations of important American and European psychologists (Boring 1950; Lambertini 1995). Having graduated in medicine in 1856 from the University of Heidelberg, Wundt began his academic career in the laboratory of the physiologist and anatomist Johannes Peter Müller (1801–1858) in Berlin, after a short interim working as a physician in a local clinic. Two years later he returned to Heidelberg and became an assistant to one of Müller's most important disciples, the physicist and physiologist Hermann von Helmholtz (1821–1894), the so-called ``Imperial Chancellor of Physics'' because of the influence of his ideas. Here, young Wundt was able to familiarize himself with the current methods and knowledge of physiology. As a consequence of his training in Helmholtz's laboratory, Wundt published a ground-breaking two-volume book on the principles of physiological psychology in 1874 (Wundt 1874). Whereas Helmholtz was more focussed on physiological questions, Wundt developed a specific interest in the psychophysiological ``fringe area'' of the field, where exact and objective physiological mechanisms were – at least from Helmholtz's perspective – distorted by hazy and fuzzy psychological processes (Krüger 1994). Wundt gradually shifted his focus of interest from physiology to psychology (Ziche 1999). Nevertheless, the two scientists managed to get along for some time despite a level of scientific disagreement, and Wundt continued to work as assistant in Helmholtz's laboratory from 1858 to 1867. Remarkably, in 1871 – when Helmholtz was appointed to the prestigious Berlin chair – Wundt, a seemingly natural candidate, was bypassed for appointment to succeed his mentor in the then vacant Heidelberg chair. After this, the relationship between the two men seems to have deteriorated, and Wundt, after a period as professor of inductive philosophy at the University of Zurich, managed to obtain an appointment as full professor for philosophy in Leipzig in 1875. It is interesting to note that he was supported by Johann Zöllner (1834–82) and Gustav Fechner (1801–87), who were both sceptical of Helmholtz's positivist ideas on physics, but were rather interested in ideas associated with a more romantic world view (such as a universal metaphysical dimension *within* physics) (Heidelberger 2004). It was at the University of Leipzig that Wundt, surrounded by scholars who were disapproving of Helmholtz's anti-idealistic approach, established a psychological laboratory in 1879, where subsequent generations of young psychologists were to be trained in experimental (psychophysiological) methods. However, because Wundt perceived a narrow-mindedness in the experimental approach to explaining complex cultural phenomena, he dedicated the last 20 years of his life to devising a voluminous cultural anthropology that he called ``Völkerpsychologie`` (comparative folk psychology). Wundt was appointed as Chancellor of the University of Leipzig in 1890, and awarded honorary citizenship of the city of Leipzig in 1902. After having published more than 55,000 pages of scholarly work during his professional career, he retired from teaching in 1915 and died in 1920, shortly after finishing his autobiography (Wundt 1920).

BUILDING AN EPISTEMOLOGY FOR THE MODERN AGE: NINETEENTH CENTURY SCIENCE STRUGGLING WITH KANTIAN PHILOSOPHY

But what was the greater paradigmatic framework of Wundt´s life achievements, and in which developmental lines of the history of ideas was this embedded? Speculative ``Naturphilosophie`` (philosophy of nature) was an offspring of romanticism, asserting that all forms of life are imbued with a spiritual power that can only be grasped by means of speculative transcendental concepts. This was predominant in most scientific fields within Central Europe during the first half of the nineteenth century. In contrast, the rapidly developing field of the natural sciences was progressively grounded in an empirico rational experimental approach, and challenged the older view (Paul 1984). Consequently, the decline of ``Naturphilosophie`` in the second half of the nineteenth century made room within German academia for idealism and empiricism, two antithetical philosophical directions that were increasingly confronted with nationalistic ideas. During this time, the German scientific climate and professional environment of Wundt was preoccupied with an ongoing tension between proponents of idealism and materialism. This became gradually more apparent in most sectors of society and science (Treitel 2004).

The controversy between idealism and empiricism was viewed by the educated class as an unavoidable consequence of Kantian philosophy. Kant´s central thesis was that the possibility of human knowledge presupposes the active participation of the human mind. Despite its deceptive simplicity and seeming straightforwardness, it turned out to incur an epistemological pitfall (Pippin 2005): Kant maintained that the human mind had to operate within given categories (or as Kant termed them ``synthetic judgments a priori``). Thereby he had inevitably linked the concept of reality – or at least whether human beings could determine and perceive reality – to the human condition itself. In modern terms, Kant had moderated empirical realism with a kind of transcendental constructivism. Although this insight was seen as a large step towards an enlightened critical development within epistemology, Kant´s philosophical system also generated an insecurity regarding the question of whether we can actually perceive reality in the first place. Despite Kant´s desire to overcome the flaws of both empiricism and idealism by means of acknowledging the importance of inductive a-priori and deductive a-posteriori judgements, his philosophy was revealed to be notoriously complex to apply in detail. Correspondingly, depending on the precise interpretation, there was room for (proto-)positivist and empiricist, as well as (proto-)metaphysical, viewpoints in Kantian constructs. Specifically, the ongoing necessity to continuously renegotiate the limits of empiricism against the boundaries of idealism emerged as a weak point of Kantian philosophy. When used for demarcating the ``borders´´ of science and philosophy, Kant failed to create a viable construct that would allow valuable grounding notions. Hence, extensive debates concerning the ontological foundations of world views were inevitable as new theories of mind were formed.

NINETEENTH CENTURY PHYSICS TESTING THE LIMITS OF EMPIRICISM

In the second half of the nineteenth century, physics had become the epistemological spearhead of the natural sciences. Although, or even because, physics was primarily empirically oriented, it was also inevitably confronted with the epistemological loopholes of Kantian philosophy. In the middle of the 1860s, mathematicians, physicists, and philosophers were starting to debate the question of ``geometric epistemology´´. This scientific question may sound quite innocuous at first glance; however, it had an explosive effect on the *Zeitgeist*. In realizing its full scope, it is important to recognize that the discourse over non-Euclidean geometry, and the issues about the certainty of knowledge and limits of empiricism, tended to aggravate the relationship between science and (Christian) spirituality (Valente 2004). In other words, an important pillar of idealism was actually at risk of being overthrown by empiricism. The pivotal question within mathematics and physics was whether Kant´s a priori of time and space was the final border that had to be nominally defined by means of transcendental axioms (a priori), or whether n-dimensional spaces could be formally devised by means of empirical observation. The latter would allow for determining the metric structure of the dimensions by means of empirical data, which would be (and as a matter of fact actually is) an important prerequisite for modern physics. Specifically, non-Euclidian, Riemannian geometry contradicted not only the Kantian a priori of space, but also challenged the view of the transcendent nature of such a-priori categories. It is equally important to note that this epistemological debate was not merely of interest to mathematicians and physicists, but also the educated public, primarily for its implications regarding idealistic and transcendental philosophy. Edwin Abbott's 1884 novel *Flatland* provides an example of the epistemological importance of addressing the spiritual aspects of this debate (Abbott 1991).

As the root of the problem was associated with an important aspect of transcendental philosophy, it is not surprising that German physicists were also divided over this question. Hermann von Helmholtz was seen as a leading figure of what was regarded as a modern, anti-metaphysical, empirically oriented positivistic physics. On the other hand, at the University of Leipzig was Johann Karl Zöllner, an expert in astrophysics, under the influence of Gustav Fechner, both of whom were keen on reconciling speculative and metaphysical natural philosophy with empirical physics (Heidelberger 2004). Although both scientists agreed that n-dimensional spaces could exist, they had diverging ideas about the cosmologic, ontologic, and epistemologic consequences.

To understand this complex issue, let us first consider Helmholtz's point of view. In the course of working on his *Physiological Optics*, Helmholtz contested the Platonic assumption, upheld by Kant, that the axioms of Euclidean geometry are simply given as necessary, transcendental forms of intuition, existing a priori. In other words, Helmholtz was questioning the thesis that Euclidean metrics are ``innate'' to the human mind in such a way that they that cannot be resolved by further psychological processes (Kaku 1995). Helmholtz argued that the perception of a fourth dimension could potentially be learned, but only if this level could also be phenomenologically (i.e. experientially) accessed by human beings. To make his point, Helmholtz devised a thought experiment and posited a fictitious species that he named ``surface dwellers''. According to this thought experiment, the ``surface dwellers'' were restricted to living in a two-dimensional space and correspondingly could not think of an object moving along a third dimension. For them, an object allowed to move into a third dimension would simply appear to have vanished (Stromberg 1989). According to Helmholtz, human beings are in a position comparable to the ``surface dwellers'' when it comes to perceiving a fourth dimension. Thus, although Helmholtz argued that the conceptualization of Euclidean geometry may be attributed to learning processes (Richards 1977), he did not hold that the potentially possible n-dimensional space could overlap with the ordinary real world, and interact with its objects. That is to say that, according to Hemholtz, although n-dimensional spaces are potentially possible, there was (in his opinion) no need to postulate such a fourth dimension, at least not until empirical evidence could show that three-dimensional bodies can escape the three-dimensional space. Hence, he correctly assumed in accordance with Riemann´s theorem, that there would be a distinct barrier between the abstract metrics of non-Euclidean geometry and the concrete phenomena of the natural world.

Zöllner used the same argument as originally developed by Helmholtz in his thought experiment about the ``surface dwellers´´ for demonstrating the possibility of a fourth transcendental dimension, although in a contrary manner and without crediting Hemholtz for devising the idea (Zöllner 1879). Whereas Helmholtz believed that the existence of a non-Euclidean fourth dimension might be (in principle) empirically inferable, Zöllner deemed it to be not only experimentally verifiable, but also tangible. Thus, Zöllner assumed that the fourth dimension could physically overlap and interact with the three-dimensional Euclidean-based common sense reality of the ordinary world. It is noteworthy that Zöllner´s conviction about the substanti-ality of the fourth dimension was probably fanned by a small work called *Space has Four Dimensions*, written in 1846 by Fechner under the pseudonym ``Dr. Mises´´ (Heidelberger 2004). In this ironical essay, Fechner – arguing in the tradition of idealistic–romantic science – tried to save the idea of a unifying metaphysical background principle (that subserves the phenomena of empirical physics) by introducing a fourth transcendental dimension (Ellenberger 1970).

So, whereas Hemholtz interpreted the fourth dimension as an abstract concept, Zöllner thought this to be a concrete space capable of hosting Euclidean objects. The only thing Zöllner had to do was to provide experimental proof for the existence of a fourth dimension by means of an ``experimentum crucis´´. He claimed to have found such an experimental approach by the means of spiritualistic séances.

THE SCHOLARLY DISPUTE ON SPIRITISM IN LEIPZIG 1877

In central Europe during the second half of the nineteenth century, spiritualistic ideas co-existed with the modern secular world view as derived from science, despite the sharp contrast in method (Sawicki 2002). In short, spiritists or spiritualists believed – in accordance with an important pillar of Christian faith – in the survival of the soul beyond the body and the possibility of communicating with it, for example by means of a séance. They would sometimes call themselves ``radical idealists'' (Benedikter 2001; Thissen 2000).

Leipzig was particularly well known for a somewhat anti-modern disposition, and for a certain occult flair. The latter had been enthused by the Oswald-Mutze-Verlag, a very active publishing house specializing in spiritualist and occult literature, established in 1872 (Linse 1999). Apart from Victorian literature on spiritism, Mutze also published the works of German ``avantgarde spiritists'' such as Carl du Prel (1839–1899) and Baron Lazarus Hellenbach (1827–87). Thus, it seems to be possible that when Wundt was appointed as a young professor at the University of Leipzig, his happiness may have been slightly diminished by the fact that he actually found himself to be in the lions' den of late romantic, ``radical idealistic'' occultism.

When an American psychic of questionable reputation, Henry Slade (1839–1909), began a tour of Europe in 1877, Leipzig seemed to be a reasonable starting point. The American medium, who had been sentenced to three months' hard labor for deception and fraud in England and had therefore fled the country, delivered some startling exhibitions, such as the famous knot experiment (Klinckowstroem 1925). Here, Slade allegedly went into a trance, in which he was able to present strange phenomena such as communicating with spirits and asking them to tie a knot in a closed rope loop (Treitel 2004; Staubermann 2001). In other words, Slade was offering the type of experimental proof that Zöllner had been looking for. Seen from Zöllner's perspective, Slade was not only providing experimental validation of the existence of a fourth dimension and the existence of spirits, but was also demonstrating their tangible interrelation with the natural world.

Within a short time Slade managed to both attract a broad audience, and befriend Zöllner. The Leipzig academic *intellegentsia* was also attracted by the American medium, as were leading scholars at the University, such as the mathematician Wilhelm Scheibner. Fechner, Zöllner, and Weber also attended Slade's séances. On two occasions Wundt himself attended his séances (Treitel 2004). Zöllner and – at least to some degree – Fechner were thereafter convinced that the phenomena produced by Slade were genuine and could be regarded as empirical proof of the existence of a transcendental dimension.

According to Zöllner, this usually concealed dimension would be inhabited by the disincarnated spirits of the deceased, who could nevertheless be brought to interact with the world if summoned by a gifted medium (such as Slade). Zöllner skilfully devised an experimental protocol to prove that the phenomena were genuine and not artifacts of sleight-of-hand. A professor of logics, Hermann Ulrici (1806–1884), although not personally attending the séances, went so far as to make Zöllner´s experiments with Slade public by describing them in a scientific journal, in which he stated that Wundt and other professors had attended the séances (Ulrici 1879). Ulrici concluded that spiritism would be a scientific question of utmost importance as it could bring new and significant insights, empirically corroborated, to the human condition. Moreover, he urged the scholars who had attended the séances to publicly testify about what they had experienced.

When Wundt read Ulrici´s paper, he was compelled to write a harsh rejoinder (Wundt 1879). His argument against Ulrici was threefold.

> First, if the phenomena produced by Slade were true, spiritism would correspondingly violate the assumption of universal causality, which has always been, and remains one of the most important prerequisites for the empirical sciences. To quote from Wundt´s letter:

> > The natural scientist accesses his observations with an unshakable belief in the veracity of the objects he is studying. [. . .] He cannot be deceived by nature as there is neither caprice nor randomness within the natural things. However, you have to admit that one cannot speak of a distinct lawfulness with regard to the spiritual phenomena in question; quite to the contrary, it seems rather that every form of lawfulness is derided by spiritism
> >
> > Wundt 1879, pp. 8–9, translated by NK.

> Second, it is by no means clear that scientists were the best profession to be charged with judging the phenomena produced by Slade under obscure conditions, as sleight-of-hand could primarily be unveiled by trick magicians, illusionists, and similar professions more familiar with the trickery that might be potentially involved. Thus, Wundt argued that scientific observations under poor experimental conditions (as common for séance settings), would be comparable to ``. . . scrutinizing the swinging of a pendulum through a keyhole,´´ or – possibly in an allusion to Zöllner – ``recommending to an astronomer to install his telescope in the basement.´´

> Third, if spiritism was true, this would also entail a moral problem, as the spirits of the deceased would not only fall victim to a medium but also show themselves to be in a deplorable intellectual state.

Finally, Wundt stated that he could only wonder why a trained and experienced philosopher such as Ulrici had not recognized the fact that spiritism as a cultural phenomenon would only draw a distorted picture of a higher metaphysical order in a deformed materialistic manner, and correspondingly this could in turn only be seen as a sign of the ``. . . cultural barbarism of our times´´.

Having written the rejoinder, Wundt himself was then furiously attacked by Zöllner, who threatened Wundt with a formal lawsuit as he deemed his (and Slade´s) professional and private reputation damaged by the young professor of philosophy (Zöllner 1879). In his ire, Zöllner went so far as to accuse Wundt, who had insidiously been identified as ``a medium of strong power´´ by Slade, of being possessed by (evil) spirit (s) while writing his critique against spiritism. Zöllner claimed that his conversion to spiritism had actually healed him from a deep depression that he developed as a consequence of a materialistic world view. Of interest is that during the controversy Wundt was indirectly supported by Helmholtz, who had declared Zöllner to be insane (Cahan 1994). The debate gradually ceased, and ended completely after Zöllner´s sudden and unexpected death in 1882. Notably, when Wundt was made head of the commission for nominating Zöllner´s successor to the astrophysics chair, he – in clear contrast to the appointed astronomers of Leipzig Observatory – recommended *not* appointing a successor. Interestingly, as the saved budget was then bestowed upon Wundt to equip his own ``Institute for Experimental Psychology´´, the young professor could go on and develop his laboratory, which is well known to represent the birthplace of ``modern´´ experimental psychology (Bringmann & Tweney 1980; Staubermann 2001).

WUNDT´S PRAGMATIC WAY OF DEALING WITH SPIRITISM:
NARROWING THE SCOPE OF EXPERIMENTAL PSYCHOLOGY
AND SETTING UP A PROTO-``INCLUSIVE´´ CULTURAL
ANTHROPOLOGY

At first glance, one might consider the clash over spiritism, between the founding father of experimental psychology Wundt, and the astrophysicist Zöllner, to be an isolated event. However, the fact that similar clashes between proponents of spiritism and positivistic scientists also took place in Victorian Britain show that the Leipzig events were not isolated (Lamont 2004, 2005), but part of the larger picture within the modern history of ideas. This process can be understood as a consequence of converting the spiritual doctrine of the soul into a scientific theory of mind. Taken together, these events can be taken as illustrations or historical symptomatologies of how modern psychology struggled with old supernatural ideas in order to obtain a theory of mind that was allegedly free of metaphysical assumptions.

However, these can also be taken as symptoms of how deeply the battle connected with this attempt was tainted with ethical dimensions and implications. Thus, experimental psychology, the new science of the mind and behavior, as the forebear of (post)modern ``neurosciences´´, was connected with ethical questions from its very beginning. The majority of these questions have still not been resolved, but are part of the dialectic of contemporary ``neurosciences´´, and the quest for a reliable ``neuroethics´´ amid renewed controversy between (post)-idealistic and (post)-empiricist positions. However, we must ask how, and why, this has come to be.

The epistemological incompatibility between holistic science, empiricism, and positivism became ever more visible in the course of the second half of the nineteenth century, especially when spiritists claimed to have produced experimental proof for their transcendental beliefs. This is what Lamont has felicitously called the ``crisis of evidence´´ (Lamont 2004). Wundt was presumably more stunned by his older colleague´s reactions to the séances than by the experience with spiritism itself, and saw not only the scientific but also the moral problem(s) associated with spiritism as a cultural phenomenon. According to Wundt, spiritism could only be understood as a materialistically disfigured form of spirituality, mirroring the materialistic predilection of the contemporary *Zeitgeist*. However, when evaluating Wundt´s stance against spiritism, it is crucial to keep in mind that he considered himself to be not only a scientist but also a politically and socially engaged philosopher (Bringmann & Tweney 1980; Lambertini 1995). Thus, Wundt saw probably not only the scientific but also the social and moral problems that would inevitably emerge as a consequence of spiritism.

It is thereby noteworthy to remember that Wundt had been receiving scientific training from Helmholtz, who considered his anti-speculative positivistic program not only a scientific, but also a social necessity in order to transfer the values of humanism into an increasingly technological German culture (Paul 1984). Thus, despite his antipathy to speculation, Wundt should actually be recognized as a protector of the humanistic cultural tradition, as he saw – together with others – the necessity for overcoming the speculative approach of holistic science in order to make progress, but at the same time the need to maintain certain humanistic values. Correspondingly, although he saw society's spiritual needs and demands, he viewed these as deformed by spiritism, and opposed spiritism not only for scientific, but also for moral reasons in order to enable intellectual and social progress. Hence, Wundt's fight against spiritism as well as his firm belief in scientific and intellectual and moral progress may (at least from our contemporary perspective) actually be interpreted as a ``negative'' defence of moral and humanistic values. In this light, one could speculate that whereas Wundt rejected a materialistically distorted, regressive form of spirituality, he may have actually intended to pave the way for a progressive, more ``rational'' form of spirituality. In Wundt's rejection of spiritism and the possibility of metaphysical components influencing or producing conscious phenomena, he not only defined consciousness as a natural phenomenon but also paved the way for the development of secular inquiry into human consciousness through the use of experimental methods.

For Wundt, the only pragmatic way of saving the experimental approach to secular theories of mind was by removing studies of altered states of consciousness from the research agenda. This is exactly what Wundt did when he wrote a book on hypnotism and suggestion in 1892, in which he stated that hypnosis (together with other dubious altered states of consciousness) should be regarded as epistemologically more or less inconsequential, and from the viewpoint of mental hygiene even as perilous states (Wundt 1892). In sum, Wundt's conclusion was twofold. First, as one cannot seriously build an academic psychology on the basis of altered states such as trance, somnambulism, and hypnotism, experimental psychology should restrict its research scope to ``ordinary'' states of consciousness. Second, as altered states of consciousness can in principle be dangerous, they do not belong in a psychological laboratory but rather in the hands of specially trained psychiatrists.

By allocating the study of altered states of consciousness to the field of medicine, the groundwork for the separation of experimental psychology (as an epistemological science) and clinical psychology (as an applied field) was established. Altered states of consciousness and their importance in medical contexts were scrutinized by means of clinical concepts that were developed by scientists like Bernheim, Charcot, Breuer, Freud, and Janet.

In other words, as is frequently the case at an early stage in the evolution of complex biological, social and conceptual systems, an important pediment was established within the secular theory of mind. Within clinical psychology, in order to be able to explain extraordinary states and the concomitant phenomenon of being influenced by intrusive, strange and alien and unexplainable sensations, emotions, thoughts and associations, concepts such as ``unconsciousness'' or ``subconscious processes'' were frequently harnessed, whereas Wundt's experimental psychology focused more on the activity of the subject and correspondingly paved the way for his theory of voluntarism (Kohls 2004; Kohls & Sommer 2006). With regard to the construct of the ``unconscious consciousness'' Wundt stated in the second edition of *Hypnotism and Suggestion* that this oxymoron reminded him of a key principle of mysticisms, the ``coincidence of opposites'' (``*coincidentia oppositorum*''). Accordingly, as Wundt reveals in a footnote of this treatise, from his perspective Freud's ideas ``*touch on occult theories associated with the medical natural philosophy of the Schelling school at the beginning of the 19th century*''. Experimental psychology, in contrast, was restricted for a long time to the examination of ordinary states of consciousness and their concomitant psychological, predominantly conscious, cognitive processes, in accordance with Wundt's pragmatic decision.

It is, however, important to note that Wundt was far from considering himself to be a disbeliever in a divine principle. He actually reveals in his last work that although he had personally experienced phenomena that he would not hesitate to label as mystical, he simply could not support the view that non-causal, metaphysical factors are involved in conscious processes (Wundt 1920). The epitaph on his grave in Leipzig summarizes his creed in a concise way: ``God is spirit, and those who worship Him, have to venerate him both in spirit and in truth.''[1]

WUNDT'S PARTITIONING OF CONSCIOUSNESS STATES AT A TURNING POINT IN THE HISTORY OF THE SUBJECT AND ITS IMPRINT ON THE CANON OF MODERN NEUROSCIENCE

The proposed partitioning of consciousness into subversive extraordinary states and potentially normal ordinary states may be seen not only as the inception of academic psychology, but also as a turning point in the history of the subject that paved the way for a

---

[1] German original: ``Gott ist Geist und die ihn anbeten, müssen ihn im Geiste und der Wahrheit anbeten.''

two-fold conceptualization of a secular theory of mind that has since then been divided into an experimental and a clinical field. As a matter of fact, this has influenced not only the cognitive, but also the moral image of academic psychology and neuroscience up to the present. Let us briefly consider three important, interrelated aspects.

1 An integrative approach of neuroscience striving to overcome Wundt´s twofold (Kantian) solution to the problem of consciousness

Although Wundt´s work has unfortunately been mostly confined to his contributions to experimental psychology, his actual scientific program was much broader. Wundt held the opinion that experimental approaches within psychology would be restricted to the exploration of the inferior mental processes, and in order to explain the superior mental processes, he dedicated the last twenty years of his life to the development of a complex cultural anthropology that he called ``völkerpsychologie``. It is in this voluminous part of Wundt´s work, where he deals with the complex cultural phenomena that also embrace occult and mystical phenomena, not in an empirical way, but from a cultural–anthropological perspective. Interestingly, whereas Wundt treated his two approaches as methodologically distinct but epistemologically necessary if not complementary orientations, modern neuroscience strives towards combining them by means of an integrative but neuroscientifically grounded perspective, which must take the complex interaction between genetic, physiological, psychological and social variables into account in order to provide the best explanatory model for the human condition. Although the demarcation line that separated neuroscience from other disciplines (such as philosophy) has been gradually extended, (cognitive) neuroscience, in contrast to Wundt´s experimental psychology is no longer restricted to scrutinizing inferior mental processes; this discipline seems to have developed a rather inclusive self-concept. Nevertheless, one of the questions that remain unsolved is associated with how inclusive neuroscience can actually be without falling prey to producing categorical errors. For example, one controversy is whether neuroscience is capable of providing a basic epistemological foundation that is fully or only partly able to explain the phenomenon of consciousness, as well as embrace questions of philosophy, theology, and ethics.

2 Psychophysiological paralellism as a non-reductionist basis for a secular theory of mind

Wundt did not believe in materialist reductionism, or in Cartesian interactionism, and correspondingly he had to find a middle ground. Hence, he was willing to assume that brain and mind states are two independent yet synchronized layers of description that are both necessary in order to understand and describe consciousness in a complementary way. In other words, he assumed that conscious processes are associated with brain functions, although both bodily processes and mental processes appear to have a ``causality´´ of their own. Thus while thinking along the lines of the Leibnizian idea of a pre-established harmony, as well as Spinozian concept of psychophysical parallelism as possible explanation for the synchronization of the physical and the mental realm, Wundt introduced his appealing idea of a psychophysical parallelism of consciousness processes in the brain as a pragmatic working hypothesis. It is thereby noteworthy that the postulated mechanism responsible for the synchronization of the two layers ``brain and mind´´ still – at least implicitly – requires a metaphysical construct similar to Leibnitz´s monadology, unless one is willing to accept monism. Thus, as one can easily see the idea of physiological parallelism immediately created (and still creates) problems associated with the question of free will. In short, if there is no such metaphysical entity as a soul or homunculus (dualistic theories) on the one hand, and no strict mechanical causality of brain functions producing respective mental phenomena on the other (reductionistic theories), how can the connection between the realm of mind and body, as well as their interaction, be conceived? Either, as it is assumed within emergentism, consciousness emerges as a result of complex brain functions, which would – at least partly – support determinism and cast doubt on the concept of free will and freedom of choice, or alternatively, if it is assumed that mental processes may have impact upon brain functions, then the contemporary physical worldview would be incomplete at best.

3 The triumphant structuralistic approach and its focus on the experimental investigation of substantive states of consciousness

Wundt adopted the experimental approach utilized by early psychophysiologists like Fechner. This had proven to be successful in studying sensory perception by manipulating stimuli and having subjects trained in the method of introspection report their sensations and inner experiences.[2] Hence, as conscious processes (i.e. sensations above the subliminal threshold of consciousness) can only be empirically observed by means of introspection, Wundt understood experimental psychology as the analysis of the structure of stable states of conscious experience that are tangible and expressible; according to this line of thought, direct observation of unconscious processes – and consequentially analysis of content free thinking – would be impossible. Wundt's aim was to find the ``basic elements'' of conscious experience by systematically breaking mental processes into the most basic but still perceivable components by means of introspection. This structuralistic approach, by focusing on the tangible ``substantive'' (i.e. verbally expressible) elements of consciousness has had major impact on the development of the later course of psychology, and particularly cognitivism, as this paradigm allowed the application of an efficient form of rationally oriented (psycho) logics (Kohls 2004; Kohls & Sommer 2006). This is supported by the fact that the emotional aspects of conscious processes were neglected for a long time within cognitivism, very likely owing to emotional phenomena of consciousness being frequently ambiguous with regard to meaning, and correspondingly semantically difficult to describe.

Yet it is important to recall that the American counterpart (amd perhaps also antithesis) of Wundt, the psychologist and philosopher William James, championed functionalism as the opposing position to structuralism and he was – in contrast to Wundt – willing to take the radical empiricist position that nature and experience can never be captured by absolute and objective analysis, as they are naturally dependent on the mind(set) of the observer. Thus, for James, consciousness may be described not only by means of its tangible (verbal) content but also as a process that he dubbed ``stream of consciousness''. This term is supposed to embrace the full range of thoughts, emotions, and sentiments as complex inner sensations, and not only verbally expressible thoughts. In other words, James held the opinion that in addition to substantive states, transitive states – ``*flights to conclusions*'' as he called them – as the instable states, between substantive mental states, although not tangible and directly perceptible, are important for the understanding of consciousness. Hence, it does not come as a

---

[2] Wundt understood introspection not as a naïve way of self-perception but rather as a method for the examination of one's own thoughts and feelings that had to be systematically trained in order for an individual to become a skilled introspector.

surprise that James was not only interested in scientifically scrutinizing the ``stable´´ ordinary, but also ``unstable´´ extraordinary states of
consciousness. To be more specific, James´ broad approach left a venue
for researching spiritual, religious, and meditative experiences, and by
focusing on the experiential side of transcendental experiences and
their impact upon health, James thereby did important work in both
philosophy and psychology of religion. Moreover, James was convinced
that altered states of consciousness could be epistemologically useful
to explain certain aspects of consciousness.

Whereas Wundt restricted the scope of experimental psychology
to scrutinizing the ordinary (``conscious´´) states of everyday consciousness, he made certain assumptions concerning the epistemology,
scope, and methodology of academic psychology and in this way also
defined its boundaries and limits. His concept left no leeway for har-
boring spiritual aspects, at least within consciousness. Admittedly
Wundt´s approach was swiftly assailed and partly overcome by other
approaches developed by his students and immediate successors, such
as Gestalt psychology and the movement known as the Würzburg
School, and was eventually superseded by behaviorism and functionalism at the beginning of the 1920s (Kohls 2004; Kohls & Sommer
2006). However, as history has shown, some basic aspects of the
structuralistic line of thought described by Wundt have prevailed over
functionalism and other rival approaches, and Wundt´s work has certainly left an imprint on the scope and methods of experimental
psychology, as well as (cognitive) neuroscience, and thus determined
the image of academic psychology to the present. As the counterdraft
of experimental psychology, holistic psychology in the tradition of
William James has not managed to achieve the status of an academ-
ically well-respected discipline, and has been relegated to scientifically
less respected fields such as parapsychology, humanistic psychology, or
transpersonal psychology.

THE RETURN OF THE DISPUTE ON A ``POSTMODERN´´ SCALE SINCE 1990 AND SINCE 2002

It is important to realize how much of the debate that took place in
Leipzig some 140 years ago is still present as a background to today´s
cultural and scientific discussion about studying consciousness and
related phenomena in an inclusive way. The dialectic between
empiricism and idealism, and between physiological, psychological,

and "spiritual" dimensions of consciousness, still exerts an influence upon the contemporary debate associated with "neuroethics", at least indirectly by means of *implicit* connotations of concepts such as "psyche", "mind" and being. Let us here provide some brief examples.

1. The current debate about the "easy and the hard problems" of consciousness, (i.e. the relationship between the physical brain and the immediate self-awareness called "I" or "self" (Pinker 2007)), centers around "empirical" and "idealistic" viewpoints and hypotheses. One currently influential group, predominantly composed of secular philosophers and experimental psychologists and scientists, offers rejection of any metaphysical assumptions about the nature of consciousness. Whereas Wundt saw the necessity of upholding (1) the dialectics between an irreducible psychophysiological parallelism for explaining inferior mental processes and a cultural–anthropological approach for understanding higher mental processes as well as (2) social conventions and ethical standards, there are those in contemporary neuroscience (i.e. the materialists) who maintain that the physical brain is the monocausal evolutionary origin of consciousness. The apparent self-givenness of the "I" or the "self" usually does not include an immediate awareness of physiological brain processes; for materialists, consciousness seems to be little more than an epiphenomenon of neuronal activity. Seen from the viewpoint of the history of ideas, this group follows a newly "purified" paradigm of physiological reductionism, which is clearly similar to the one developed by the young science of experimental psychophysiology in the second half of the nineteenth century, but to a certain extent is even more radical. Compared with Wundt, this group of contemporary thinkers tends to a much more "transhumanist" or "posthumanist" position. Interestingly, one of the main reasons for monocausalism seems to be a "negative" experience with metaphysics and its moral ideas as such. Steven Pinker, for example, addressed different strands of such traditions (Pinker 2007) and seems to have adopted a view that indistinctly associates *every* metaphysical dimension with a kind of speculative or anti-scientific attitude. This is actually not far from the pivotal reason why Wundt rejected spiritism.

Another group, perhaps less influential but still publicly present, is led mainly by philosophers and humanists such as Colin McGinn, and holds exactly the inverse opinion. The apparent self-givenness of the "I-feeling" or the "I-experience" should be regarded as a primary empirical fact, explicitly comparable to brain processes. Moreover, the fact of the so-called "conscious mind" – understood not as a *passive entity*, but as an *active* and *in actu* process of self-awareness – precedes the fact of the brain

(McGinn 2007). What is the rationale for that statement? A key argument is that the mere concept of "the brain" (i.e. the interpretation of a perception and the creation of a sentence such as "the brain is the primary cause of the I-feeling, and it creates the I-feeling") is only possible because it has been produced by an "I-feeling", i.e. by an immediate self-givenness of a subject (or a first-person, subjective experience) who acts as the rational concept-builder. In other words, the self-givenness is, from a strictly experiential–empirical standpoint, a contextual prerequisite necessary for every statement about the brain. Therefore, for this group of "neo-humanists", from a logical and phenomenological–empirical standpoint, *the "I" must be the primary cause on which the concept of the "brain" is always already dependent.* Thus, this "I" must be regarded – at least to a certain extent – as a "meta physical origin in itself" that cannot be reduced to an epiphenomenon (Gebser 1985). To state the matter differently, seen from this perspective, the "I" is the fountain-head of the self and the world alike, and correspondingly the phenomenal origin of everything else: every experienced phenomenon, be it a perception, sensation, thought, or higher-level interpretations, as well as the origin of the perception itself. It seems to be obvious from this line of thought that this immediate "self-givenness" of the "I" or "self" cannot be reduced to a secondary phenomenon associated with the physical brain by means of monocausal relations. However, in order to be able to fully acknowledge the reality of the conscious self-givenness associated with the "I", it seems necessary to recognize it by a different or even complementary form of empiricism. One of the different forms of empiricism fully able to grasp this "other", rather metaphysical or even idealistic "spiritual" origin of the self seems to be a neo-idealistic form of introspection. Possibly, this may be interpreted as a first sign of a realignment of the methodological approach to an examination of (self) with empirical–experimental methods. It is important to recall that this tradition was largely abandoned in Europe after the first half of the twentieth century (Benedikter 2005).

2. In the debate between post- and neo-humanistic paradigms mentioned above, an ideological but largely unnoticed tension currently manifests itself in the current content of "neuroethics". Although the "spiritual" aspects of the mind–matter problem seem to be a side-bar to the research agenda (Walach 2007), these aspects seem to be "indirectly" at work behind very basic world views of the major participants on both sides of the discussion. For example, some of the arguments brought forward by Pinker as well as by McGinn seem to indirectly hinge on certain conceptualizations of "metaphysical"

aspects of the brain-self question. These may be "negative" arguments, and we refer to the notion "negative" in order to address our observation that domains that have been assigned to spiritual realms (within non-secular theories of the mind) are usually not directly addressed within contemporary scientific theories of mind in a positive way, but are only "negatively" defined by means of their exclusion from the scientific debate. In order to illustrate this point, let us briefly consider the psychological function of dissociation and its contemporary and past interpretations.

Dissociative processes are usually considered to be natural psycho-physiological events that functionally exhibit a defocussing effect on the conscious mind. From a clinical perspective, they are regarded as subconscious processes for managing powerful negative emotions. However, depending on the severity of the symptoms, dissociative processes may also be regarded both as a psychological coping mechanism and/or as a psychopathological experience. Historically (in medieval times), psychological dissociation may have been interpreted in a more positive way: a medieval mystic, for example, may have regarded dissociation as a powerful tool for systematically diminishing the "I" in order to allow a "universal truth" to emanate in the realm of consciousness. Within this world view, regular practice of specific introspective practices such as meditation or contemplation – potentially eliciting dissociative processes – may have been interpreted as a venue for voluntarily melting down the self in a systematic manner. Observe that this interpretation might not be feasible from a secular epistemology in a similar way, because from a phenomenological perspective there is no more basic entity than the "I". Thus, it seems that the implicitly positive connotation of dissociative processes must only be possible in world views where the "I" is not seen as the epistemological starting point (Kohls 2004). To draw a line, it seems that at least some conscious phenomena that can – at least potentially – be looked upon favorably within more spiritual world views, may have very different connotations when interpreted within a secular framework. This is both a cultural and an epistemic issue, particularly given that the scientific debate around the mind–matter problem has conjoined certain theological perspectives. This is important given that spiritual and religious beliefs and experiences are basic practices of many individuals and cultures; therefore, a scientific theory to explain human experience and behavior would need, at the very least, to address the human need and desire for spirituality and the cultural manifestations of these beliefs and practices.

3. The debate about the ``easy and the hard problems´´ of the mind–matter relation is increasingly influenced by a tendency that has been called ``the global renaissance of religion´´ since the fall of the Berlin wall in 1989, the collapse of Communism in 1991, and the terror attacks on the World Trade Center on September 11, 2001. The contemporary renaissance of religion adds a strictly metaphysical, if not spirito political aspect to the debate, that may be seen as a counterpart of the radically materialistic concept of consciousness brought forward by the first group mentioned (i.e. Pinker *et al.*). This radicalized ``spiritual´´ concept of the origin of the self is the concept of the ``immortal soul´´ (Joseph Ratzinger, Elio Sgreccia (cf. Benedikter 2008b)) that is totally independent of the physical brain. The advocates of this position add this concept to the current debate as a ``forgotten´´ aspect of the true nature and origin of consciousness (beyond all its restrictions and reductions at the hands of contemporary scientific research). Admittedly, this concept is not identical to the spiritistic assumptions of Zöllner in the debate with Wundt, but it cannot be doubted that, from Zöllner´s viewpoint, a similar line of thought was the main inspiration for his scientific experiments with the medium Slade: materialism and reductionism can be depressing world views. It is therefore not a surprise that in the current debate between (1) radically monocausal, objectivistic, and materialistic views (e.g. Pinker), (2) empirically subjectivistic and neo-idealistic views (e.g. McGinn), and (3) radically monocausal, objectivistic, and ``spiritual´´ concepts of brain, mind, and self-experience there will be problems similar to those that arose in the debate between Wundt and Zöllner. In the main, these pertain to the relationship between physiological, psychological, and spiritual transcendent aspects of the complex and often paradoxical nature of consciousness, which have remained unresolved since debated by Wundt and Zöllner in Leipzig, 1877–79 (Benedikter 2008b).

4. Thus, the debate between ``materialistic´´ and ``spiritual´´ aspects of the ``easy and the hard problems´´ seems to have generated an epistemological controversy *within* the currently dominant ``postmodern philosophies´´, paradigms, and world views of the Western open societies, as well as in the humanities in general. The impact of this epistemologic tension on the future paradigmatic orientation of Western societies can hardly be overestimated.

It is noteworthy that many leading philosophers of so-called ``postmodern´´ or ``mature modern´´ contemporary philosophy who conceive of themselves as the ``principal thinkers´´ of the epoch (e.g. Jean-Francois Lyotard, Jacques Derrida, Paul Feyerabend, Helene Cixous,

Jürgen Habermas), have opened up their earlier, rather radically secular-materialistic paradigm of the mind–matter debate to a "neo-spiritual" dimension in their late works. In the years after 1990, the majority of these thinkers – if in very different ways and forms – began to ponder the necessity of introducing an enlarged, "empirical–idealistic", "subjective–objective" or "rationally spiritual" paradigm in order to fit the requirements of the new epoch, which emerged after the collapse of the old polar ideologies of the post-war world. However, the majority of them, possibly owing to their post-WWII and post-1968 critical education, seemed not to have been well prepared for dealing with the "return" of spiritual and religious dimensions to the world stage. This may be the reason why many of these leading thinkers seem to have fallen prey to the temptation to adhere to old proto- or para-"spiritual", if not proto-"spiritistic", concepts of the metaphysical dimension connected with the immediate self-awareness of the "I". Nevertheless, in their last years, they all seem to have experienced a certain uncertainty, in which they were deeply divided by the apparent contradiction between an empirical–materialistic framework of their ideas, and the eruption of a new metaphysical awareness. It was the latter that led many to embark on a (sometimes desperate and in many regards mainly "negative; cf. (Benedikter 2008b; Lyotard 2001) search for a dimension of "spiritually enlightened" or "rationally spiritual" consciousness, which has for example been called the "realm of the Not-I" by Jean-Francois Lyotard (2001).

To draw a line, we believe that the dichotomy between Wundt and Zöllner can be found again in the last works of the main postmodern thinkers mentioned previously. Although the split between materialistic–empirical and "proto-spirititual" aspects of consciousness seems to be irreconcilable within the limits of "postmodern" concepts of these thinkers, those ideas are still dominating the Western humanities and the mainstream of current academic philosophical thinking (Benedikter 2008b). This rift, as identified by the aforementioned "postmodern" thinkers, could only be bridged by "negative" means (i.e. by developing fruitful tensions pointing towards an enlarged concept of the "I" and its inherent psychological dimensions). However, the inability to reconcile "empirical" and "idealistic" dimensions of the self *in a positive way* can not only be found in the leading postmodern concepts, but also manifests itself in the contemporary debate(s) associated with core issues of neurosciences and neuroethics. We opine that the bisection within late "postmodern" mainstream philosophical and cultural thinking sketched above is similar to the dichotomous viewpoints that are currently debated by ``physiological empiricists´´ (Pinker *et al.*), ``subjectivistic neo-idealists´´ (McGinn *et al.*), and ``radical metaphysicists´´ (Elio Sgreccia *et al.*) and that this debate may shape the form and content of ``neuroethics´´ in the Western hemisphere.

CONCLUSION: ELEMENTS FOR FURTHER DISCUSSION

Distinct problems are associated with efforts to study consciousness. At some level, these seem to repeat debates that occurred in a rather primordial form in the nineteenth century. Perhaps the unresolved fundamental problem can be stated as: how can metaphysical (or ``idealistic´´) and physical (or empirical–materialistic) aspects associated with the ``easy and hard problems´´ of modern neuroscientific research be properly related? The study of the history of ideas of the nineteenth century, and especially of the early rise of modern psychology as an emerging science, might assist our understanding of the conceptual and practical complexity of this problem. From such reflection upon debates of the nineteenth and those we face in the twenty-first century, some conclusions can be drawn.

1. Both the necessity and the desire for scrutinizing, explaining, and interpreting consciousness is unquestionably a constant in the history of modernity. One might speculate that this has probably been a matter of utmost importance for the self-concept and the historical evolution of modernity (and later postmodernity) as such. Yet, the modern field of consciousness studies is usually only seen as having commenced at the eve of Enlightenment. However, Hermann Ebbinghaus´ famous and concise remark that psychology ``has had a long past and only a short history´´ reminds us that its cultural roots are much older and that this needs to be acknowledged in order to be able to consider the tacit transcendental (and perhaps spiritual) undercurrent inevitably associated with the mind–matter problem.

2. One of the most influential European ``post-humanists´´ of the second half of the twentieth century, Martin Heidegger, has described how technology transforms not only our orientation towards the concept of the world, but also our understanding of it. Owing to a process that Heidegger called ``enframing´´, human beings are revealed as orderers of their environments, and consequentially other entities of the world are revealed as being ordered. Thus, one might surmise that a theory of mind as a modern tool for explaining consciousness is also affected by this process of enframing within the modern history

of ideas. To be sure, there has probably always been a certain tendency to explain consciousness in congruence with the most important contemporary epistemological concepts. However, with the advancement of technical methods and processes, technology has increasingly been used as both a metaphorical and a literal model for interpreting consciousness.

One of the most important examples of this is the ``cognitive revolution'' in the 1950s. Interestingly, after the inception of the computer era, computational metaphors for explaining important aspects of brain–mind function were instrumental in paving the way for the field of cognitive neuroscience. In a similar vein, the nineteenth century spiritism might be regarded as an important example of wedding technological concepts to idealistic theories of mind (Noakes 1999). Remarkably, a decade after the first commercial electrical telegraph was constructed and put into operation on the Great Western Railway in Britain, the basic idea of spiritism arose that telegraph-like communication with the spirits by means of raps would be possible (Noakes 1999). The clash between Wundt and Zöllner on the question of spiritism can be seen as an example of the durable struggle between the old psychology, which was upholding and defending a dualistic theory of mind, and a new, modern, scientific model of consciousness, which has been advocating a non-dualistic, more monistic explanation.

3. Although it may appear odd at first glance, it is interesting to compare the structural and functional similarities and differences between the ``cognitive revolution'' and ``spiritism''. First, both concepts harness technological concepts for explaining distinct features of consciousness. Intriguingly, whereas advocates of spiritism used telegraphy as a communicative vector for interacting with spirits dwelling in a transcendental realm, several proponents of the cognitive revolution assume that by studying and developing procedural algorithms in artificial intelligence and computer science it will actually be possible to devise empirically testable theories about human mental processes (if not to create such processes themselves). In other words, whereas spiritists assumed that they had provided empirical evidence for the structural existence of a soul, some cognitive scientists believe that they could draw conclusions from artificial intelligence to human beings or evoke ``human cognition'' in a machine.

It might be noteworthy to realize that the term ``functional'' insulates the scientific perspective of modern cognitive neuroscience. Had this term not been used, then it might not be such a stretch to regard the panpsychological inclination of cognitive neuroscience as roughly comparable to the radical idealistic ideas of spiritism. *Deus ex machina est Deus ex machina.*

4. It is important to note that the debate between Wundt and Zöllner has not ended but only shifted its center of gravity away from psychology. Three examples might suffice by way of illustration: (a) the controversy between Einstein and Bohr concerning the question of determinism in the context of the Copenhagen interpretation of quantum mechanics (Held 1998; Whitaker 1996); (b) the question of the ontological status of a transcencental realm with regard to the ordinary *Lebenswelt* (the everyday world), as addressed by linguistic philosophy in the mid-1920s of the Vienna Circle (specifically, as addressed by Ludwig Wittgenstein in the *Tractatus Logico-Philosophicus*); and (c) emergentism – one of the most promising non-reductionist theories to explain consciousness – which is based on a layered view of nature, and the assumption that higher-order properties supervene upon lower levels without direct causal interaction. Within these approaches, nature has been conceptualized as imbued with a non-causal principle of transgression; surely this would have amazed Zöllner, who was desperately trying to prove the connection between transcendental and ordinary dimensions.

In conclusion, the debate about how to explain consciousness is structurally comparable to the debate between Wundt and Zöllner: although the mind–body–spirit problem has been reduced to the mind–body problem (Walach 2007), there is still a tendency to use black box concepts in order to fill explanatory gaps. Similar to the days of Wundt and Zöllner, the intricacies of physics in light of quantum mechanics provides a current example of the schism between empiricism and idealism. Some scientists, such as the late John Eccles or Roger Penrose, assume that quantum processes might be involved in consciousness in order to defend a non-materialist position (Eccles 1980; Penrose 1994). Others hold that the mind, and correspondingly the self, is a pure epiphenomenon of the brain, and that the self (and free will) should be regarded as a persistent illusion (Metzinger 2004).

Suspiciously, there remains room for spiritual thought in all these beliefs – be it that the soul is an immortal entity as suggested by Abrahamic tradition, or that our ego persona is simply an illusion, as suggested by Buddhist philosophy. It would be difficult to affirm which thought is more or less spiritual. In any case, the idea derived from the Enlightenment that superstition, religion, and spirituality would finally be swept away by science is a rather naïve, if not likewise superstitious assumption. Rather, it seems that these domains that we label as spiritual or mystical (Forman 1998) adapt as reaction(s) to the mainstream *Zeitgeist* and paradigm(s). This needs to be taken into account within neuroethics, if this endeavor wants to be fully aware of and accountable for its complex and conflict-ridden origins. As a field, neuroethics must confront the reality that these debates not only cause tensions and problems, but concomitantly carry the unparalleled potential for scientific progress and cultural inclusion.

ACKNOWLEDGMENTS

We thank Prof Dr. Harald Walach, University of Northampton, UK, for continuous support and critical contribution to this chapter.

REFERENCES

Abbott, E. A. 1991. *Flatland: A Romance of Many Dimensions*. Princeton, NJ: Princeton University Press.

Benedikter, R. 2001. *Die Beurteilung Rudolf Steiners durch Julius Evola. Ein Hinweis auf die Unvereinbarkeit von Faschismus und Anthroposophie*. In Ravagli, L. (ed.) *Jahrbuch für anthroposophische Kritik*. Munich: Trithemius Verlag, pp. 66–193.

Benedikter, R. 2001. *Einführung in das postmaterialistische Denken*, Vol. 1. Vienna: Passagen Verlag.

Benedikter, R. 2005. Die wissenschaftliche Wiederentdeckung der Introspektion. *Das Goetheanum, Wochenschrift für Anthroposophie* **84**(5): 6–7.

Benedikter, R. 2005. *Perspektiven postmaterialistischen Denkens*, vol. 7. Vienna: Passagen Verlag.

Benedikter, R. 2008a. *Postmodern Spirituality. Orifices of Late Postmodern Thought. Approaches towards a "Rational Spirituality" in the late works of some Leading "Postmodern" Thinkers as an Alternative to the Global "Renaissance of Religions": Jacques Derrida, Jean-Francois Lyotard, Michel Foucault, Paul Feyerabend and Others.* (In press)

Benedikter, R. 2008b. The recent Italian debate about the nature of consciousness between secular and metaphysicist approaches – and its perspectives for the development of an inclusive viewpoint. In Benedikter, R. (ed.) *Consciousness – Individuality – Freedom. Dimensions and Perspectives of the Paradigms of the new Neurosciences*. Vienna (In press).

Boring, E. G. 1950. *A History of Experimental Psychology*. New York: Appleton-Century-Crofts.

Bringmann, W. G. & Tweney, R. D. 1980. *Wundt Studies*. Toronto: Hogrefe.

Cahan, D. 1994. Anti-Helmholtz, anti-Dühring, anti-Zöllner: the politics and values of Science in Germany during the 1870s. In Krüger, L. (ed.) *Universalgenie Helmholtz: Rückblick nach 100 Jahren*. Berlin: Akademie-Verlag, pp. 330–44.

Caputo, J. 2005. The experience of God and the axiology of the impossible. In Hart, K. & Wall, B. E. (eds.) *The Experience of God: A Postmodern Response*. New York: Fordham University Press, pp. 20–41.

Eccles, J.C. 1980. *The Human Psyche*. Berlin: Springer.

Ellenberger, H. F. 1970. *The Discovery of the Unconscious. The History and Evolution of Dynamic Psychiatry*. New York: Basic Books.

Forman, R. K. C. 1998. *The Innate Capacity: Mysticism, Psychology, and Philosophy*: Oxford University Press.

Gebser, J. 1985. *The Ever-Present Origin*. Athens, OH: Ohio University Press.

Gulat-Wellenburg, W. Von, Klinckowstroem, C. Von, & Rosenbusch, H. 1925. *Der Okkultismus in Urkunden Bd.2. Der Physikalische Mediumismus*. Berlin: Ullstein Verlag.

Heidelberger, M. 2004. *Nature From Within: Gustav Theodor Fechner and his Psychophysical Worldview*. Pittsburgh, PA: University of Pittsburgh Press.

Held, C. 1998. *Die Bohr-Einstein-Debatte: Quantenmechanik und Physikalische Wirklichkeit*. Paderborn: Ferdinand Schöningh.

Kaku, M. 1995. *Hyperspace: A Scientific Odyssey Through Parallel Universes, Time Warps, and the Tenth Dimension*. Oxford: Oxford University Press.

Kohls, N. 2004. *Aussergewöhnliche Erfahrungen – Blinder Fleck der Psychologie? Eine Auseinandersetzung mit aussergewöhnlichen Erfahrungen und ihrem Zusammenhang mit geistiger Gesundheit*. Münster: Lit-Verlag.

Kohls, N. & Sommer, A. 2006. *Die akademische Psychologie am Scheideweg: Positivistische Experimentalpsychologie und die Nemesis der Transzendenz*. In: Büssing, A., Ostermann, T., Glöckler, M. *et al.* (eds.) *Spiritualität, Krankheit und Heilung – Bedeutung und Ausdrucksformen der Spiritualität in der Medizin – Perspektiven, Schriften zur Pluralität in der Medizin und Komplementärmedizin*. Frankfurt: Verlag für Akademische Schriften.

Krüger, L. 1994. *Universalgenie Helmholtz. Rückblick nach 100 Jahren*. Berlin: Akademie.

Lambertini, G. 1995. *Wilhelm Maximilian Wundt (1832 – 1920) – Leben, Werk und Persönlichkeit in Bildern und Texten*. Bonn: Deutscher Psychologen Verlag.

Lamont, P. 2004. Spiritualism and a mid-Victorian crisis of evidence. *The Historical Journal* **47**: 897–920.

Lamont, P. 2005. *The First Psychic: The Peculiar Mystery of a Notorious Victorian Wizard*. London: Little, Brown.

Linse, U. 1999. ``Das Buch der Wunder und Geheimwissenschaften´´. Der spiritistische Verlag Oswald Mutze in Leipzig im Rahmen der spiritistischen Bewegung Sachsens. In Lehmstedt, M. & Herzog, A. (eds.) *Das bewegte Buch. Buchwesen und Soziale, Nationale und Kulturelle Bewegungen um 1900*, vol. 12. Wiesbaden: Harrassowitz.

Lyotard, J. F. 2001. *The Soundproof Room. Malraux´ Anti-Aesthetics*. Stanford, CA: Stanford University Press.

McGinn, C. 2007. An unbridgeable gulf. *Time Magazine* (February 12): 42.

Metzinger, T. 2004. *Being No One: the Self-Model Theory of Subjectivity*. Cambridge, MA: MIT Press.

Noakes, R. J. 1999. Telegraphy is an occult art: Cromwell Fleetwood Varley and the diffusion of electricity to the other world. *British Journal for the History of Science* **32**(04): 421–59.

Paul, R. 1984. German Academic Science and the Mandarin Ethos, 1850–1880. *British Journal for the History of Science* **17**(1): 1–29.

Penrose, R. 1994. *Shadows of the Mind*. Oxford: Oxford University Press.

Pinker, S. 2007. The mystery of consciousness. *Time Magazine* (February 12): 38–46.

Pippin, R. B. 2005. *The Persistence of Subjectivity: On the Kantian Aftermath*. Cambridge: Cambridge University Press.

Richards, J. L. 1977. The evolution of Empiricism: Hermann von Helmholtz and the foundations of geometry. *The British Journal for the Philosophy of Science* **28**: 235–53.

Sawicki, D. 2002. *Leben mit den Toten. Geisterglauben und die Entstehung des Spiritismus in Deutschland 1770-1900*. Paderborn: Ferdinand Schöningh.

Staubermann, K. B. 2001. Tying the knot: skill, judgement and authority in the 1870s Leipzig spiritistic experiments. *British Journal for the History of Science* **34**(1): 67–79.

Stromberg, W. H. 1989. Helmholtz and Zoellner: nineteenth-century empiricism, spiritism, and the theory of space perception. *Journal of the History of the Behavioural Science* **25**: 371–83.

Thissen, S. 2000. *De spinozisten. Wijsgerige beweging in Nederland 1850–1907*. Den Haag: SDU Uitgevers.

Treitel, C. 2004. *A Science for the Soul. Occultism and the Genesis of the German Modern*. Baltimore & London: Johns Hopkins University Press.

Ulrici, H. 1879. Der sogenannte Spiritismus eine wissenschaftliche Frage. *Zeitschrift für Philosophie und Philosophische Kritik* **74**: 245.

Valente, K. G. 2004. Transgression and Transcendence: Flatland as a Response to "A New Philosophy". *Nineteenth Century Contexts* **26**: 61–77.

Walach, H. 2007. Mind – Body – Spirit. *Mind & Matter* **5**(2): 215–39.

Whitaker, A. 1996. *Einstein, Bohr, and the Quantum Dilemma*. Cambridge: Cambridge University Press.

Wundt, W. 1874. *Grundzüge der physiologischen Psychologie*. Leipzig: Engelmann.

Wundt, W. 1879. *Der Spiritismus – Eine sogenannte wissenschaftliche Frage*. Leipzig: Engelmann.

Wundt, W. 1892. *Hypnotismus und Suggestion*. Leipzig: Engelmann.

Wundt, W. 1920. *Erlebtes und Erkanntes*. Leipzig: Kröner.

Ziche, P. 1999. Neuroscience in its context. Neuroscience and psychology in the work of Wilhelm Wundt. Physis. *Rivista Internazionale Di Storia Della Sczienzia. Indici* **36**(2): 407–29.

Zöllner, K. F. 1897. *Die Transcendentale Physik und die sogenannte Philosophie: eine Deutsche Antwort auf eine sogenannte wissenschaftliche Frage*. Leipzig: Commissionsverlag von L. Staackmann.

3

On the cusp
The hard problem of neuroscience and its practical implications

R. D. ELLIS

INTRODUCTION

When David Chalmers introduced the notion of the "hard problem of consciousness" (1995), he contributed to a revolution in the neuroscience of consciousness and cognition as well as in the philosophy of mind. The main point of the hard problem is that, even if we could discover the "neural correlates of consciousness," we still would not have answered the "harder" question: *Why* do those physical events exhibit the property of consciousness, whereas other physical events do not?

I acknowledge that this "hard problem" notion should not be construed as an argument for mind–body dualism, or as a reason to reject physicalism. (More on that later.) None the less, Chalmers' point has important implications for neuroscience in general, as well as cognitive science in particular. There is a tendency in neuroscience to assume that if a brain process B correlates with a mental process M, then B is the physical process that produces M. But this reasoning can lead to gross oversimplifications. There may be a much more complicated process, P, that causes both B and M to occur, and therefore causes B and M to correlate with each other. To be sure, P may very well be a purely *physical* process. My point is that P often may be a more *complicated* physical process than just B. In some cases, it may turn out that B is actually a somewhat minor or even peripheral part of the

Scientific and Philosophical Perspectives in Neuroethics, ed. J. J. Giordano & B. Gordijn. Published by Cambridge University Press. © Cambridge University Press 2010.

more complicated process P that causes B and M to correlate. Yet there may be a strong temptation to focus on B as the physical ``explanation'' for M, simply because of the correlation that is accessible from the observations that our current instruments enable us to make. Whenever this is the situation, we may be tempted to jump to a hasty conclusion. And in that case, we may find our explanations dictated by the prejudices created by our current instrumentation and currently fashionable research paradigms.

For example, I shall argue that the fMRI (functional magnetic resonance imaging) technique for correlating brain areas with mental processes leads to a cortical bias and less attention to the role of subcortical processes. The brain area that ``lights up'' may only be playing a role in a much larger process that includes cortical and subcortical elements, and in which timing is crucial. (Besides picking up mainly on cortical rather than subcortical activity, fMRI is notoriously insensitive to the *timing* of brain processes.) Too much focus on the observed correlation with an fMRI image thus plays into the hands of a theory of consciousness and cognition that treats them as less active and self-organizational, thus more passive and piecemeal processes, than they really are. The attempt to view either cognition or the brain primarily in terms of receiving information, ironically, then blocks us from what is needed to answer Chalmers´ ``hard problem of consciousness.'' Instead of seeing specific brain mechanisms as parts of a larger dynamical system, we try unsuccessfully to see the isolated brain mechanisms as a processor of received inputs. We therefore systematically neglect and marginalize theories in which consciousness results from a self-organizing organism´s attempts to *act upon* its environment rather than merely receiving information *from* the environment.

Finally, in the last section of the chapter, I shall show how such a self-organizational approach can avoid the errors of mere ``explanation by correlation.'' By doing so, such an approach can both provide more coherent accounts of observed mental–physical correlations, and address the ``hard problem,'' which can never be answered as long as we confine ourselves to explanation by correlation.

THE HARD PROBLEM: PRACTICAL IMPLICATIONS?

In a way, it is regrettable that so many discussions of the ``hard problem of consciousness'' take such an ultra-abstract form. The hard problem actually has very practical implications for what is happening right now in the neurosciences and cognitive theory. It is not merely about whether, if in some utopian future we were to know absolutely everything about the brain, consciousness would then have been ``explained.'' What is important and practical about the hard problem is that it can help direct us toward more coherent theories to explain *why* certain conscious states correlate with the specific physical processes with which they are associated.

The abstract statement of the hard problem is that, even if we were to know that a conscious state is either caused by or identical with a brain process B, we still would not have explained *why* B causes that conscious state or has the property of being conscious (Chalmers 1995). But a more down-to-earth purpose of the hard problem is to highlight how vulnerable cognitive science is to some serious difficulties with what I call ``explanation by correlation.'' Here is what I mean: Suppose we observe that events A and B regularly correlate. In many such cases, there will be a temptation to focus on whether A ``explains'' B, when in fact the true explanation as to why A and B correlate may be more complicated than either A or B, and must appeal to a deeper layer of theory. But the credibility of that theory in turn will require that it also explain in a coherent way many *other* facts besides just A and B. Moreover, if some underlying mechanism, X, causes A and B to correlate, then we cannot even correctly say that A causes B. X may be more complex than either A or B in isolation.

For example, it is known that, at least in the US, Bible sales and liquor sales significantly correlate, both historically and geographically. But no one would jump to the conclusion that Bible sales ``explain'' liquor sales, or that the two phenomena are identical or bear a direct causal relation. Of course, there probably *is a causal explanation* for the correlation – but it is bound to be a complex and messy one. If we were simply to assume that Bible sales ``explain'' liquor sales, we would never find the real explanation. Nor do we do much better merely by mincing words and saying that Bible sales ``predict'' liquor sales, or ``are associated with'' liquor sales. We are still avoiding the fundamental question as to what *causes* Bible sales and liquor sales to correlate.

In the neuroscientific context, we often say that the amygdala ``lights up'' in an fMRI study when the subject feels anger, or that the anterior cingulate cortex lights up when the subject pays attention to a stimulus. It is then tempting simply to say that amygdala activation *causes* anger, or that the anterior cingulate is the substrate for the direction of attention. At a very practical level, the hard problem reminds us to reformulate the question in something like the following way: *Why* does amygdala activation correlate with anger? Framing the question in this more open-ended way leaves open the possibility that there may be a third factor that causes anger and at the same time, for a more complex reason, also correlates with amygdala activation. This more complex question must also make room for an understanding as to why the particular brain mechanism in question should have the property of consciousness.

When LeDoux first observed the correlation between anger and amygdala activation, he did not frame the question in this more open-ended way, and the results were correspondingly misleading (LeDoux 1996). Everyone began speaking of the amygdala as ``the seat´´ of anger and fear, just because its activation systematically correlated with them (Goleman 1994). It remained for a few maverick neuroscientists, such as Panksepp (1998, 2000), to keep insisting that amygdala activation was not the substrate of anger, but instead might correlate with anger only because it played an important role in learning and remembering *which stimuli* should elicit anger. Panksepp´s view is that the periaqueductal grey area (PAG) deep in the subcortex is the most crucial part of a complex anger circuit involving many brain areas other than the amygdala. It may even be that anger could be felt without any amygdala activation, but that in this case the anger would be indiscriminately directed. That is, the anger would not be elicited by a specific stimulus. The anger circuit is much more complicated than what LeDoux observed about the amygdala, because he did not go further than to note the correlation (see Ellis 2005). This sheer correlation prompted him to speak in his book as if the amygdala is the essential brain area whose activation produces anger. By contrast, Panksepp and others show that the anger circuit is much more extensive in the brain, and the amygdala plays only a modest role in it. The amygdala allows us to learn and remember which stimuli to *associate with* our anger.

The hard problem is more than a mere warning against the familiar ``correlation proves causation´´ fallacy. We often think that to jump from correlation to causation is dangerous only because not enough extraneous variables have been *controlled for* in the particular study. For example, the fact that child abuse correlates with later criminal activity on the part of the abused child does not prove that child abuse is a *cause* of the criminal activity, because there are other possible causal explanations for the correlation. For instance, there may be a violent gene that is passed along from parent to child, and the parent´s abusive behavior, like the child´s subsequent criminal behavior, may be only an expression of this gene. Or it may be that low-income parents are more likely to abuse their children.

But in this type of situation, the competing explanation can easily be eliminated by controlling for the relevant variables. For example, we can look at the correlation between child abuse and crime in foster children, who do not share genes with the abusive foster parent. And we can show that the correlation between child abuse and crime holds up irrespective of socioeconomic status. When we have ruled out *all* of the plausible competing explanations for the correlation, it seems that the correlation *can* establish a causal relation after all.

The hard problem, by contrast, is not gotten around so easily. No matter how tight our controls are, the correlation between conscious state C and brain event B still does not explain *why* B should have the property of C. What is missing here is a theory that could make sense of the relationship between C and B, beyond merely noting their correlation. The theory, T, in conjunction with B, would then become the fuller explanation of C. T, if we can ever discover it, would have to be at a level of even greater complexity than the explanation as to why liquor sales correlate with Bible sales.

THE HARD PROBLEM FURTHER COMPLICATED BY PHILOSOPHICAL PARADOXES

One reason for greater complexity in the case of conscious and mental states is that they raise philosophical problems that do not come into play when the phenomena to be connected have similar ontological status or if the epistemological methods of observing and measuring them are similar. In the case of liquor and Bible sales, both phenomena are empirically observable and straightforwardly ``physical.´´ (That is, they can be directly observed through the empirical research methods of the physical sciences.) The correlations between them do not raise the kind of logical paradoxes that are raised by theories that would attempt to explain the correlations between mental and brain processes.

The fact that theories about consciousness raise not only scientific but also philosophical puzzles highlights one of the most obvious differences between philosophical and scientific theorizing. In science, we typically have an array of empirical observations that can be equally well explained by a variety of competing theories, and the problem is how to devise a way to choose from among the many possible theoretical explanations. In a sense, there are *too many* possible explanatory theories from which to choose. In philosophy, the typical scenario is just the opposite: it turns out that every theory we can think of to explain the phenomena ends up leading to one or another paradox or self-contradiction, or cannot simultaneously reconcile itself with solutions to all aspects of the problem at stake – for example, the mind–body problem. So the problem is that we cannot find *even one* coherent and consistent theory capable of explaining all the data.

For example, theories that propose that states of consciousness either are or are not identical with the brain states that correlate with them will end up entailing paradoxes of one type or another. There will be problems either way.

If we posit that conscious states and their brain correlates are literally identical with each other, we are faced with several difficulties. In the first place, psychophysical identity theories seem not to explain what Jackson (1986) calls the ``knowledge argument.'' Simply stated, even if a neurophysiologist knows all about the brain, this knowledge by itself would not tell the scientist what it ``is like'' to experience the particular conscious state that the subject is experiencing. Phenomenologists had long been aware of this problem before Jackson called it to the attention of empirically oriented thinkers (see Ellis 2007). If a conscious state and its brain correlates were *literally the same entity,* then whatever is predicated of the one should also be predicated of the other. One thing that can be predicated of a subject's brain states is that a scientist can know all about them through empirical–scientific observation alone. But this same predicate (the predicate of being empirically observable) cannot be attributed to the phenomenal feel of the subject's states. The phenomenal feel, or ``what it's like'' to experience the state in question, is *not* empirically observable from an objective perspective. It seems to follow that the phenomenal feel – the subjective, conscious experience with its qualitative, ``what it's like'' aspects – cannot be the same as the brain states that are empirically observable. If the two were literally identical, it would seem that they both should be equally empirically observable.

I do not wish to argue that this problem is irresolvable. The point is that an adequate coherent theory of the relationship between the mental and the physical must provide a resolution for the paradox. It must explain why what is predicated of the brain states (for example, that they are empirically observable from an objective perspective) does not seem predicable of the conscious state and vice versa.

And this explanation will not be achieved any more easily by positing that mental and physical states are *not* identical. An example of a major difficulty with that approach is that it seems incapable of accounting for the problem of mental causation. Simply stated, the mental causation problem is that, if my conscious choice to move my hand plays a causal role in getting the hand to go up, then the conscious choice has causal power. But the hand going up can also be *completely* accounted for by previous *physical and chemical* events. And if the movement is completely accounted for by previous physical and chemical events, then that leaves *no* causal power for the *mental choice* – unless, of course, the mental event is somehow *exactly identical with* the physical and chemical ones. But as we have just seen, that too would be problematic because of the knowledge argument. In other words, the mental event is not completely empirically observable, whereas the physical and chemical ones are – seeming to imply that the mental and the physical/chemical are *not* exactly identical. We are damned if we say that mental and physical/chemical are identical, and damned if we don´t.

To the extent that we want to explain the apparent causal power of mental or conscious states, it would seem that we *must* equate them with physical ones. And this raises a serious difficulty for non-physicalist theories. Perhaps a non-physicalist can provide a coherent explanation of the problem of mental causation, but a coherent theoretical explanation must be reconcilable with this dilemma in one way or another, and it must explain why this paradox exists. Moreover, such a theory must explain what the ontological status of conscious states are, if they are not physical. What kind of event or property could be non-physical, and why should one non-physical property be differentiatiable from any other?

Correlations between physical and mental events require coherent theories for their explanation, and those theories must account for philosophical as well as scientific problems. The most important point of the ``hard problem,´´ for practical purposes, is that it highlights the need to leave open the question: *Why* does physical event P correlate with conscious event C? It seems that no purely empirical observation can answer this question, because the empirical account can tell us only *that* P is accompanied by consciousness, not *why* it is.

THE GOOD HARD PROBLEM VERSUS
THE BAD HARD PROBLEM

A plethora of books and articles have been addressed to refuting Chalmers´s ``hard problem´´ argument. But it is seldom acknowledged that there are actually two hard problem arguments, even as early as Chalmers´s (1995) paper introducing the notion. I have suggested that the simple version of the hard problem outlined above is valid and legitimate. This version is actually similar to Joseph Levine's (1983) ``explanatory gap'' argument. Levine posited that, if conscious event C really were equivalent with some physiological event P, then we should be able to deduce, by means of some logical inference, from the P to all the properties of C, including its subjective ``what it's like'' qualities. But we cannot. As I have said, this problem has serious practical implications for the way neuroscience and cognitive theory are carried out. We could call this the ``epistemological'' version of the hard problem argument.

On the other hand, when Chalmers begins talking about zombies and twin earths, he is getting into a more ``ontological'' version of the argument, which is rightly criticized (see Ellis & Newton 2005; also Ellis & Newton 2009). In this ontological type of ``hard problem'' argument, Chalmers is insisting that we can imagine zombies (or creatures on twin earths) behaving exactly the way *we* do, including our information-processing capacities, without being *conscious* while they engage in these behaviors. Because we can imagine such things, they are possible. And this proves, Chalmers thinks, that it is possible for beings to be physically exactly like us, but without being conscious. Therefore, Chalmers concludes that whatever makes us conscious cannot be explained by our physical properties. Thus consciousness is *ontologically* distinguished from our physical properties.

This ontological argument is a ``harder'' version of the hard problem, insisting that the hard problem cannot ever be solved. But, as I have discussed elsewhere (for example, Ellis 2005), this argument is analogous to claiming that, because we can ``imagine'' Clark Kent not being Superman, this proves that whatever makes him Superman must be independent of the being Clark Kent, whom we have imagined as not being Superman; therefore, Kent cannot be equivalent with Superman. Obviously, such an argument cannot be valid, because Superman just *is* Kent, no matter how well we think we can imagine Kent as *not* being Superman.

The simpler, merely epistemological version of the hard problem, nonetheless, is a legitimate problem with which we must grapple. In other words, even when we have explained all the neurophysiological correlates of consciousness, we still would not have explained why they have the property of consciousness. What makes the problem hard is that this dilemma will remain no matter how successful or complete our physical explanations become, and seems to apply in principle to any sheerly physical or empirical explanation.

The beginning of the current Kuhnian revolutionary situation in the philosophy of mind coincided with Chalmers's popularizing the concept of the hard problem of consciousness. In 1994, Chalmers's keynote address at the Tucson *Toward a Science of Consciousness* conference was also published in the newly launched *Journal of Consciousness Studies,* which in turn was a co-sponsor of the conference. The argument Chalmers presented actually had already been developed by Levine (1983) under the rubric of the ``explanatory gap´´ argument, but Levine was slightly ahead of his time, so the argument attracted less attention from neuroscientists and cognitive theorists, who were not yet ready to give up on the computer metaphor, and therefore were not yet casting around for alternative approaches. Chalmers's ``hard problem´´ lecture both showed *why* the old approaches were inadequate, and also helped an audience already dissatisfied to see where the crucial problem lay, and in general what demands would need to be satisfied by an alternative approach.

Perhaps because of the pervasive Kuhnian revolutionary fervor, there has been a tendency to conflate the two versions of the ``hard problem´´ concept. This is especially unfortunate because the epistemological one is much more logically compelling than the ontological one. I shall refer to the two versions as the ``good hard problem´´ and the ``bad hard problem´´ – or alternatively, the valid and the invalid hard problem arguments. We should not permit the numerous legitimate critiques of the bad hard problem to distract our attention from the important implications of the good one. The good hard problem can be helpful in avoiding simplistic explanations. For example, as we have seen, the hard problem warns us against some subtle yet crucial instances of ``explanation by correlation.´´

The good hard problem also forces us to think seriously about what we are asking for when we ask for an ``explanation´´ of consciousness. What do we mean by ``explanation´´ in the context of ``explaining´´ consciousness? We could either mean (1) a statement of all the physical antecedents that will causally bring about the phenomenon in question; or (2) a demonstration of *why* the phenomenon in question *must* be just the way it is and no other way, given its causal antecedents and given a coherent theory of how the phenomena interconnect. Chalmers's good hard problem argument obviously is valid in the sense that explanations of type (1) do not necessarily yield explanations of type (2); but this should not lead people to assert, equivocally, that consciousness simply ``cannot be explained´´ by physical antecedents. If this is what Chalmers means, then he is equivocating the term ``explanation.´´

On the other hand, Chalmers's bad hard problem argument is invalid for the reasons just mentioned. Imagining Kent as not being Superman doesn't show that he is not Superman. What neuroscientists must be careful to keep in mind, though, is that we want to give an explanation of type (2) of consciousness, not merely an explanation of type (1). There actually is no ``explanatory gap'' in sense (1) of ``explanatory.'' If all we want is to show the necessary and sufficient antecedents of consciousness, this can be done by means of empirical research. But with regard to sense (2) of ``explanation,'' the explanatory gap argument implies that we should never expect to be able to *deduce* a property like subjective consciousness from sheer empirical observation of the elements that combine to produce it. We can empirically show *that* the lower-level properties give rise to the subjective, conscious ones, but showing *why* they do will require a more elaborate strategy. We can never deduce the qualitative features of consciousness from its empirically observable components alone. A coherent general theory is needed to make sense of why those components *should* lead to the unique qualities of consciousness when combined in that way.

If what we mean by ``explain'' is ``state necessary and sufficient causal preconditions,'' then to explain the physical substrates of consciousness *is* to explain consciousness. But the problem is that, in order to discover *just the right* physical processes that subserve consciousness will require discovering, not merely that certain physical processes, P, *correlate* with conscious ones, C. We also need to ask *why* that P correlates with that C. And this will require a fuller coherent general theory – an explanation of type (2).

For example, the theory of psychophysical identity is not a thesis that needs to be deducible from a specific P–C correlation. The identity of consciousness with some physical process must be justified independently of the explanation of the physical processes themselves, by showing that any other ontological relation between consciousness and the physical entails insurmountable logical contradictions, paradoxes, and inconsistencies with fact. So, in sense (1) of ``explanation'' (causally explaining physical events XYZ), one can perfectly well ``explain'' consciousness. But we still want an explanation as to why those physical causal antecedents could not have resulted in those physical consequents *in the absence of consciousness*. In that sense, it may be that we have not yet discovered the explanation because we have been trying to get the wrong *type* of ``explanation'' to do the job – an empirical–scientific explanation, which is able to explain only *what* the necessary and sufficient causal antecedents of XYZ are, not *why they should have the property of consciousness.*

Notice that, when X and Y are identical, this does not mean that Y has to be deductively inferrable from X. Clark Kent and Superman are identical, but we cannot deduce from the fact that Kent is present to the conclusion that Superman is present – unless we *already* know that they are identical *on other grounds*. In this latter case, of course, we would also have to *define* Kent in terms of *all* of his properties, including the (presumably known) fact that he is Superman. In that case, of course, we *could* deduce Superman from Kent (i.e. from the totality of Kent's properties, including the properties that make him Superman). This would require, however, that we already have known all the Superman-ish properties of Kent prior to making the inference from Kent to Superman.

Analogously, if we already know that XYZ brain process is identical to consciousness, then of course we can deduce the presence of consciousness from the presence of XYZ. However, there is no way to deduce from the presence of Kent (without already knowing that he is Superman) the fact that he must be Superman. Similarly, Chalmers (in spite of all his other mistakes) rightly points out that we cannot deduce consciousness from brain process XYZ, unless we already know that XYZ is identical with consciousness. There is nothing about Kent, in his ``essence´´ (as Kripke would put it), that would imply that he *must* be Superman. But of course this still does not imply that he *cannot be* Superman, and we know on independent grounds that he is; analogously, we may know on independent grounds that consciousness is physical – so Chalmers is wrong to use this version of the ``hard problem´´ as an argument against physicalism.

It should be obvious that this distinction between the two different senses of ``explanation´´ have important implications for the theory and neurophysiology of consciousness. Explanations in sense (2) must be full-fledged *theories,* and they must include both scientific and philosophical considerations. Some of their justifications will be not merely that they are consistent with certain empirically observable correlations, but also that they avoid the self-contradictions and other problems entailed by certain philosophical positions. A general theory of this kind is not deducible from the facts it must explain. On the contrary, we conclude *inductively* that it is the best available theory to explain the totality of facts that need to be explained.

The bad hard problem argument tries to require science to do what can be done only with the help of philosophy. It asks for a scientific explanation as to why consciousness must be physical, when in fact only a theory that takes philosophical arguments and problems into account could explain why consciousness must be physical: the explanation – if there is such an explanation – will require showing that every competing theory of the mind–body relation is untenable, either by leading to logical contradictions, or by contradicting easily established empirical and phenomenological facts. And finally, it must show that the theory advocated is consistent with all those facts and resolves all those logical problems. As we have seen, it is difficult for a theory of psychophysical identity to resolve all the problems, because it still must face the Charybdis of the problem of mental causation and the Scylla of Jackson's ``knowledge argument.''

Moreover, such a general theory also must provide an explanation for the problem of ``multiple realizability'' – that is, the problem that the same mental event might be realizable by several alternative brain sequences. The problem is that if the mental event could be realized by several alternative brain processes, then it would be difficult simply to equate it with one of those alternative processes. To do so would be analogous to defining Tchaikovsky's Sixth Symphony as one particular performance of the symphony by one particular orchestra. Also, the successful theory must show why some physical systems are not conscious whereas others are. And it must explain the ability of consciousness, as a biological phenomenon, to initiate action (as all biological systems do, in a minimal sense of ``action'') as opposed only to reacting to inputs.

Surmounting all these constraints simultaneously and without internal contradiction is a tall order, but it is not, as Chalmers sometimes suggests, unattainable in principle. In fact, the constraints imposed by these difficulties can actually help us reject untenable theories of consciousness, and point us toward better ones.

As a question about the interrelations between explanations of types (1) and (2), the good hard problem has crucially important consequences for contemporary neuroscience. Suppose we do avoid simple ``explanations by correlation'' and instead look for a coherent explanation for the correlation at a deeper level. Philosophy has a great deal to contribute toward helping direct this line of research. The important point is that any relation between a physical and a psychical phenomenon requires a general theory for its explanation. Simply noting a correlation, or even a whole series of correlations, will not get us there.

THE SEARCH FOR A GENERAL THEORY OF CONSCIOUS
PROCESSES

When we acknowledge the importance of general theories in accounting for the correlations between mental and physical events, we are more prone to admit that no *single* mental phenomenon can really be explained except with reference to a general theory that is also capable of explaining *all the other* mental phenomena. A theory that can explain only a few phenomena is not a general theory at all, but instead is merely an ``explanation by correlation.``

Theories at the level of generality needed to satisfy the ``hard problem`` will therefore be subject to all the Kuhnian problems with the sociology of theory acceptance and rejection (Kuhn 1962). Scientists will tend to adopt a theory that can explain the ``normal problems`` with which they are immediately concerned, and ignore the kinds of problems that this theory cannot explain. The questions asked will be the ones prompted by current instrumentation and research paradigms, and the going paradigms and instrumentation will tend to lead scientists to focus on observations that confirm the theory they prefer. Questions unanswerable by the going theory will tend to be ignored for as long as possible, and ad hoc explanations proposed. Only when some important practical problem cannot be solved, after extensive attempts, will the old theory be thrown into question.

This is what the problem of consciousness did to the computational paradigm, or computer analogy, in the 1990s. Computationalist cognitive theorists promised to construct a conscious machine by the year 2000. When the 1990s came, everyone realized that this achievement was no closer than ever, and the field was thrown into a Kuhnian ``revolutionary situation`` comparable to Russia in 1917: the old order was disrupted, and it was unclear what might replace it.

Instrumentation plays an important role in establishing Kuhnian paradigms. Theorists find themselves drawn to metaphors based on the latest technology – levers in the Renaissance, electricity in the early twentieth century, computers in the late twentieth century. In addition, the ability to conduct experiments is determined by what kinds of instrument are available. During the 1990s, EEG technology gave way to fMRI as the latest method of observing brain events. EEG measures timing precisely, but not location; fMRI is just the opposite. Also, fMRI measures changes in blood flow. But subcortical processes require only tiny changes in blood flow to achieve their normal mental/ emotional effects, whereas cortical events involve substantial blood flow changes. So cortical areas light up much more readily in fMRI studies, and the fMRI instrumentation naturally leads to a cortical bias. Explanations of mental and conscious events tend to center on cortical areas, and to de-emphasize subcortical ones.

The cortical bias of fMRI, along with its inability to measure the precise timing of neural events, in turn leads to a de-emphasis of the importance of emotional and action-initiating processes in various kinds of mental and conscious phenomena, since those are initiated primarily at the subcortical level and require exact timing. Subcortical processes tend to be *action-initiating,* whereas cortical ones tend to be *information-receiving.* As a result, the fMRI instrumentation encourages passive-receiving models of mental processes, rather than action-initiating models. Many cognitive theorists simply scratch their heads when they hear someone proposing that action-initiating circuits are involved in all consciousness, as suggested by Merleau-Ponty (1941, 1942), Newton (1982, 1993, 1996), and Varela *et al.* (1991). Such ``enactive'' proposals (as they are now sometimes called) sound strange to corticocentric neuro-scientists, because corticocentricity encourages seeing mental processes as input-receiving states, like the areas of the cortex themselves. I will say more later about the enactive model. I believe it can address the hard problem of neuroscience by providing explanations of correlations within a coherent theory that also accommodates the philosophical paradoxes of the mind–body problem.

Sometimes instrumentation not only biases the direction of research, but also forms unlucky interactions with going theoretical predispositions that were passed down from the immediately preceding period. In the case of consciousness, the previous period had been heavily influenced by the computer metaphor, which tried to look at consciousness in terms of *information processing.* Moreover, it saw the brain primarily as a *receiver* more than a *sender* of information, because this information-receiving bias had been picked up by the stimulus–response paradigm of the *earlier* twentieth century.

So the corticocentric bias of the fMRI, combined with the information-receiving model, has led scientists to explain consciousness in terms of cortical processing of received inputs. Moreover, the experimental situation itself encourages such a bias. In the psychology laboratory, it is easy to deliver a *stimulus* and then observe the brain's *reaction* – especially if our instrumentation leads us to take ``the brain'' to mean ``the cortex.''

The upshot is that we find ourselves more than ever tempted to explain consciousness in terms of correlations with what happens in the *cortex* when it *receives* certain inputs. We are then all the more seduced into a passive-receiving model of consciousness and the mental, in which not only are emotional and action-initiating sub-cortically based processes overlooked, but so are the complexities that inevitably form the real basis for the simple correlations that we *can* observe.

And here again, we find ourselves dangerously close to an ``a-theoretical´´ attitude. Instead of looking for coherent theories capable of explaining why A correlates with B, we content ourselves with proceeding as if A already *were* the explanation of B. It is just as if we were to think that an increase in Bible sales *explains* the increase in liquor sales, rather than looking for the more complex system of relations that could explain why the correlation exists.

SELF-ORGANIZATION THEORY AS A COHERENT EXPLANATORY RESPONSE TO THE HARD PROBLEM

EEG patterns, CT scans, and other measures of neural activity in various parts of the brain have now been extensively correlated with conscious acts such as feelings of elation and depression (Ahern & Schwartz 1985; Damasio & Van Hoesen 1983); remembering (Damasio 1989; Damasio *et al.* 1985); attention (Posner & Rothbart 1992; Cohen *et a.l* 1988); consciousness involving both sensory and memory elements as integrated via frontal lobe activity (Nauta 1971); obses-sional thought patterns (Gibson & Kennedy 1960); hysterical condi-tions (Flor-Henry *et al.* 1979); conscious word recognition (Petersen *et al.* 1989); and many other such consciousness/brain-electrical correlations.

I want to focus on one possible way to make sense out of these correlations, while at the same time allowing for an understanding as to *why* consciousness should accompany some neural processes and not others. The problem can be sharpened by asking this question: What is the difference between instances of information-processing that are conscious and those that are not conscious? The difference cannot be found by examining what is required to process information, as the previous generation of computationally inspired computer-metaphor theories had hoped.

The difference, in my view, is that only *self-organizing* systems can process information in a conscious way. The reason is that self-organizing systems *act* upon their environment rather than merely *react*. Beings that act must contact their environment by sending self-initiated, *efferent* nervous signals, as opposed to merely receiving *afferent* signals. Efferent signals flow *away* from the initiating brain areas, such as in action commands, which originate deep in the sub-cortex and are then refined as they travel through the brain's inter-neuron system and finally to the body's extremities. Afferent signals flow *inward* from the body's extremities, for example from the optic nerve, and are transformed and reorganized as the brain interprets their meaning and then responds.

The point I wish to emphasize about afferent and efferent path-ways is that many neuroscientists attempt to explain vision, emotion, etc. by means of receiving *afferent* signals, *from* the sense organs or *from* the viscera of the body. (For emotions, this information would be in the form of ``proprioception'' of the body's viscera.) But such an account, in principle, *cannot address the hard problem*. It cannot explain the difference between conscious and non-conscious information processing. Afferent data can be received on a *non-conscious* basis, both in computers and in human nervous systems – as in blindsight, inattentional blindness, and so on.

A self-organizational account that makes conscious processing contingent on *efferent* nervous impulses will fare better with the hard problem. On the one hand, such an account does not require an anti-physicalist view of the ontology of consciousness. Such a theory can distinguish between a *process* and the physical micro-constituents that *make up* the process. So the overall process can be physical, and yet may not be identical with the mere collection of physical micro-constituents that make it up, any more than Tchaikovsky's Sixth Symphony is defined by the mere collection of notes that make it up. The same notes may be in Beethoven's Third Symphony, but arranged in a different pattern. Different notes could have made up Tchaikovsky's Sixth (espe-cially if it were transposed to a different key), but it would still be the same symphony, as long as the notes are in the same *relation* to each other. Certainly, not the same *token performances* of those notes are needed to make up Tchaikovsky's Sixth.

On the other hand, a self-organizational theory grounded in efferent processes can also explain Jackson's ``knowledge argument.'' Jackson's question is: If consciousness is equivalent with a brain pro-cess, and the brain process is completely knowable by an objective observer, then why isn't the ``what it's like'' dimension of conscious-ness revealed by means of objective observations? An approach that emphasizes efferent action commands as the basis of consciousness can answer this question. The answer is that, if consciousness is an *action* that I perform, by sending efferent action commands in order to imagine how I could act relative to my environment, then it is not surprising that someone else cannot observe what my consciousness is like by receiving afferent nervous signals from *their perception* of my actions. That would be like saying that someone could know what it is like for me to dance by observing me dancing. To be conscious is to act, not merely to *observe* an action. We know our world in terms of how we could act relative to it.

To be sure, we need not act to be conscious. A paralyzed person can be conscious. But a paralyzed person can *imagine* acting relative to the environment. When we imagine acting, as Jeannerod (1997) and many others have shown, we send action commands just as we would in overtly acting; but at the same time, we frontally inhibit the action commands at the level of the motor, premotor, and supplementary motor areas even while continuing to send the command. This process is efferent in the sense that we initiate the signal ourselves as opposed to receiving it through afferent pathways. (This efferent/afferent distinction is spelled out more fully in Ellis 1995, 2005.) Only complex self-organizing systems can imagine acting relative to the environment, because only self-organizing systems can act per se. Understanding action affordances (imagining what actions would be possible and which are impossible) is the way in which complex self-organizing creatures ``understand´´ their environment (Newton 1996). As Newton explains, this is precisely the sense of ``understanding´´ in which Searle's famous ``Chinese Room´´ is fed translations and then spits them out, but without actually ``understanding´´ Chinese. So Newton's concept of ``understanding´´ differentiates non-conscious information processing from the kind of processing that conscious beings perform.

A self-organizing system is a thermodynamic system that exchanges energy and materials with its environment while maintaining a relative constancy in its own pattern of activity (Kauffman 1993; Newton 2000). Rather than an epiphenomenon of the causal interactions of its micro-constituents, it has the ability, because of the way it is structured, to appropriate and replace substratum elements as needed to perpetuate the pattern of the overall process (Ellis 1986). This is what biological systems do. Even though they obey the principles of chemistry as in any inorganic system, they also are structured so as to rearrange the background conditions needed in order for a given micro-level causal mechanism to occur in a particular context at the substratum level. For example, in stroke recovery, the brain recruits new micro-level causal mechanisms – cells and synapses – to do the work of the destroyed cells and synapses.

Self-organization is a structuring of a system such that certain outcomes will be achieved, in the interest of maintaining the system, even if achieving this outcome means rearranging, replacing or recombining the substratum elements that, all together, make up the system. Food metabolism and the re-routing of damaged synapses are obvious examples. The ability of a system to maintain its own patterns relative to environmental perturbations distinguishes action from mere reaction.

In the context of the philosophy of mind, this theory makes possible the notion of a process that is clearly distinguishable from the sum of its own components – indeed, has a kind of causal power *over* its own components in the sense that it appropriates, replaces, and rearranges them as needed. Thus it may be possible to model a self-organizing system that engages in phenomenal consciousness, where the consciousness is a self-organizing feature of the system, yet cannot be known by an objective observer who is not in a position to actively *execute* the organismic processes whose execution would constitute knowledge of what the person´s consciousness ``is like.´´ In this way, we can avoid a non-physicalist dualism that would violate physical causal closure, yet satisfy Jackson´s demand that consciousness be irreducible to any combination of events that can be empirically observed.

If we distinguish between ``physical´´ and ``empirically observable,´´ the import of Jackson´s knowledge argument is only to show, not that consciousness is not a *physical* process, but rather that it is not identical with an *empirically observable* process. Even showing this much makes psychophysical identity theories problematic, if we assume that the physical events with which consciousness is to be identified occur at an empirically observable level (i.e. discrete neurophysiological events), because consciousness itself notoriously is in principle *not* empirically observable from an objective, external perspective. If we are to avoid metaphysical dualism, with all its well-known logical problems, then consciousness can still be a kind of physical process that is distinguishable from the lower-level physical constituents of the process because the process is realizable by alternative sets of physical constituents. This is, in fact, the hallmark of self-organizational systems, and is remarkably consistent with the fact that all currently known conscious systems are biological organisms, and therefore are self-organizing systems in the sense defined above.

HOW SELF-ORGANIZATION CAN RESOLVE
THE MIND–BODY PROBLEM

The physical sciences *empirically* identify predictable patterns of brain events that are as explainable by currently available physical/chemical principles as any other physical/chemical system. In this sense, sequences of brain events are sufficient causal sequences, observed to obey the same causal laws as everything else in nature. The brain is not full of mysterious violations of the principles of physics or chemistry. But if so, then some combination of physical *and empirically observable* events in the brain, labeled "P1" (see Figure 3.1, below), is causally necessary and sufficient for subsequent physical and empirically observable event P2. And we know that, in numerous well-documented instances, a conscious event, C1, is of a type that correlates regularly with and is somehow associated with P1, and some subsequent C2 correlates with and is somehow associated with P2.

```
C1 - - - > C2
 |          |
P1 - - - > P2
```

Figure 3.1 Relationships between conscious and physical events.

If P1 and C1 were identical, then it would make sense that both of them can be necessary and sufficient for some subsequent event. But if not, then we seem to be left with two options: P1 causes (or "realizes") C1 (epiphenomenalism); or C1 causes P1 (reverse epiphenomenalism) – or some combination of the two (interactionism, of the Popper & Eccles 1977 variety).

But all these alternative options seem untenable. Epiphenomenalism is untenable because to say that P1 causes C1 implies that P1 and C1 are different events, since a cause is not the same thing as its effect; and if C1 is different from P1, the question arises whether C1 is physical or non-physical. Most epiphenomenalists admit that C1 cannot be non-physical, because this would entail all the problems of dualism, such as the problem of mental causation, which we discussed earlier. But if C1 is a physical property of P1 (or "realized by" P1), the resulting physicalist epiphenomenalism does not explain why consciousness should be in principle empirically unobservable, whereas most physical properties are empirically observable, at least in principle (Kim 1993).

Some people argue for an ``interactionism´´ form of epiphenomenalism, in which P1 might cause C1, which causes C2, which causes P2, which then causes P3, etc. (as in Popper and Eccles 1977). The problem here is that the failure of P1 to work as a necessary and sufficient cause of P2 would violate what we know about the regular behavior of the physical events in the brain. We do not find the continual ruptures of the principles of physics or chemistry that would be entailed by this kind of ``interactionism.´´

But, as we have already seen, there is a remaining option: C1 may be related to P1, not as cause to effect, but in the way that a process relates to the various elements of the physical substratum for that process (Ellis 1986, 1995). For example, a transverse wave takes certain physical particles, and discrete movements of these physical particles, as its substratum when the wave passes through that particular material medium (a sound wave through a wooden door, for example), but the wave is not identical with the door, nor is it caused by the door. There is an important sense in which the wave could have been ``the same´´ wave it is even if some other material medium (for example, a different door, or a volume of air) had been in a position to serve as its substratum. (However, the sense in which this is true requires some philosophical clarification, since there is another sense in which two waves having the same pattern are not numerically ``the same wave.´´ See Ellis 2005.)

In a self-organizing system, in the sense defined above, the overall pattern of the process – a relational pattern, which we could label R – can be realized by alternative substrata, P(a) or P(b). R will readjust certain components of its own organization if that is what is necessary in order to use P(b) as its necessary and sufficient substratum whenever P(a) is not available to be used. The relation R is arranged in such a way that it changes some of its component actions in order to maintain the overall relation R across a variety of possible P-elements, depending on which P-elements are available to be used as substrata for R.

The temperature of a gas in a chamber, while multiply realizable (because a variety of combinations of particle motions *could have* yielded the same temperature), is not multiply realizable in this self-organizing way. Whether the same temperature is maintained is not determined by organizational properties of the gas in the chamber, but by antecedent conditions *external* to the current behavior of the gas in the chamber. Whether the gas particles move this way or that way is a result of the causal antecedents that cause each particle to move in the way it does, and the temperature is a result of the totality of these antecedents.

An analogous case involving a *self-organizing* system would be one in which an organism is functioning to maintain pattern R, while maintaining R requires maintaining temperature T. Even if all antecedents external to R remain the same, but P(a) is not available as a substratum for T, R will *readjust other aspects of itself* in order to make it possible for P(b) to be used as a substratum for T; furthermore, R's organization sets up a strong tendency for T and the now-altered elements within R to still interrelate so as to preserve the overall pattern R. A standard thermostat does not fit this description because it is not a self-organizing system to begin with. But our own bodies *are*, among other things, self-organizing, living thermostats. (For other specific biological examples, see Monod 1971; Merleau-Ponty 1941).

If consciousness is associated with such self-organizing processes, then consciousness can appropriate and replace substratum elements needed to perform its functions, rather than merely being a consequence *of* those elements. None of this entails that R itself does not have perfectly necessary and sufficient causal antecedents. The point is that, once the pattern of R has been set up, *then* R is capable of using either P(a) or P(b) as its substratum, without any antecedent factors having been different, except of course for those needed to bring it about that P(b) is available whereas P(a) is not. Self-organizing processes are thus ``free'' in that they are not completely determined by anything that is *currently* external to themselves. But this does not entail that the organization of R itself is not the result of *earlier* causal antecedents of some sort. Self-organization does not contradict the regular, deterministic nature of physical processes.

The notion of self-organization offers a solution both to the mental causation problem and to the knowledge argument simultaneously. According to the self-organization approach, consciousness is an embodied process, taking ``body'' to refer to a type of self-organizing system whose tendency to maintain its structure becomes elaborated in terms of motivationally and emotionally relevant purposes. If phenomenal consciousness must always have an embodied, motivational aspect, then in order to know what a state of consciousness ``is like'' or ``feels like,'' one would have to inhabit the same *body* that serves as substratum for that conscious process, because the embodied, emotional motivations for the anticipation of cognitive content is a vital part of what the consciousness ``is like.'' On this view, consciousness would be a higher-order process constituted by certain relations between the body, the brain, and the organism's environment. Only by *being* an organism in some such relation could one be conscious of anything; thus only by being the organism that is in such a relation could one ``know what it is like'' to be in that relation. Yet the lower-order substratum elements that are used as the *relata* for the relation would still be empirically observable, and could be studied by means of empirical–scientific methods.

What reasons are there for believing that all phenomenal consciousness must be motivated by organismic purposes? Recent trends in neuroscience suggest an increased importance for the role of emotion and self-organization in consciousness (Posner & Rothbart 1992; Alexander & Globus 1996; Watt 1998, 2000; Freeman 1987; Panksepp 1998, 2000). A mere computational registering and processing of sensory signals (e.g. in the occipital lobes for vision) by itself does *not* result in perceptual *consciousness* of the relevant information (Aurell 1989; Posner & Rothbart 1992). Instead, midbrain-orchestrated emotional processes are crucial for phenomenal consciousness: frontal areas such as the anterior cingulate must be activated in order to direct conscious attention, and these frontal areas are activated in turn by stimulation of the limbic, thalamic, and midbrain areas associated with transmitting emotional motivations of the whole organism to brain areas that bring the emotions into consciousness and also allow them to direct the processes of attention, imaging, and activation of abstract concepts (Luria 1980; Posner 1980; Segal 1971). Emotional processes are thus a necessary component for consciousness.

In conscious processing, unlike non-conscious processing in digital computers that passively respond to input, motivational purposes must precede any registering of sensory data in consciousness. The *afferent* brain areas (those that *receive* stimulation from external sources) – such as the occipital lobe – can be completely activated, in just the way they are in a perception, but with no perceptual *consciousness* of the object occurring (Luria 1980; Posner & Rothbart 1992). Consciousness occurs only when the *efference*-activating system, beginning with the emotional midbrain/limbic area, prompts the frontal lobe to start looking *for* environmental items that might be of *interest* to the organism, and activates neurotransmitters to catalyze the corticothalamic loops needed to enhance important signals and direct either voluntary or involuntary attention to them (Ellis 1995; Ellis & Newton 1998).

If the organism is motivated to look *for* a certain kind of item, but the item is not present in the perceptual field, what occurs is a mere mental *image* of that kind of item. For example, when subjects are told to look *for* blue triangles to be flashed on a screen, interspersed with other items of no interest, the subject forms a mental image of that which is to be looked for, and this enables her to see it when it is presented and to ignore the other items (Corbetta *et al.* 1990; Hanze & Hesse 1993;

Rhodes & Tremewan 1993). This "looking-for" process, which consti-tutes the mental image of the non-present object, is accomplished by *efferent* (internally generated) brain processes occurring in the thalamus, amygdala, frontal cortex, and efferent aspects of the parietal and occipital lobes (Luria 1980). This motivated efferent activity, absent afferent input, is sufficient to create the mental image.

If a corresponding object *is* present in the perceptual field, and leads to *afferent* activity (in posterior cortical areas such as the occipital lobe), and if this afferent activity resonates with already occurring *efferent* activity (as the organism looks *for* emotionally interesting items), only then does an image occur which seems to the subject like a perceptual image of an actually existing object. The image is phe-nomenally similar to a mere mental image (although perhaps more "vivid"), but now becomes the image of an actually present object.

When subjects selectively pay attention to a given type of image flashed on a screen, the process of "looking for" that type of object leads to a mental image or "concept" of the object in consciousness. The subject's interest in seeing the object can be experienced phenomeno-logically as leading to an imaginary consciousness of the idea of the object, even before the object is actually presented. This perceptual "priming" effect has been replicated in thousands of different contexts.

RESPONSES TO OBJECTIONS

Someone might think that emphasizing an emotional or motivational component to *all* phenomenal experience is an overgeneralization. It might be argued that, when I am just "vegging" in front of a TV commercial, I have no emotional or motivational interest in the commercial, yet I see it none the less. But the fact is that our organisms are designed to direct conscious attention more toward types of objects that are *generally likely* to be important – moving objects in the per-iphery and unusual lights, for example – because those *kinds* of objects do often turn out to be important.

It might still be objected that we often are aware of objects that are not even members of some general class of objects that are par-ticularly *likely* to be important for the organism's purposes. But *any* type of object might be important under *some* circumstances. This is why Panksepp's "seeking system" (Panksepp 1998, Chapter 8) is not directed toward any particular type of stimulus; it motivates us simply to explore the environment in general. Curiosity, in fact, is one of the most basic motivating emotions (hence the title *Curious Emotions* for my 2005 book).

I readily grant that the kind of complex self-organization that makes motivation possible is a necessary but not sufficient condition for consciousness. Some complex self-organizing systems are not conscious. The subset of such systems that do exhibit consciousness seems to include those that combine emotional motivations and anticipations with an additional capacity – the capacity to represent the environment by means of fairly precise estimates of the action affordances of various environmental situations. This requires the ability not only to be motivated and to receive input, but also the ability to imagine doing things that one is not now doing. When a self-organizing system can represent merely possible scenarios (for example, in mental imagery or abstract concepts) as well as actual ones – by imagining actions through the inhibition of the relevant action commands, based on a motivated interest in the present or merely imagined situation – then the being is conscious (see Ellis & Newton 1998, 2005).

Still another objection against this use of motivation and emotion to distinguish conscious from non-conscious processing is that emotions and motivations are already the kinds of things of which people normally can be conscious; thus explaining consciousness as a result of them seems circular. But what has just been said about the role of emotions does not depend on defining ``emotions´´ and ``motivations´´ as necessarily conscious phenomena. Emotions and motivations are characterized by purposive strivings, and there do seem to be non-conscious yet purposive phenomena in nature, especially in biological organisms. For example, the human organism purposely does what is necessary to regulate its heartbeat and blood pressure, yet normally is not *conscious* of doing so. As phenomenologists are quick to point out, there is such a thing as purposeful but non-conscious action (Ellis 1986).

How would such an emphasis on a motivational and emotional component for all consciousness enable self-organization theory to resolve the problem of the empirical unobservability of consciousness as reflected in the knowledge argument? The theory of self-organization, with its emphasis on embodiment and organismic motivation in all consciousness, can explain this paradox on the basis that an objective or external observer, such as Jackson´s color-blind neuroscientist Mary, can survey everything empirically observable about my neurophysiological processes and yet not be inhabiting the self-organizing system that is *my body*. Even if not color-blind, she still would not have the *emotionally interested anticipations* that, for me, are crucial for *generating* the phenomenal character of what a given state of consciousness is like *for me* (Posner & Rothbart 1992; Luria 1980; Ellis 1995; Sedikides 1992; Hanze & Hesse 1993). She cannot enact the actions of my body. When she observes the relationship between my brain, my body, and the object of my consciousness, she must always feel what it is like to have the phenomenal character of her experience determined by the interested anticipations that arise from *her* body. If she understands enough about biological organisms, then she could possibly observe *that* my organism had emotional interests, but she still would not know *what* the emotional interests ``are like'' because to know what a state of consciousness ``is like'' requires being emotionally motivated to ``look for'' certain patterns of incoming stimuli. The ``what it's like'' aspect requires *having* the emotionally interested anticipations that would cause it to ``feel'' a certain way. The only way a person could know what a phenomenal state is like would be to be emotionally motivated to *enact* that state (Varela *et al.* 1991/1993), because the emotional motivation *is* the most crucial element in the *knowledge* of ``what it's like.'' The only way the objective observer could enact those emotions would be to *have* the body that generates them (and not merely look *at* that body).

This point helps clarify the mystery as to what strange kind of relation there could be that cannot be empirically observed. The relation in question can be ``observed'' only by *enacting* the particular emotionally interested anticipations that are *constitutive* of the requisite ``observations.'' Knowing what an object looks like to me requires *having* my motivations, not just *knowing* that I have certain brain correlates of motivations, because knowing, like any state of consciousness, always requires embodiment, and is always from someone's embodied point of view. The having of the motivations which lead to the anticipations that shape phenomenal experience is an embodied activity that requires *being in* the body – or more simply, *being* the body – that enacts them.

To say that one can know what the consciousness is like only from a certain perspective is to say that one can know what it is like only by *being* or *enacting* the relation in question. Thus phenomenal consciousness is both (a) ontologically distinguishable from its empirically observable substrata, and (b) inaccessible to empirical observation (i.e. from an external perspective), even though its substrata *are* accessible to such empirical observation. None of this entails that consciousness is non-physical. In fact, even if consciousness is a thoroughly physical process, it can very well be irreducible to its empirically observable substrata; it can be a pattern of activity that makes use of those substrata, while the way it does so must be enacted rather than externally observed in order to know "what it is like."

This entire discussion illustrates the benefits of opening rather than prematurely closing the question as to *why* XYZ correlates with a conscious state. Opening this question not only prompts us to consider that the explanation might be more complicated than XYZ itself, but it also forces us to consider the full range of restraints on the possible coherent answers to the question. We are forced to consider general theories of consciousness in light of *all* the evidence, not just the particular correlation we initially wanted to explain.

CONCLUSION

The hard problem reminds us not to confine ourselves to the "easy problems." For example, "What are the mechanisms of neural signaling?" "How are visual signals transferred from the thalamus to the occipital lobe?" The hard problem runs deeper: even when we have successfully explained all the physical mechanisms and their causes, the question remains, why does physical mechanism XYZ exhibit the peculiar property of consciousness, whereas physical mechanism ABC does not? And why is XYZ the substrate of *that* particular conscious state, rather than some other conscious state, or no conscious state at all? Both XYZ and the conscious state may be aspects of a more complicated scenario. Why this scenario should give rise to both XYZ and the consciousness will never be discovered if we content ourselves with noting the correlation between XYZ and the consciousness. If we say that XYZ "explains" the conscious state in question, we not only succumb to a facile "explanation by correlation," but we also obscure the most important questions about why XYZ correlates with a conscious state.

I have hinted at the direction I think such a general theory would have to take. If the theory is to withstand philosophical as well as scientific problems, then it must attack the hard problem head-on. Only a self-organizational theory of consciousness can hope to do this, because non-self-organizational theories always remain at a loss to explain why information processing is never conscious in machines that are constructed on a non-self-organizational basis. The question as to *why* brain process B should correlate with mental state M cannot be answered unless we first have a general theory that spells out the difference between conscious and non-conscious processes per se. At that point, we realize that B correlates with M, not because B is simply the cause of M, but because B plays a role in a larger self-organizing process, all of which is needed to explain why M can be mental and/or conscious. The most important lesson of the hard problem, then, is: Beware of explanation by correlation!

REFERENCES

Ahern, G. L. & Schwartz, G. E. 1985. Differential lateralization for positive and negative emotion in the human brain: EEG spectral analysis. *Neuropsychologia* **23**: 745–55.

Alexander, D. & Globus, G. 1996. Edge of chaos dynamics in recursively organized neural systems. In MacCormac, E. & Stamenov, M. (eds.) *Fractals of Brain, Fractals of Mind*. Amsterdam: John Benjamins, pp. 31–74.

Aurell, C. G. 1989. Man´s triune conscious mind. *Perceptual and Motor Skills* **68**: 747–54.

Chalmers, D. 1995. Facing up to the hard problem of consciousness. *Journal of Consciousness Studies* **2**: 200–19.

Cohen, R. M., Semple, W. E., Gross, M. *et al.* 1988. Functional localization of sustained attention. *Neuropsychiatry, Neuropsychology and Behavioral Neurology* **1**: 3–20.

Corbetta, M., Meizen, F. M., Dobmeyer, S., Schulman, G. L. & Petersen, S. E. 1990. Selective attention modulates neural processing of shape, color and velocity in humans. *Science* **248**: 1556–9.

Damasio, A. 1989. Time-locked multiregional retroactivation: a systems level proposal for the neural substrate of recall and recognition. *Cognition* **33**: 25–62.

Damasio, A. & Van Hoesen, G. W. 1983. Emotional disturbances associated with focal lesions of the limbic frontal lobe. In Heilman, K. & Satz, P. (eds) *Neuropsychology of Human Emotion*. New York: Guilford Press, pp. 85–108.

Damasio, A., Eslinger, P. J., Damasio, H., Van Hoesen G. W. & Cornell, S. 1985. Multimodal amnesic syndrome following bilateral temporal and basal forebrain damage. *Archives of Neurology* **42**: 252–9.

Ellis, R. D. 1986. *An Ontology of Consciousness*. Dordrecht: Kluwer/Martinus Nijhoff.

Ellis, R. D. 1995. *Questioning Consciousness: The Interplay of Imagery, Cognition and Emotion in the Human Brain*. Amsterdam: John Benjamins.

Ellis, R. D. 2000. Three elements of causation: biconditionality, asymmetry, and experimental manipulability. *Philosophia* **29**: 1–21.

Ellis, R. D. 2005. *Curious Emotions: Roots of Consciousness and Personality in Motivated Action*. Amsterdam: John Benjamins.

Ellis, R. D. 2007. Phenomenology-friendly neuroscience: the return to Merleau-Ponty as psychologist. *Human Studies* **29**(1): 33–55.

Ellis, R. D. & Newton, N. 1998. Three paradoxes of phenomenal consciousness: bridging the explanatory gap. *Journal of Consciousness Studies* **5**: 419–42.

Ellis, R. D. & Newton, N. 2005. The unity of consciousness: an enactivist approach. *Journal of Mind and Behavior* **26**: 255–79.

Ellis, R. D. & Newton, N. 2009. *How the Mind Uses the Brain*. Chicago: Open Court.

Flor-Henry, P., Yeudall, L. T., Koles, Z. T. & Howarth, B. G. 1979. Neuropsychological and power spectral EEG investigations of the obsessive-compulsive syndrome. *Biological Psychiatry* **14**: 119–29.

Freeman, W. 1987. Simulation of chaotic EEG patterns with a dynamic model of the olfactory system. *Biological Cybernetics* **56**: 139–50.

Gibson, J. G. & Kennedy, W. A. 1960. A clinical-EEG study in a case of obsessional neurosis. *Electroencephalography and Clinical Neurology* **12**: 198–201.

Goleman, D. 1994. *Emotional Intelligence*. New York: Bantam.

Hanze, M. & Hesse, F. 1993. Emotional influences on semantic priming. *Cognition and Emotion* **7**: 195–205.

Jackson, F. 1986. What Mary didn't know. *Journal of Philosophy* **83**: 291–5.

Jeannerod, M. 1994. The representing brain: neural correlates of motor intention and imagery. *Behavioral and Brain Sciences* **17**: 187–244.

Jeannerod, M. 1997. *The Cognitive Neuroscience of Action*. Oxford: Blackwell.

Kauffman, S. 1993. *The Origins of Order*. Oxford: Oxford University Press.

Kuhn, T. 1962. *The Structure of Scientific Revolutions*. Chicago, IL: University of Chicago Press.

Kim, J. 1993. *Supervenience and Mind: Selected Philosophical Essays*. Cambridge: Cambridge University Press.

LeDoux, J. 1996. *The Emotional Brain*. New York: Simon & Schuster.

Levine, J. 1983. Materialism and qualia; the explanatory gap. *Pacific Philosophical Quarterly* **64**: 354–61.

Libet, B., Curtis, A. G., Wright, E. W. & Pearl, D. K. 1983. Time of conscious intention to act in relation to onset of cerebral activity (readiness-potential). The unconscious initiation of a freely voluntary act. *Brain* **106**: 640.

Luria, A. R. 1980. *Higher Cortical Functions in Man*, 2nd edn. New York: Basic Books.

Mackie, J. L. 1974. *The Cement of the Universe*. Oxford: Oxford University Press.

Merleau-Ponty, M. 1941/1962. *Phenomenology of Perception*, transl. C. Smith. New York: Humanities Press.

Merleau-Ponty, M. 1942/1963. *The Structure of Behavior*. Boston, MA: Beacon.

Monod, J. 1971. *Chance and Necessity*. New York: Random House.

Nauta, W. J. 1971. The problem of the frontal lobe: a reinterpretation. *Journal of Psychiatric Research* **8**: 167–87.

Newton, N. 1982. Experience and imagery. *Southern Journal of Philosophy* **20**: 475–87.

Newton, N. 1993. The sensorimotor theory of cognition. *Pragmatics and Cognition* **1**: 267–305.

Newton, N. 1996. *Foundations of Understanding*. Amsterdam: John Benjamins.

Newton, N. 2000. Conscious emotion in a dynamic system: how I can know how I feel. In Ellis, R. & Newton, N. (eds.) *The Caldron of Consciousness: Motivation, Affect, and Self-organization*. Amsterdam: John Benjamins, pp. 91–108.

Panksepp, J. 1998. *Affective Neuroscience*. New York: Oxford University Press.

Panksepp, J. 2000. The neuro-evolutionary cusp between emotions and cognitions: implications for understanding consciousness and the emergence of a unified mind science. *Consciousness and Emotion* **1**: 17–56.

Petersen, S. E., Fox, P. T., Posner, M. I., Mintum, M. & Raichle, M. E. 1989. Positron emission tomographic studies of the processing of single words. *Journal of Cognitive Neuroscience* **1**: 153–70.

Popper, K. & Eccles, J. 1977. *The Self and Its Brain*. Berlin: Springer-Verlag.

Posner, M. I. 1980. Orienting of attention. *Quarterly Journal of Experimental Psychology* **32**: 3–25.

Posner, M. I. & Rothbart, M. K. 1992. Attentional mechanisms and conscious experience. In Milner, A. D. & Rugg, M. D. (eds.) *The Neuropsychology of Consciousness*. London: Academic Press.

Rhodes, G. & Tremewan, T. 1993. The Simon then Garfunkel effect: semantic priming, sensitivity, and the modularity of face recognition. *Cognitive Psychology* **25**: 147–87.

Sedikides, C. 1992. Mood as a determinant of attentional focus. *Cognition and Emotion* **6**: 129–48.

Segal, S. 1971. *Imagery: Current Cognitive Approaches*. New York: Academic Press.

Varela, F., Thompson, E. & Rosch, E. 1991/1993. *The Embodied Mind*. Cambridge, MA: MIT Press.

Watt, D. 1998. Affect and the `hard problem´ neurodevelopmental and cortico-limbic network issues. *Consciousness Research Abstracts: Toward a Science of Consciousness, Tucson* **1998**: 91–92.

Watt, D. 2000. The centrencephalon and thalamocortical integration: neglected contributions of periaqueductal gray. *Consciousness and Emotion* **1**: 91–114.

4

The mind–body issue

D. BIRNBACHER

MIND–BODY: WHAT IS THE PROBLEM?

The mind–body problem has been under discussion for more than 2000 years, and it is still a live issue. One might even go further and say that with the advent of the neurosciences it has become a more hotly debated issue than ever. This is explained by a simple fact. Although the mind–body problem is fundamentally a philosophical one, the progress made in solving it is to a large extent dependent on the progress of neuroscientific knowledge. The philosophical debate is essentially about how to interpret the facts in the light of undisputed or at least widely accepted criteria of rationality and coherence. But these facts are primarily provided by the neurosciences. As new facts come to light, interpretations must be reconsidered. Several of the models of the mind under discussion today can be found as early as in the dialogue *Phaedo*, in which Plato defends a substantialist conception of the mind against a number of ``materialist'' conceptions that leave no room for immortality and knowledge of eternal forms. But only the remarkable progress, since its beginnings in the eighteenth century, of empirical investigations into the working of the mind and its substrate, the brain, has provided the resources necessary for a realistic assessment of these models and for leaving behind speculation and wishful thinking. Of course, the converse is also true. Facts are uncovered against a background of hypotheses, models, and preconceptions, and these are, at least to a certain degree, thought out and elaborated by philosophers. An adequate picture of our inner nature seems to be no less the product of a continued cooperation between science and

Scientific and Philosophical Perspectives in Neuroethics, ed. J. J. Giordano & B. Gordijn. Published by Cambridge University Press. © Cambridge University Press 2010.

philosophy than an adequate picture of outer nature. In locating ``the place of mind in nature'' (the title of a pioneering work by C. D. Broad (1925)) neuroscience, psychology, and philosophy of mind have to work hand in hand.

In order to understand why the mind–body issue is one of the perennial problems of Western philosophy it is important to be clear about what is meant by the term ``mind'' (or the corresponding adjective, ``mental'') and why this concept gives rise to puzzles that so stubbornly resist resolution. What is meant by ``mind'' and the ``mental'' in talking about the mind–body issue is *consciousness*, the inner life we enjoy that is hidden from public inspection, the domain of processes, states and acts of which we know by looking into ourselves. There are good reasons to doubt that there can be an illuminating and non-circular *definition* of consciousness. Consciousness seems to be so fundamental a datum that it cannot be reduced to any other thing in the world. But the meaning of ``mind'' can at least be explained by referring to some of the familiar items of which it is made up. There are essentially two kinds of items. One is the domain of what has been called *phenomenal* consciousness, containing sensations, feelings, moods, and other passive states that come and go and last for a certain time. They are, as it were, episodes in the film that is being reeled off ``in our head'' while we are awake and, during sleep, while we are dreaming. Most types of phenomenal consciousness are such that we do not only have experience of them but are also able to *introspect* what we experience, and to *reflect* on it. However, items on which we exercise this capacity usually form only a minute fraction of the myriad of items presented by phenomenal consciousness. The vast majority of items are experienced without being given any attention. The other domain is that of *intentional* acts and states like meaning something, thinking about something, desiring something, or intending to act in a certain way. The fact that they are called ``intentional'' dates back to a medieval sense of intending, according to which intending means ``being directed at something''. Differently from items of phenomenal consciousness items of intentional consciousness have objects, either of the nature of a thing or person or of the nature of a proposition. In pointing at someone or something, I mean whatever it is I am pointing at. In saying something I usually mean the proposition expressed by what I am saying. Of course, consciousness of the phenomenal and intentional type often go together, as, for example, in emotion. Whenever I am angry about someone or about something my inner state is at once a feeling-state and a state directed at something, a thing, person, or a state of affairs.

There is another aspect of the mind–body issue that needs clarifying before we go into details.

It is often assumed, especially in popular discussions, that body and mind do not exhaust the alternatives and that there is a third realm, a realm of entities uncovered and studied by ``depth psychology´´, that is neither part of our conscious life nor part of the brain processes underlying it. In contrast to this, an autonomous realm of ``unconscious´´ or ``subconscious´´ states and processes is never mentioned in philosophical debates about the mind–body problem. This is easily explained. Philosophers who restrict their attention to the binary distinction between body and mind do by no means want to deny the phenomena uncovered by depth psychology, including unconscious beliefs, desires, and motives. They interpret the language used to refer to these states and processes, however, as oblique, and potentially misleading, ways to refer to certain physical processes in the brain, i.e. to processes closely connected with the processes that underlie our phenomenal and intentional consciousness and therefore particularly suited to explain our conscious thoughts and feelings. The unconscious is no separate realm distinct from the physical realm of brain processes. What happens in becoming aware of a formerly ``unconscious´´ item is not the unearthing of something buried mid-way between the domain of the mental and the domain of the physical but the manifestation in consciousness of something that existed before only in the realm of the physical, as a neural state, structure or process. The basic ontology presupposed in the debate about the mind–body issue is the Platonic and Cartesian ontology of two, and no more, categories of entity existing in time. They and only they are assumed to constitute the essence not only of humans but of all sentient animals.

Given these explanations, what exactly is the problem? What, in philosophy, is called a ``problem´´ is not a single but a complex of problems. The ``problem´´ is made up of a great number of individual though interdependent questions. In the following, I shall concentrate on two of these questions that have not only dominated philosophical and scientific discussions but are, I think, at the root of the wonderment motivating people to philosophize about their own nature.

The first question is the *ontological* question about the status and place of the mental in the framework of the physical universe. Is the realm of the mental a substantial and independently existing entity separate from the brain (a ``soul´´), or is it something more dependent, a property or function of the body, or of the brain? Is the existence of a brain a necessary condition of the existence of a consciousness or can there be such a thing as a free-floating, disembodied consciousness (a ``spirit´´)? How can we understand the relation between the mental and the physical? Obviously, they are closely connected, but at the same time they seem to have very different natures. Items of consciousness have a location in time but they are not part of space, at least not of the space that comprises the spatial positions of physical phenomena; they are not open to public inspection as physical phenomena are; and they have specific features, such as intentionality, indeterminacy, and vagueness, unknown in standard physical objects. More puzzles come up once we take the perspective of the scientific world-view and divide the world up into the realms of primary and secondary qualities. How do things obtain their colors, sounds, and smells, which, according to the picture drawn up by the natural sciences, are not part of their objective nature but are qualities projected onto them by the mind?

The second question, much labored in recent debate, is the question of how to interpret the *correlations* between mental and neural phenomena discovered by brain science and psychology since their beginnings. Brain research suggests that there is a high degree of co-variation between mental states and brain states. Certain mental states, e.g. perceptions of the color blue, are consistently accompanied by one or more specific kinds of brain state. In some cases these brain states are specific enough to allow a scientist to diagnose that a person is seeing or visualizing something blue on the mere inspection of his brain and in the absence of reports about his inner visual state or information about his perceptual situation. How shall we account for such correlations? A conservative and non-committal way of interpreting correlations of this kind is to say that the visual impression of blue *supervenes* on the brain process that regularly occurs in looking at the unclouded sky in daylight. ``Supervenience´´ means an unspecified relation of unilateral depend-ence. Saying that the impression blue supervenes on certain brain states is to say that the impression is an invariable concomitant of brain pro-cesses of a certain specified kind. Neuroscientific evidence suggests that such supervenience relations sometimes are many–one rather than one–one relations. Mental phenomena of the same kind can be the super-venient correlates of more than one kind of brain state. Though the supervenience relation implies that two brain states of the same kind invariably have the same counterpart (if they have any), the opposite does not hold. Two indistinguishable headaches can be the correlates of brain states of two or more different kinds.

A more far-reaching interpretation of the correlations between mental states and their neural counterparts is a *causal* interpretation beyond regular concomitance and supervenience. Though regular concomitance and supervenience are compatible with a ``parallelist´´ account such as that asserted by Leibniz´s ``pre-established harmony´´ that recognizes correlations but denies interaction, it seems that nothing short of a causal account seems adequate if we want to understand what is going on in these correlations. Only a properly causal interpretation satisfies the desire for understanding. Of course, we have to make up our minds about what causality can mean in a context where our familiar conceptions of causality are no longer applicable. After all, we enter a field lying not only outside the sphere of mechanics, from which our popular conceptions of causal interaction are derived, but outside the sphere of the physical altogether.

It does not come as a surprise that the majority view of the ontological as well as the causal question in the history of philosophy corresponds rather closely to what might be called the ``common sense view´´ that has been, and still is, dominant in popular thinking on these matters. In ontological respects, this is the view that the mind is not only a separate entity of some sort but is ontologically independent to the extent that it is in principle capable of surviving the decay of the physical brain. In causal respects, this view is interactionist. It takes it as self-evident that most if not all items of consciousness are causally dependent on brain processes and that at least some bodily processes (e.g. the movements of one´s limbs in motor action) are causally dependent on items of consciousness such as acts of will. However, present philosophical and scientific discussions of the ontological and the causal questions have taken a strikingly different turn. They are clearly anti-substantialist, and they are far from unanimous in asserting causal interaction. As in other fields, intellectuals and popular ways of thinking have parted company.

THE PROS AND CONS OF DUALISM

Dualism continues to be the most popular view of the mind–body relation in ontological respects. At the same time, it continues to be the main target of criticism and even polemics on the side of neuroscientists and philosophers of mind. In fact, ``dualism´´ often serves as a shorthand for ``substance dualism´´, and substance dualism does indeed seem a rather unpromising theory of the mental.

Substance dualism´s picture of the mental is essentially that of a kind of non-material thing (the ``soul´´), sharing typical properties of material things. It persists or even remains constant during a whole life and constitutes the identity of its bearer. It is the logical subject to which mental predicates are ascribed, just as the body is the logical subject to which physical predicates are ascribed. Anti-substantialists like Wittgenstein think that "substance" or "soul" is just a projection by which the identity and continuous existence we attribute to a human body is provided with a parallel identity and continuous existence on the mental side. But of course this presupposes that substance dualism is mistaken, which has to be shown independently.

Before discussing the reasons substance dualists give for their view, it is appropriate first to make a distinction between two versions of substance dualism. These versions have different implications and face different kinds of objections. The first view postulates a persisting soul as a transcendent substance inaccessible to conscious experience, whereas the second view postulates an identity of soul and conscious experience. According to the *transcendent* view, the soul manifests itself in conscious experience but is distinct from it. According to John Eccles, one of the recent and best known representatives of this view, the "self-conscious mind" (another name for the traditional soul) causally acts on conscious experience via its action on the brain in order to coordinate its functioning, not unlike the coordination God was supposed to perform by occasionalists like Malebranche in the seventeenth century (cf. Eccles 1978). This action, however, is effectuated without consciousness. This "self-conscious mind" is (in spite of its name) not itself conscious but has to be thought of as a kind of demon manipulating the brain in such a way that it supports or generates certain conscious acts such as thinking and reflecting. According to the *identity* view, the soul is immanent rather than transcendent. Far from being inaccessible to experience, it is supposed to be the best-known entity imaginable. After all, it is the self-same thing as conscious experience. According to Descartes, the best known representative of this view, *res cogitans* is nothing but *cogitatio* itself, conscious experience. Epistemologically, this makes a world of a difference. While the transcendent view is purely speculative, the identity view is thoroughly empirical. Nothing seems more evident than the distinctness of consciousness and the physical body.

The problem with substance dualism of both the transcendent and the immanent type is that it starts from a perfectly sound intuition and goes on to draw conclusions from it that this intuition is unable to support. The underlying intuition is the familiar one that mental and physical properties are not only *logically* distinct (i.e. mental properties cannot be logically reduced to physical properties) but also *essentially* distinct in the sense that it seems implausible to identify events that involve mental properties (such as sensations and thoughts) with events that involve physical properties (such as discharges of neurons). The mental and the physical have too little in common, it seems, to reduce their duality into unity by declaring them to be one and the same, either by identifying mental and physical properties or by identifying the events involving these properties. This duality of properties is, however, by no means sufficient to justify the conclusion drawn by substance dualists. It does not show a corresponding duality of substances. What it shows is a duality of properties and no more. A theory of property dualism is perfectly sufficient to do justice to the basic intuition of the distinctness of the mental and the physical, and at the same time is much more in line with the general principle of science and metaphysics to economize as far as possible on postulates of a purely speculative nature. This criticism applies to both versions of substance dualism alike. The postulate of a transcendent soul has no basis in experience whatsoever. All phenomena that have traditionally been adduced in favour of the possibility or reality of a disembodied soul or a transmigration of souls (a priori knowledge, déjà-vu experiences, the presence of dead ancestors in dreams, the feeling of familiarity in the presence of a beloved person, supposed memories of former incarnations) can be successfully explained by psychological mechanisms that do not presuppose an independent existence of a soul.

No less problematic is Descartes´s defence of his thesis that experience itself persists during a whole lifetime along with the body. The fact Descartes frequently refers to, i.e. the fact that it is thinkable that the mind exists independently of the body, can at most show a logical possibility. It cannot demonstrate that an independent existence of the mind is possible in the world as it really is. Furthermore, Descartes´ thesis seems to imply that conscious experience continues even during dreamless sleep, narcosis, and coma, which is unsupported by experience. It must be said in Descartes´s honor, however, that he tried to be consistent. His conviction ``l´âme pense toujours´´, that the soul always thinks (letter to Gibieuf, 19.1.1642), is the price he was prepared to pay for substantialism. But the intermittent nature of the mental, the fact that the stream of consciousness is interrupted by periods of unconsciousness, and the implausibility of assuming that consciousness starts at the same stage of early embryonic development at which the life of the human body begins, are much better accommodated by a theory of property dualism than by a theory of substance dualism. All a theory of property dualism needs to accommodate intermittence is to make the mental a property of the body alongside its physical properties. According to a weakly dualistic theory of this type the appropriate ontological category for the mental is not that of substance but that of property or function. On the other hand, property dualism meets the requirement that a substantial, independently existing bearer is to be found for the mental. That means that mind is not an independent, but a dependent form of being. It does not exist of itself, as things exist, but is tied to the existence of the physical. In brief: the mind–body relation is profoundly asymmetric. Body can in principle exist without mind, but not the other way round.

Property dualism is implicit in most conceptions of the body–mind relation discussed at present, including many that are customarily subsumed under labels that suggest otherwise, such as ``non-reductive physicalism´´ or ``identity theory´´. The various versions of the theories subsumed under this category have in common that they explicitly state or implicitly assume that mental and physical properties are distinct and that mental properties cannot be reduced to physical ones, however close their relation may be in other respects. They also have in common a number of metaphysical presuppositions implied by this view, but rarely spelled out. They share a *realistic* picture of the world according to which the existence of the physical is ontologically independent of the existence and functioning of the mental, and they share a picture of the history of the universe according to which the mental is a relatively late addition to a universe that was, for billions of years, exclusively physical. This picture is incompatible with the view of panpsychists (e.g. Spinoza) that physical properties are invariably accompanied by mental properties. On the other hand, it creates the challenge to find an explanation for the sudden appearance of consciousness at some point in the evolutionary history of animals. Though shared by the vast majority of present-day philosophers, it is well known that this view did not seem satisfactory to all observers. The Austrian physicist Erwin Schrödinger was outright appalled by a world view according to which the illumination of consciousness was switched on only in the last few seconds of the day through which the universe has passed up to now. It cannot be, he thought, that the evolution of the universe had played to empty stalls for billions of years (Schrödinger 1967, pp. 100, 146). This reaction remained, on the whole, idiosyncratic. The ontological and temporal priority of the physical has become firmly embedded in the world-view of scientists as well as philosophers. There is near unanimity that the existence of the mental is dependent on a certain degree of functional complexity of the animal brain, both in phylogenetic and ontogenetic respects.

DUALISTIC AND MONISTIC VARIANTS OF PHYSICALISM

Later generations will presumably have difficulties in understanding why ``physicalism´´ has been a label so much appreciated during the past fifty years. Various conceptions have been eager to classify themselves as oblique variants of ``physicalism´´ (like ``non-reductive physicalism´´) though they have made every effort necessary to do justice to the fundamentally dualist intuition that mental properties are irreducible to physical ones. One possible explanation is that the term ``dualism´´ had fallen so much into disrepute in certain circles that the self-interpretation as some kind of ``physicalism´´ was the only way to keep up one´s intellectual self-respect. Another is that physicalism is the secret ideal to which these conceptions aspire, and that the concessions made to dualism are seen as a burdensome heritage of tradition of which one should get rid at the earliest possible occasion.

Is physicalism such an ideal? This may well be doubted. Physicalism proper, or *reductive* physicalism, is the radical view that mental properties are identical with physical properties and that all the differences they may be thought to exhibit are only apparent. The fact that we tend to assume the irreducibility of these properties is, according to physicalists, explained by popular misconceptions (``folk psychology´´) as well as by the different kinds of language used to describe mental states and brain processes. Headaches may *seem* to be fundamentally different from C-fibre activations, but this is due to familiar but fundamentally mistaken ways of thinking and to the obvious differences in vocabulary used by psychologists and physiologists. According to physicalism, these differences conceal a fundamental identity. Once this identity is recognized it will become evident that mental states conceived as entities *sui generis* are just as mythical as witches and sorcerers and will be looked upon as equally antiquated by future and more enlightened generations. If mental states can claim any kind of existence at all, then it is only as *intentional* objects of certain ways of thinking. Existence as an intentional object is, however, a rather weak form of existence. Mental states would enjoy no other kind of existence than that enjoyed by unicorns and griffins.

Reductive physicalism is the heir of older forms of materialism and shares with them a radical simplification of the ontology of our world. By reducing the mental to the physical it overcomes the ``bifurcation of nature'' that has confused the philosophical world view since antiquity. It maximizes theoretical economy and is superior to dualist conceptions in bridging the gap between philosophy and neuroscience. These undisputed achievements, however, come with a price. The reduction of mental properties to physical properties is something only few would intuitively accept. Physicalism leaves open an ``explanatory gap'' (Levine 1983), especially with respect to the qualitative nature of phenomenal consciousness (``qualia''). One is even tempted to say that if anything is distinct from anything, then mental events like pains or thought processes are distinct from the neural processes with which they are correlated. The sense of distinctness in question here is, admittedly, pre-theoretical. But that does not mean that it can be eliminated without loss at the level of philosophical or scientific theory. On the contrary, any theory that denies the fundamental difference between mental and physical properties seems to deny an essential condition of its own intelligibility.

It does not matter, as far as the ontological assessment of reductive physicalism is concerned, whether mental properties are identified with ``simple'' physical properties like neural discharges or with the properties of whole neural circuits, networks, and systems. A theory that identifies mental properties with the properties of neural systems may be empirically preferable to others (since mental events do in fact seem to be correlated with properties of extended cortical areas rather than with events in individual neurons). Ontologically, however, such adjustments make no real difference. Even *functionalist* conceptions postulating an equivalence of mental states with physical states exemplifying a certain function are in the same boat with non-functionalist versions. They offer the same advantages in theoretical economy and suffer from the same deficiencies in adequacy. By identifying mental properties with functional properties rather than material properties, functionalist versions of physicalism allow for a considerably more generous metaphysics of the mental. Mental properties are no longer tied to the specificities of the physical universe as we know it but might be exemplified in universes of radically different kinds, provided the components of these universes realize the same patterns of functioning as neurons do in our world. Mentality, on a functionalist view, depends on software rather than hardware. Structures, functions, and programs are essential, whereas it is contingent in which kind of medium these are realized. One conclusion of this approach is that even computers or robots mimicking the neural complexity of the brain have to be ascribed mentality in a non-metaphorical sense, including sensations and feelings – in unashamed opposition to the widely held belief that ``only living creatures can literally have feelings´´ (Ziff 1959, p. 64). Of course, a functionalist view of the physical substrate of the mental can also be integrated into a dualist framework. It then assumes that the mental is causally dependent on the exemplification of certain patterns and functions in the underlying physical medium, regardless of its exact nature (cf. Chalmers 1996, part III).

Ultimately, however, physicalist functionalism shares with reductive functionalisms the essential weakness that it does not preserve the intuitive distinction between the mental and the physical and that it is unable to explain why there is an ontological mind–body problem at all. According to physicalism, this issue rests on a grandiose misunderstanding, possibly induced by our forms of speech. But even philosophers who are scientifically minded enough to have a priori sympathies for physicalism often hesitate when it comes to eliminating the mental altogether from our picture of the world.

These philosophers sometimes take recourse to one of the less radical forms of physicalism, the most wellknown of which is the *identity theory*, first proposed within the philosophy of mind by Herbert Feigl (1958) and Jack Smart (1959) but already part of the philosophy of Schopenhauer in the early nineteenth century (Schopenhauer 1819). The identity of the mental and the physical that the identity theory proposes is a *contingent* identity instead of the logical or semantic identity of reductive physicalism. Differently from reductive physicalism it maintains the logical distinctness of mental and physical properties and thus preserves the duality of languages with which we refer to mental states and to their neural correlates. This duality is as irreducible for the identity theory as for other brands of property dualism. Instead of identifying *properties* it identifies the *events* of which these properties are elements. Although the property of having a headache is different from the property of having a C-fibre activation in one´s brain, there is only one event happening, an event, however, with two very different components.

There is more than one way of defining events, and whether it is possible to distinguish between an identification of properties and an identification of events depends on what kind of definition is presupposed. If two events are the same only if all their descriptions are equivalent, then an event exemplifying one or more mental properties cannot possibly be identical with an event exemplifying one or more physical properties. In this case, the identity theory collapses into physicalism. On a more liberal definition of event, i.e. if events are defined as constellations of things, properties, and relations that can be described in more than one way (cf. Davidson 1980) the distinctness of the theories is preserved. This does not prevent us from asking, however, what the specific merits of the identity theory are, especially if compared to a theory of property dualism that simply asserts the correlation of every mental event with a neural event without identifying them (Brandt 1961, 67). The merits attributed to this theory by its adherents are essentially twofold. (1) Events are the relata of causal relations, and by identifying mental with physical events the identity theory allows for a causal role of mental events, which might seem problematic without identity. (2) By reducing the number of entities, the theory allows for greater theoretical economy. The first argument will be considered later in the context of the question of causal interaction. The second argument is certainly a point in favor of the identity theory. However, the simplification of our picture of the mind–body relation achieved by the identity theory is severely limited by the facts of multiple realization. Since many types of mental events do not seem to be correlated with just one type of physical event but with more than one, the identity theory can at best assert the identity of individual mental events with *individual* physical events (``token identity´´). Any identification of *types* of mental event with types of physical event (``type identity´´) is impossible, given multiple realization, by virtue of the transitivity of identity that prevents one event being identical with two events that are not themselves identical. It has to be doubted, therefore, whether the theoretical economy achieved by the identity theory is substantial enough to make it attractive as an alternative to reductive physicalism. It remains to be seen how it fares under the second crucial aspect of the mind–body issue, the question of causal interaction.

INTERACTION OR ONE-WAY ACTION?

The common-sense view of the causal relations between mental events and events in the human brain follows the lines of Descartes´s classical interactionism: mind acts on body, and body acts on mind. Even the way in which the areas of respective causal influence are distributed is conceived roughly along Cartesian lines: mind acts on body whenever a mental event contains an element of willing, and body acts on mind whenever we have sensations or emotions. In sensing and feeling, the mind is passive, it is ``affected´´ by the body (the sense organs, the brain, the organism as a whole), in willing and acting it is active, it ``affects´´ the body (via the brain) and is the proper author and controlling agent of our actions (outer and inner) in so far as these are voluntary and uncoerced.

This view, however familiar, raises more questions than it tends to be aware of, and I shall pick out just three of them. (1) If causal relations are at all possible in a transphysical context how do they have to be conceived? (2) How far are ``passive´´ mental events causally dependent on brain processes? (3) How far are ``active´´ mental events causally relevant to brain events? Whereas the first question is largely a challenge to philosophical analysis, the two other questions are a challenge, and an opportunity, for a coordinated effort of all contributing disciplines, including the neurosciences.

How has causality to be conceived to make it applicable to relations between physical events and mental events as well as to relations between mental events? Obviously, only a few candidates qualify. A mere regularity analysis according to which c is the cause of effect e if events of type c are regularly accompanied by events of type e will not do because this condition is fulfilled by regular successions such as that between night and day and by the various symptoms of one identical underlying cause, such as fever and spots with measles. The relation between cause and effect is stronger than the regularity view allows for. Furthermore, the regularity analysis fails to provide a framework within which to distinguish between the standard dualist positions competing in this field: interactionism (two-way interaction), epiphenomenalism (one-way action), and parallelism (no interaction). On the other hand, causal relations cannot be characterized by features inherently limited to the physical sphere, such as the transfer of energy from cause to effect. The concept of energy involved in the idea of a transfer of energy is *physical* energy, and this concept cannot coherently be applied to mental events. The only candidates that remain are two closely connected ones: a *nomological* analysis of causality that defines causal action as the instantiation of a causal law, i.e. a law of nature that meets certain further conditions such as the temporal precedence of the cause; and a *counterfactual* analysis that defines causality by the truth of certain hypothetical conditionals. According to the first analysis c is a (complete) cause of e if e invariably follows upon c, and there is a natural law to the effect that all instances of c are followed by instances of e; according to the second analysis, c is a (complete) cause of e if c is in fact followed by e and would be followed by e in all possible worlds sufficiently similar to the actual world. These analyses are closely related because at least some conceptions of what makes a natural regularity a natural law implicitly or explicitly contain the requirement of counterfactual validity. There is, however, no agreement, at the present stage of discussion, as to whether this condition is strictly necessary.

It emerges that on both analyses the conditions for interpreting a correlation between mental events and other events (physical or mental) as a causal relation are fairly stringent, and far more stringent than is assumed in the common-sense view. First, the condition that the relation between c and e must be nomological, i.e. be covered by a law of nature, does not seem to be fulfilled for quite a number of events which are commonly invoked as causes and effects of psychophysical interactions. Psychological and psychophysical laws are more often than not tendency laws with an irreducible statistical element and do not provide relations of successions in which the cause is invariably followed by the effect. Often, a great number of causal factors is involved in producing a certain sensation or emotion, and even if both common sense and neuroscience assume that what happens follows natural laws it is often impossible to actually state the laws involved in the process. Second, the standard definition of causality requires that causes are sufficient conditions of their effects, i.e. that the effect is inevitable once its cause is instantiated. This, again, is a very stringent condition. Neuroscientists and philosophers of mind agree with common sense that physical events are *necessary* causal conditions of mental events and that sensing, feeling, and thinking are impossible, at least in this world, without causal contributions from the body. No single mental event has been discovered so far that can be assumed to be causally independent from processes in the central nervous system. Even those near-death experiences that many people are tempted to interpret as harbingers of what awaits them beyond the ultimate decay of their bodies causally depend on the residual activity of their physical brains. There is disagreement, however, about whether brain processes are also causally *sufficient* to produce these mental events. Some people have great difficulties in accepting that their innermost feelings, e.g. in the domain of spirituality, are the causal products of brain processes and that it is possible to generate these feelings at will by appropriate stimulation. Paradoxically, it has proved to be a lot easier to discover the causally sufficient conditions of these apparently sublime feelings (and even to generate them by brain stimulation) than to discover the corresponding conditions of even fairly simple thoughts (cf. Persinger 1987). If there are, as most neuroscientists and some philosophers of mind assume, causally sufficient physical conditions for all individual mental events, then there should be at least as many different physical events as there are different thoughts. So far, however, it is still completely obscure how the enormous variety of contents people can make the objects of their thoughts can have sufficient conditions in brain processes specific enough to explain them one by one. While this question is still unanswered, other questions have been successfully clarified. It has become clear, for example, that not only the great majority of brain processes but even the great majority of brain processes on which our conscious life causally depends are inaccessible to consciousness. It is impossible to discover the causal precedents of our conscious experiences and acts by introspection. Another thing that has become clear is that there does not seem to be a convergence point, comparable to Descartes´s pineal gland, at which the causal lines running between mind and brain intersect. There seems to be no central node of interaction in the brain. Consciousness seems to be a field phenomenon rather than a local phenomenon. It cannot strictly be localized, but is a result of certain resonances between larger complexes of neurons, comparable to tones of a certain pitch resulting from the undulations of a string of iron.

If the assumption made by many neuroscientists that brain events are causally sufficient for mental events is true, this is of some importance for our general world view and especially for the account given of the origin of consciousness in the history of the physical universe. It implies that the physical is sufficient to generate the mental and that a further causal contribution (e.g. of something supernatural) is not called for. Although the causal sufficiency of the physical cannot rule out a supernatural influence categorically, such an influence would be redundant. It would not be needed to explain the existence and functioning of the mind.

What is problematic about the *causal action of body on mind* is that though its existence seems self-evident to nearly everyone it raises serious difficulties of verification. For a large domain of mental events (such as thoughts and beliefs) the underlying causal conditions are largely unknown. The methods of brain stimulation available at present enable a scientist to stimulate a person´s brain in such a way that he or she *visualizes* something blue, but they do not enable the scientist to stimulate the brain in such a way that the person thinks the *thought* that the sky is blue. What is problematic about *causal action of mind on body* is that though it seems no less self-evident to nearly everyone it raises even more severe difficulties. In this case, the difficulty is not one of verification but one of integration into the causal structure of the universe. For most people, it is intuitively certain that in voluntary action their thoughts and intentions causally influence their bodily movements. This is what voluntary action seems to *mean*. Of course, nobody assumes that thoughts and intentions are by themselves able to innervate the appropriate muscles. But the will, a purely mental act, is at least felt to take the initiative and to trigger a causal chain that with the help of physical factors such as the efferent nerves ultimately leads to the purely physical event of a moving limb. The arm *goes up* because it is *raised* by the person as an autonomous agent.

Besides its intuitive appeal, there is a deeper reason why mind–body interaction seems to be ineliminable. It is difficult to understand why evolution produced the mental at all if this were an ontological luxury that contributed nothing to survival. If the mental were unable to have a causal influence on the physical there would be obvious difficulties in explaining why the mind survived in nature since natural selection proceeds only via the physical sphere. The only explanation of the survival of mind that remained would be that consciousness is so closely tied up with behavioural capacities useful for survival (such as practical intelligence and behavioral flexibility) that the conscious life of higher animals is preserved through the millennia as a mere by-product.

The challenge of integrating the possibility of mental causation into the overall picture of the workings of the mind is no doubt one of the chief motivations to prefer physicalism to any version of dualism. Physicalism, indeed, has no problems whatsoever with mental caus-ation because for physicalism the sphere of the mental exists only as a language game, as a (possibly inevitable) myth generated by deeply entrenched ways of thinking about ourselves. Objectively, the mental is in all respects identical with the physical, so that mental causation is just a particular form of physical causation. This does not mean that causal action of mental events on physical events is completely without problems even for the physicalist. The difficulty remains that the physical properties into which mental properties can be ``translated´´ are often too complex to apply the laws of physics directly to the kind of events into which these properties enter. It might well be that these properties have to be decomposed into their constituent micro-properties (e.g. at the molecular level) to allow explanations via the laws of physiology. One has to admit that this is a difficulty that is in no way peculiar to physicalism but is shared by all sciences dealing with macroproperties whose functioning is more easily described by statistical regularities than by strict natural laws. However, the inability of physicalism to do justice to the facts deprives us of this easy way out of the dilemmas of mental causation.

What exactly are these dilemmas? The first dilemma is generated by the assumption, widespread among natural scientists, that the physical world is causally closed, at least at the level of the medium-sized entities relevant for mental causation (cells and molecules). Causal closure in the physical domain means that every physical event that has a (sufficient) cause has a (sufficient) physical cause. The principle of *strong* causal closure means that every physical event that has a (sufficient) cause has *only* (sufficient) physical causes. The principle of *weak* causal closure is the more generous principle that every physical event that has a (sufficient) cause has *at least one* (sufficient) physical cause, leaving open the possibility that there may be additional sufficient causes that are not purely physical but involve mental properties. It is clear why this principle causes a dilemma for any version of dualism that wants to maintain the possibility of mental causation. Whoever holds the principle of strong causal closure must deny the possibility of mental causation, and whoever holds the weaker principle can admit mental causation only as a remote and problematic possibility. Since causal closure even in its weak form implies that every physical event has a sufficient physical cause, any physical event for which there is, in addition, a sufficient mental cause is causally overdetermined, with the consequence that the mental cause is redundant. The causal nature of mental causes would be safeguarded, but at the cost of their causal irrelevance. The fact that an act of will is among the causal precedents of an innervation of the efferent nerves leading to muscle contraction would not make any difference to the innervation because its physical causes are perfectly sufficient to explain its occurrence. If causal overdetermination is a real possibility (which is controversial), mental causation is compatible at least with a principle of weak causal closure. But the redundancy of any mental cause implied even by the weak principle makes this solution of the dilemma appear unattractive.

The second dilemma is generated by another principle firmly entrenched in the scientific world view, the principle of the conservation of energy. According to this principle, changes in the physical states of neurons require some amount of physical energy. Whence does this energy come if the causes of the respective change are, as interactionists assume for the case of voluntary action, purely mental?

Furthermore, the energy content of the brain would to have to increase with every act of voluntary action unless compensated by the energy losses due to causal processes in the other direction. It is well known that Descartes, who was acutely aware of the problem, attempted to circumvent it by postulating that the effects of volition in the pineal gland (according to him the locus of interaction) consist entirely of changes in the direction and not in changes of the velocities of material particles (cf. Williams 1978, p. 281). But this was no real solution because according to the laws of mechanics even changes of direction require an impulse, i.e. a form of energy.

There are several strategies to deal with these dilemmas, and each of these has been explored in one or the other of the dualist theories discussed in recent debate. A simple way out is to call into question the universal validity of either or both of the principles of the scientific world-view generating the dilemmas, the principle of causal closure and the principle of the conservation of energy. As long as there is no independent evidence for their restricted validity from other quarters, however, these moves look too desperate to appear satisfactory. Another, no less simple way out is to accept epiphenomenalism and to assert the illusory character of mental causation. Epiphenomenalism is the view, first developed by Thomas H. Huxley (Huxley 1874), that mental properties are a by-product of neural properties and incapable of causal action. They are produced by physical conditions but are unable to react on them. This is the view favored, among others, by the present author (cf. Bieri 1992; Birnbacher 1998, 2006; Robinson 1999).

The epiphenomenologist strategy escapes the dilemmas posed by the scientific world view, but again, at a price. One of its consequences is that it makes the normal self-ascription of the ability to initiate changes in the world by conscious willing appear as one huge illusion. According to epiphenomenalism, this is in fact an illusion, even if possibly an inevitable one. A person who believes that it pushes, rather than that it is pushed, is less likely to have its will to self-assertion paralysed than a person whose beliefs were through and through fatalistic. This person will be more likely to survive in a world that sets a high premium on the ``will to power´´ in its various forms. Another implication of epiphenomenalism is the above-mentioned difficulty in explaining the maintenance of consciousness in biological evolution, first mentioned by William James (1879) and later elaborated by Karl Popper (Popper & Eccles 1977). We normally assume that it is advantageous for an organism to react to (for instance) collisions with obstacles with felt pain. Animals that react to collisions not just physically, but also mentally, are, we think, better or quicker at learning to avoid such obstacles than those that do not. For epiphenomenalists, however, consciousness has no independent survival value. It is nothing but a symptom of the possession of physical capacities that add to the survival chances of certain animals. If creatures endowed with consciousness (including humans) have been selected in the course of evolution, this is exclusively due to their corresponding superior physical capacities.

Interesting attempts have been made recently to put the causal activity of consciousness to test and to devise experimental set-ups by which a causal contribution of consciousness might be empirically validated (cf. Gray 2004, p. 114f.). The experiments carried out so far, however, are far from conclusive, mainly owing to the fact that causality is a matter of interpretation rather than of measurement. Experiments that show that persons react differently to certain situations whenever a certain stimulus has been consciously (instead of unconsciously) perceived and that, consequently, consciousness makes a difference to behavior, can nearly always be given an interpretation along epiphenomenalist lines. The epiphenomenalist can argue that according to the general framework assumption of modern dualism mental properties are supervenient upon physical properties. As a consequence, the physical conditions underlying conscious and unconscious perception are different, so that the differences in behavioral effects can with equal justification be attributed to these.

The strategy most common among dualists to integrate mental causation is to take recourse to the assumption of supervenience and to assert that mental events are causally active *via* their physical correlates, or, in the case of the identity theory, *via* the physical events with which they are identical. This assertion presupposes, of course, that the correlation in question is sufficiently strong to meet the stringent conditions of causal interaction. This requires, first, that the physical event underlying the act of will in voluntary action is of the appropriate kind to figure in a law that is needed to make the succession of events in the neural domain a genuinely causal relation. It requires, second, that the correlation of the act of will with its neural correlate is itself based on a (psychophysical) law. Only under these conditions a causal interpretation of the relation between act of will and subsequent innervation is justified. Alternatively (according to the counterfactual analysis) there must be sufficient grounds to assume that the physical effect would follow the mental cause even in the absence of irrelevant factors.

Although this strategy to overcome the dilemmas of mental causation is favored by a large variety of dualist approaches, it can be questioned whether it succeeds in giving an account of mental causation compatible with causal closure and conservation of energy. The problem is that by postulating that mental events are active via their physical counterparts this strategy seems to meet the requirements of genuine causality but sacrifices the *causal relevance* of the mental events. If the causal relations between mental causes and physical effects are construed in the way most variants of the theories of property dualism do, it seems to make no difference at all to the physical effect whether it is preceded by the respective mental event or not, because the physical correlate of the mental event is itself assumed to be causally sufficient for the effect (cf. Birnbacher 2006). Whether the mental event is interpreted as a correlate of or as identical with the physical event, in neither case is its causal efficacy dependent on its being connected with a mental event. We are again faced with a diagnosis of redundancy. A mental event whose causal efficacy is mediated by a physical event that is itself sufficient to produce the effect is strictly redundant even in cases in which it is true to say that the physical event would not have occurred unless the mental event had occurred.

WHENCE CONSCIOUSNESS?

A metaphysically deep question that is left open by nearly all present discussions of the relations between mind and body is why there is a thing like consciousness in the physical universe at all. Perhaps the fact that it is so rarely asked can be explained by the feeling that this question is fruitless, if not downright meaningless. But it is certainly a question that cannot be left aside. It arises naturally from the naturalistic framework of present-day analysis of the mind–body issue and constitutes a problem for any account that postulates an inherent duality of body and mind, independently of whether consciousness is assigned a function (as in interactionism) or whether it is regarded as a by-product (as in epiphenomenalism). Natural selection by itself cannot explain the advent of consciousness. It can at most explain why it has been preserved during evolution from the time when it first emerged. The most plausible account is certainly that the mental did not arise by chance but by nomological necessity so that, given the existence of psychophysical natural laws, it was inevitable that consciousness made its appearance as soon as biological evolution had progressed so far as to produce the complex neural networks to be found in the brains of higher animals. The difficulty is to understand that a chance mutation should have been sufficient to produce something like sensations and thoughts that seem to belong to a category of being so radically different from everything within the world of physics. At this point we seem to arrive at one of the limits set to human understanding. We do not seem to be able, from the narrow human perspective, to understand the origin (and, possibly, the function) of the mental in its totality. This is the meaning of the famous ``Ignorabimus´´ that one of the pioneers of neurophysiology, Emil Du Bois-Reymond, proclaimed in his lecture on the limits of natural philosophy in 1872 (Du Bois-Reymond 1974, 65). Even if the relations between mental and physical events were as transparent to human knowledge as we could possibly wish, the higher-order question as to why there is such a relation at all would still be without an answer.

REFERENCES

Bieri, P. 1992. Trying out epiphenomenalism. *Erkenntnis* **36**: 283–309.
Birnbacher, D. 1998. Epiphenomenalism as a solution to the ontological mind-body problem. *Ratio* (n.s.) **1**: 17–32.
Birnbacher, D. 2006. Causal interpretations of correlations between neural and conscious events. *Journal of Consciousness Studies* **13**: 115–28.
Brandt, R. 1961. Doubts about the identity theory. In S. Hook (ed.) *Dimensions of Mind*. New York: New York University Press, pp. 33–44.
Broad, C. D. 1925. *The Mind and Its Place in Nature*. London: Routledge & Kegan Paul.
Chalmers, D. J. 1996. *The Conscious Mind: In Search of a Fundamental Theory*. Oxford: Oxford University Press.
Davidson, D. 1980. The individuation of events. In Davidson, D. *Essays on Actions and Events*. Oxford: Clarendon Press, pp. 163–180.
Du Bois-Reymond, E. 1974. Über die Grenzen der Naturerkenntnis. In Du Bois-Reymond, E. (ed.) *Vorträge über Philosophie und Gesellschaft*. Hamburg: Meiner, pp. 54–78.
Eccles, J. C. 1978. *The Human Mystery*. New York: Springer.
Feigl, H. 1958. The ``Mental´´ and the ``Physical´´. In Feigl, H. *et al.* (eds.) *Concepts, Theories ,and the Mind-Body Problem*. Minneapolis: University of Minnesota Press, pp. 370–497.
Gray, J. 2004. *Consciousness: Creeping up on the Hard Problem*. Oxford: Oxford University Press.
Huxley, T. H. 1874. *On the Hypothesis that Animals are Automata and its History*. London: Macmillan.
James, W. 1879. Are we automata? *Mind* **4**: 1–22.
Levine, J. 1983. Materialism and qualia: the explanatory gap. *Pacific Philosophical Quarterly* **64**: 354–61.
Persinger, M. A. 1987. *Neuropsychological Bases of God Beliefs*. New York: Praeger.
Popper, K. R. & Eccles, J. C. 1977. *The Self and its Brain. An Argument for Interactionism*. London/New York: Springer.

Robinson, W. S. 1999. ``Epiphenomenalism´´. Article in *Stanford Encyclopedia of Philosophy*, archive edition of March 31, 1999. Available at http://plato.stanford.edu/entries/epiphenomenalism.

Schopenhauer, A. 1819. *Die Welt als Wille und Vorstellung*. Leipzig: Brockhaus.

Schrödinger, E. 1967. Mind and matter. In Schrödinger, E. (ed.) *What is Life?/Mind and Matter*. Cambridge: Cambridge University Press, pp. 99–178.

Smart, J. J. C. 1959. Sensations and brain processes. *Philosophical Review* **68**: 141–56.

Williams, B. 1978. *Descartes. The Project of Pure Enquiry*. Harmondsworth: Penguin.

Ziff, P. 1959. The feelings of robots. *Analysis* **19**: 64–8.

5

Personal identity and the nature of the self

P. COSTA

We all of us, grave or light, get our thoughts entangled in metaphors, and act fatally on the strength of them.

G. Eliot, *Middlemarch*

What is a person? What is the self? These are tough questions, indeed. They are so tricky that it is difficult even to imagine what answering them would look like. A person, a self, is not something in the objective world that we could point our finger at. Look at that: a self! That sounds queer. We need a theory of the self – and a very special theory, too – in order to speak about something that lies exactly on the border between inner and outer, value and fact, subjective and objective. As selves, we make acquaintance with the interface between different logical spaces and we come out of this experience baffled. As Augustine used to say about time, we do not have trouble with such familiar notions until someone prompts us to make explicit sense of them. Then, we get stuck in a tangle of doubts. I know that I am a self. (I am myself! My very language is compelling me to admit it.) But I do not know much more about it. Well, of course, I understand that it is me the person who is writing the first tortuous lines of a chapter that will force me to come out into the open and take sides on subject matters that put our intellectual faculties to a hard test. Somewhere in the back of my mind I know that *I* am committing myself to something and that I shall be held accountable for it. But who is that me? How long will it exist? What is its consistency? And where exactly is it? Maybe, I am deluding myself. But, then, how revisionary could or should a different view of my Self be?

Scientific and Philosophical Perspectives in Neuroethics, ed. J. J. Giordano & B. Gordijn. Published by Cambridge University Press. © Cambridge University Press 2010.

117

As Paul Ricoeur once said, ``la question de l´identité constitue un lieu privilégié d´apories´´ (Ricoeur 1990, p. 161). Moreover, it is the ideal field for those philosophical gigantomachies which have been characteristic of our Western intellectual tradition since the very beginning. The clash between Parmenides and Heraclitus jumps to mind, here, as the model of all the following discussions. What really changes and what remains the same in our ordinary experience of reality? Is it actually all a matter of an eternal and changeless Being or, vice versa, of an erratic Becoming? We do not have any clear or compelling answer to such basic questions, let alone the legendary knock-down arguments for which philosophers of every age have searched in vain.

As a matter of fact, personal identity is something that cannot be fixed or pinpointed, and still enjoys a somewhat paradoxical existence. It is a sort of sameness without substance or, to quote Ricoeur again, an ``ipseité´´ – a capacity more than an actuality: the ability to commit oneself and carry out one´s commitments (Larmore 2004). But, although the self does not have the sturdy and dense consistency of a medium-sized physical object, its dynamical and relational nature will not necessarily end up in a myriad of unrelated avatars. Its dynamism turns on a virtual hinge, which is the locus of a personal appropriation that makes it reasonable to say ``mine!´´, as when we convincingly claim that ``this is my body´´ or ``this is my view´´. Accordingly, the self consists in a reflexive practical relationship which is not suspended in the void, but takes place within a space of impersonal reasons, a pre-existing horizon of meaning, an idiosyncratic emotional universe, a web of stories, and a host of meaningful relationships. Hence, an internal, although vague, bond (with its own ``inner alterity´´) can become the source of an interminable ``work of reflexive reappropriation´´ (Gauchet 2004, p. 254).

In the following, I shall try to explore, against this general theoretical background, the historical roots of contemporary anxieties over the impact that the novel neurotechnologies and the new, rapidly accumulating scientific knowledge of the brain may have on our sense of self. My conclusion will be that the allegedly novel situation is not so novel, after all, and that, in fact, we are still moving along a track opened long ago by early-modern transformations in Western culture. This, of course, does not mean that we are not going to face serious problems, but only that we already have the intellectual resources to cope with them effectively (in so far as we consider them to be manageable issues). In the end, neuroethical dilemmas will turn out to be another variety of modern metaphysical and moral quandaries.

THE MODERN PREDICAMENT

While the topic of identity has traditionally been a source of endless metaphysical perplexities, personal identity can be seen as the modern problem *par excellence*. This is not due to purely conceptual reasons, but stems from deeper and more tangible social, religious, and economic changes. The modern emphasis upon the individual, its rights, powers, and freedoms, is contingent upon a new view of subjectivity – not only *personal* subjectivity – that set the stage for a radicalization of the common and understandable concern for one's own fate (Gauchet 2004, chapter 9). What is really salient about the reflective stance of almost all modern thinkers is that it first of all embodies a creative reaction to the early modern shift of attitude towards order and disorder, finitude and infinity, shape and shapelessness, substance and function, stability and variety, normality and pathology (Costa 2007, pp. 22–7). The disruption of boundaries and the parallel disclosure of new possibilities, which are a distinctive feature of modern culture, brought about, on the ``subjective'' side of experience, a vibrant relation between different and, until then, unsuspected parts of the inner life. As a result, the modern self emerged from the world picture's shifting balance more as a locus of conflict than as a harmonious ``pack'' (Seigel 2005).

In fact, identity matters in the modern age mainly because of its precarious and elusive status. Few things count as much as it does. Not accidentally, the hero of the modern novel is usually engaged in a quest for self, even though his or her life is the most ordinary one. Authenticity, even more than sincerity, is the key word of the age (Trilling 1972). A strong need is felt, for the first time in history, to be one and the same with one's inmost thoughts. A feeling of disembeddedment and out-of-balanceness is the emotional counterpart of the disclosure of an alterity within the self which sets the modern search in motion and, at the same time, makes it interminable. This is the reason why Parfit's renowned dictum – ``personal identity is not what matters'' (Parfit 1987, p. 245) – still causes sensation and, at first, strikes the reader's eye as a pun or a witticism. How can personal identity be irrelevant in our lives? What else counts, if it does not? And how can it be so, if almost all the social practices we are engaged in turn on the apparently simple fact that we are separate, autonomous and responsible beings – ``centers of action and consciousness'' (Seigel 2005, p. 5)? As a matter of fact, this kind of sweeping rejection of the modern quest for self actually looks more like a rejoinder to the modern obsession with self, rather than a genuine intellectual move: just another of the innumerable modern attempts (clothed in scientific garb) to ``épater le bourgeois'', by stating a totally counter intuitive thesis. Thus, ironically, Parfit's claim sounds to most of his readers like an invitation to get rid of a cumbersome sense of self in order to live a fuller personal life, rather than as a real refutation of the modern search for authenticity. It's Buddha dressed in Marcel Duchamp's or Andy Warhol's robes, as it were. What really matters now is not identity *per se*, but the *metamorphoses* of identity.[1]

All this, of course, does not mean that Parfit's subtle philosophical arguments against any substantive or Non-Reductionist view of personal identity are unwarranted or have no point at all. Whatever our opinion of the reliability of his account of our self-experience (see Ricoeur 1990, chapter 6) may be, Parfit's theoretical efforts draw the last consequences of the modern scenario by sketching a detailed picture of the difficulties which any view of personal identity that makes it a matter of all-or-nothing finally runs into. The acknowledgment that ``a person never coincides with his qualities'' – that ``we always possess an `inner difference' from the way we are at any given moment'' (Larmore 1998, p. 459) – can be seen as one of the most significant outcomes of modern attempts to come to terms with the question of selfhood. Once we accept this view, the self may actually begin to appear as a vanishing point, a sort of placeless place, even a ``mystery'' or a paradox. But, in fact, it is so only if we buy into a very narrow view of reality and suppose that, in order to be real, the self must be ``a separate entity standing behind its qualities, enjoying some independent, quality-less, `transcendental' existence'' (Larmore 1998, p. 459). Yet, this is not the case at all.

One of the most striking philosophical ambiguities of the Scientific World View, which dominates the contemporary intellectual landscape under a naturalistic disguise, comes from a failure to do

---

[1] See Parfit 1987, pp. 281–2 and Nietzsche's quotation (*Gay Science*, §343: *The Meaning of our Cheerfulness*) used as the epigraph for his book: ``At last the horizon appears free to us again, even granted that it is not bright; at last our ships may venture out again, venture out to face any danger; all the daring of the lover of knowledge is permitted again; the sea, *our sea*, lies open again; perhaps there has never yet been such an `open sea''' (significantly, Nietzsche is talking here about the sense of relief and exhilaration provided by the news that ``the old god is dead''). As to the fact that demoting the self can serve to affirm ``a mode of self-existence far more powerful and unrestricted than the one it sets out to dismiss (. . .) *a vision of transcendent freedom*'', see Seigel 2005, pp. 4–5 (italics mine).

justice to both the first-person and the third-person access to our worldly experience (Nagel 1986, chapter 1). Since we have an inner life and we enjoy a vision of reality from within, a truly "comprehensive" view should also be fair to this additional dimension of our thinking life by making something of it. This is the most salient lesson to be drawn from the Scientific Revolution and the one that better matches the twofold attitude of modern science: its anti-metaphysical, empiricist stance (along with common sense) and its fiercely revisionist bent (Costa 2007, pp. 191–203). But, of course, in the Modern Age, there has always been a deeply entrenched temptation to unilaterally emphasize the objectifying power of the scientific gaze. After all, it is exactly in virtue of the ability to reach this detached stance towards reality that modern science has managed to yield a knowledge of "out-of-order" things, rising far above our ability to directly experience them and, sometimes, also to make sense of them. This capacity to achieve an Archimedean point, which soars well beyond our common life-experience, rests, however, on a blind spot. For, in order to grasp the world objectively, the knowing subject must, as it were, leave the scene, disappear, fade into an unconditioned standpoint. As a result, it withdraws into the kingdom of truth (or thought, normativity, reason, spontaneity, freedom, value, purpose, beauty) – things that apparently cannot be fitted into the deterministic realm of scientific laws. But, then, what is the ontological status of this "ideal" space? What kind of relations does it entertain with the natural world? And, since the knowing subject is, of course, a "subject," what is the link between this thinking "I" and the real, finite selves that we are? And, last but not least, who is competent enough to answer such tough questions? Can we scientifically know the very source of our scientific knowledge?

These are the sort of conundrums that neuroscientists are also bound to come across on their way towards an objective knowledge of the brain, to the extent that the latter is understood as the site of consciousness, knowledge, and personal identity (Chalmers 1996; Searle 2007). As far as the self is concerned, an interesting ambivalence can be detected in modern science. For, while it discloses the possibility of reflecting on the self's peculiar nature by seeing it as a gap, a "crevice", an activity, rather than a separate substance, the new outlook is simultaneously at considerable pains to include it in its own ontological and epistemological framework. This is not necessarily a bad thing. Acknowledging a theoretical ambivalence can be fruitful, when it does not immediately lead to, or end in a claim of mystery. And, plainly, the self cannot be a mystery, because it is one of the most familiar things, if not the most familiar thing in the world. (Although, of course, it can be turned into a mystery once its conditions of intelligibility are not fully respected.) Yet, the riddle remains: how can we at least approximately figure out the conditions of intelligibility of personal identity?

THE SELF: EMBODIMENT, ARTICULACY, AND COMMITMENT

As a provisional definition, we can characterize personal identity as a (basically) mental phenomenon hanging on a web of relations, rather than on a substantial sameness. This relative lack of consistency (or non-coincidence with self) must not be understood as a sort of negative identity, but as a preliminary condition for self-relatedness. Otherwise put, the self's inner alterity is the source of an articulating activity and a pursuit of cohesion which primarily realizes itself through the undertaking of a chain of commitments that are both objectively and personally binding.

What view of the self can underpin such an intricate notion of personal identity? Clearly, a detailed account of the nature of the self cannot be given here (and perhaps nowhere else), but it can be useful at least to try to sketch out in rough lines the basic features of a plausible view of selfhood. If we agree that a convincing theory of self must do justice both to the core elements of our first-order self-understanding and to the relevant objective pieces of information about our ``inner´´ (and hidden) life which are increasingly supplied by the various natural sciences,[2] it seems reasonable to start off from the assumption that the self is a multi-dimensional rather than one-dimensional reality, and a dynamic rather than a static one – in other words, a matter of relatedness more than of substance. Things being so, we might usefully describe the self as a field of relations with a predominant centre of gravity that enable his or her bearer to say justifiably (even though not always correctly) ``mine´´. This justifiable appropriation claim comes out of three different facts about the self. First, it derives from its embodiment in a lived body (*le corps propre*), which is a center of action and signification (Merleau-Ponty 1945), and not merely an inert thing devoid of any kind of inwardness (or subjective standpoint). Secondly,

---

[2] This is especially true for the activity of one of the phenomenologically most secret organs of all: the brain. See Ricoeur (1990, p. 159), who speaks of an ``intériorité non vécue´´ (non-lived inwardness).

it rests on a tendency toward psychological cohesion which is contingent on the need for an experiential and practical unity that is part and parcel of being a self, in so far as it is a *living being's* self and hence a center of experience and action that we are talking about. After all, the kind of selves we are acquainted with must all lead a life and their beliefs, perceptions, emotions, are causally and intentionally related to *a* world that, although multilayered, amounts, in the end, to a unified field (Wollheim 1984). We can rightly see, then, the mental or psychological self as an *articulated whole*. "Articulated" means, here, heterogeneous, but not dissociated. The self is by and large a field of contrasts, but it cannot be the site of a war of all against all. Beliefs, emotions, and perceptions are different and sometimes conflicting forms of articulacy that belong, however, to an unitary space: the mental space of the self. (We could also call it character or personality.) When this arrangement of conflicting cooperation oversteps its "physiological" or, better, constitutive limits, the self is bound to crumble.

Thirdly and finally, the self chiefly actualizes itself in a reflective relationship, i.e. in taking a distance from its own determinations and standing back, at least ideally and temporarily, from the very centre of gravity of its existence (Taylor 1976). This act of self-distancing, however, does not occur in the void and is not prompted by a purely cognitive concern, but it is aimed at a series of commitments that only the self can undertake. Thus, the enduring self makes its appearance as it takes a stand in light of external grounds or reasons that it manages to make its own by responding to their "normative" force. There is no room here for a solipsistic or voluntaristic self-creation *ex nihilo*. We become fully fledged agents, first and foremost, by taking upon ourselves the normative implications of our own beliefs and desires. We do not discover or "make" our identity in a detached attitude, but we practically experience it through a series of personal resolutions or "attestations" (Ricoeur 1990), as when we reflectively comply with our mental contents. Reflexivity is therefore a special kind of intimacy with self (*présence à soi*) – a practical one. This amounts to saying that we do not necessarily know ourselves very well, but we cannot help but bear a responsibility for self in the broad sense that only we can undertake (or endure) the normative commitments which more or less robustly shape our personhood. This feat involves a reflexive (i.e. self-distancing or de-centering) relationship, although not always an overtly reflective one.[3]

---

[3] On the distinction between "reflectivity" (voluntary) and "reflexivity" (preconscious), see Seigel (2005, pp. 12–13).

As Charles Larmore (2006, p. 41) has aptly noted, ``reflection is essentially problem-oriented, driven by the need to straighten out the conflicts that have disrupted the ordinary course of our lives´´ and, for that reason, it cannot ``stand back from experience as a whole´´ (see also Larmore 2004, pp. 120, 214). In other words, the reflecting self manages to solve specific dissonances by activating a basic and standing capacity to take a distance from its mental contents and to focus on them. In this sense, an act of explicit reflection always implies an original self-relatedness, i.e. the subject´s non-coincidence with self (which does not mean self-estrangement). To quote Larmore again: ``There is an essential `care of the self´ (*souci de soi*) in the self (*moi*), that reflection does nothing but develop explicitly´´ (Larmore 2004, p. 184).

In a way, the reflective stance consists of actualizing a potentiality that is implicit in every acting being and finds its most peculiar expression in humans. We could call it the urge to self-reliance or self-determination. This must be meant in a very minimal sense, namely that it is up to the self to live its own life. Nobody can live it in its stead. While it might sound like a truism, this is a fact which is full of consequences, since, for an agent, living means essentially to commit oneself and, therefore, to have (more or less conscious or explicit) access to the space of reasons and grounds, i.e. to normativity. This reasons-disclosing capability is multiform and multilevelled. It does not necessarily need to be self-conscious or linguistically articulated, and so it should be better understood as a kind of positioning against a pre-given ``proto-normative´´ horizon which also serves as an enabling condition for triggering – already at the level of the lived body (Wrathall 2005) – the self-relation in which a person is essentially engaged. To the extent that some of the necessary preconditions for legitimately saying ``mine´´ are not a personal possession at all, the self is never independent or autonomous, but structurally open and relational. This is one of the main reasons why emotions are such a crucial element in personal identity, for they embody – at a both physical and mental level – our natural propensity to take a stand and judge the world in relation to our well-being, by distinguishing significant and non-significant aspects of reality and establishing a precarious balancing point between the inner and the outer world (Nussbaum 2001).

If the self is to be firstly understood as the dynamical product of a related series of acts of positioning against a space of motives and reasons, which ought to be seen not as a Platonic world of ideas, but as a web of normative relations that enjoys only a relative independence – and no separate existence – from the physical reality, then it clearly cannot be described as a self-enclosed entity amenable to a purely external account. The self is not an entity, but a process that Jerrold Seigel (2005, p. 31) has fittingly portrayed as ``a self-in-formation, living in the space between what it has been able to become and what it or others think it might be´´. Things being so, the self cannot be reduced to a matter of all-or-nothing. Different varieties of the self and different levels and degrees of personal identity – more or less fulfilled, more or less damaged or impaired, more or less vigorous – can be detected, even though there is no room left here for the idea of an archetypical identity. Not accidentally, the thread of an individual's life is mainly woven out of a puzzling and deeply disturbing question: ``*Who* am I?´´ (Wollheim 1980).

WHAT WE REALLY HAVE TO FEAR

But what kind of relevance do the preceding considerations have to the general topic discussed in this book? Is our sense of self really threatened by emerging neuroscientific developments?

To begin with, and as a corollary of what has been argued before, we are at least entitled to cultivate the idea that our accounts of the self as a mental phenomenon cannot be reduced below a basic level of complexity. Otherwise put, in order to get a minimal grip on this most peculiar entity, we cannot explain away the first-person order of experience where the lived body, the connectedness of mental life and the responsive activity of committing oneself find their common ground. The same idea can also be couched in slightly different terms, by resorting to an old label: ``saving the phenomena´´ (Costa 2005, section 2). Let me try to elucidate why and how.

If, as W. V. O. Quine (1966, p. 220) once remarked, ``science itself is a continuation of common sense´´, the same might be said of philosophy which has been struggling, as much as science, to come to terms with *sensus communis* since its origins. And exactly because they have been sharing a common field of interest, a struggle for hegemony could arise. As a result, the risk has always been that rivalry might degenerate into a zero sum game, whose inevitable upshot would be either a complete ``naturalization´´ of philosophy or the subjection of science to the transcendental authority of *philosophia prima*. But, fortunately, this is not the only game in town. For we may substantially agree with the empiricist critique of the transcendental claims of philosophical foundationalism – of the inane ambition to preliminarily delimit the spheres of competence of the various kinds of knowledge through conceptual analysis or epistemological foundation – without thereby a priori denying the possibility of having a fruitful cooperation or ``dialectic'' between science and philosophy. And precisely in order to clarify this aim, we may turn to the old catchphrase ``*sozein ta phenomena*''.

In some essays that go back to the 1970s, Charles Taylor (1971, 1973) has convincingly argued for a ``peaceful coexistence'' among the different scientific approaches to reality – especially human reality. According to him, any mechanistic (i.e. merely physiological) explanation of human behavior has to satisfy some basic (empirical) conditions of significance or intelligibility, which demands that the theory ``be rich enough to incorporate the basis of a very wide range of distinctions which, at present, mark the intentional world of human agents and which are essential to understand their behaviour'' (Taylor 1971, p. 177). In other words, the usual revisionary attitude of natural scientists should not go so far as to do away with the phenomenon they purport to make sense of scientifically. Bernard Williams (1995, p. 85) has pithily summarized this basic requirement, claiming that ``no science can eliminate what has to exist if there is to be anything for it to explain''.

This is how we should understand the updated meaning of the old adage ``saving the phenomena'', where the emphasis ought to fall on the noun rather than on the verb. The saying does not entail any request to lay a priori external constraints on scientific inquiry, but only hints at an ideal boundary, beyond which any scientific approach runs the serious risk of losing contact with its object. Acknowledging this restriction does not rule out the possibility that a systematic coordination may occur between mechanistic explanations and the ``phenomenological'' understanding of the investigated objects, states or events, in the long run. Taylor (1971, p. 182) dubbed this long-term scenario ``the convergence hypothesis'', whereby he proposed to replace the picture of a scientific explanation, which is successful only when it manages to systematically reduce complex phenomena to their basic elements and linear causal links, with the circular image of a plurality of approaches to reality that are mutually clarifying and variously coordinated (high–low, low–high, high–high, low–low), fostering feedback relations among the different explanatory levels (Midgley 1994). As a matter of fact, it would be an oddly unscientific policy to unconditionally support an investigative method which should stubbornly favor an explanatory strategy that, just because it proved successful before, would be entitled to deny the very existence of the *explanandum* once it turns out to be fruitless or meets obstacles that it is unable to overcome by itself.

Clearly, the requirement of compatibility sketched above does not always and in any case support the common sense explanations. It only draws attention to the fact that no revisionary explanation can ever go so far as to deny *in toto* the shape of our experience and the very logic of the terms that we use to make sense of it (getting wholly rid, for instance, of the intentional vocabulary with which we describe and understand our actions).[4] It is right to conclude, therefore, that even the most radical revisions of our experience must remain within the ``appearances´´ in an incessant adjustment play where the objectifying stance can never wholly dispose of the subjective standpoint. To this extent, reality can be scientifically explained without dismantling or systematically disavowing our first-person understanding of it. Which means, otherwise put, that we have to somehow come to terms with those inescapable features of our common sense experience which are essential preconditions also for the most revisionary theory of our mental life. To save the phenomena amounts, hence, to explaining them *fully*, avoiding the risk of being stripped, sooner or later, of the very foundation of our thought (Stroud 1996, p. 27–8). The end goal is to reach a sort of reflective equilibrium between the competences acquired through our ongoing engagement with reality and what we manage to learn by means of a far more detached stance toward it.

In this sense, the plea to save the phenomena works as an antidote against too quick a closing of explanations, especially when the latter is surreptitiously furthered by some tacit ``metaphysical´´ assumptions (Taylor 1971, p. 186). The principle of simplicity or parsimony is thus supplemented by that of preserving a basic and irreducible level of phenomenological complexity. This requirement, however, does not operate in the name of an abstraction – ``complexity´´ – but in the name of the selfsame experience, the variety of its articulations and the conditions of its intelligibility and recognizability. Hence, it would be more appropriate to speak of an empirical standard of significance, rather than of a transcendental veto. What I am gesturing to, here, is the idea of a condition of intelligibility that must be continually brought back to the very fact of the matter. In other words, the reassessment of our self and world experience may come about only through an ongoing refinement and readjustment of the appearances and of their

---

[4] See Taylor (1971, pp. 169, 170, 175, 177), where the idea ``that we have been talking nonsense all these millennia´´ is rejected as ``too much to swallow´´.

relationship of mutual confirmation, and not by way of a sudden and systematic replacement of one global standpoint with another.

What we need, therefore, is a suitable understanding of our common sense experience that does not sacrifice its richness of detail for the sake of a narrow view of scientific knowledge or of an abstract and one-dimensional method of enquiry (or, worse, of non-generalizable historical analogies, which gradually turn into conditioned reflexes).[5] In order to do this, we first have to underline the significance and oddness of the simple fact that we experience a reality that discloses itself to our senses and is accessible to our understanding (Chalmers 1996, p. xi). Being aware of how complex is the riddle that lies behind the sheer "presence" of the world (Olafson 1995) is the first step toward recognizing the need to save the appearances (Nussbaum 1986, chapter 8). It is thus crucial that this awareness not be impoverished, let alone eliminated, in and by the scientific investigation which, on the contrary, can greatly contribute to its elucidation.

This is the challenge lurking in the anything but quietist idea of a convergence among different ways of investigating reality in the name of a neither aprioristic nor stubborn defence of "appearances". According to this view, different scientific approaches can and ought to be applied in our study of human beings, but they have to give up any more or less explicit imperialistic claim, and never stop to correlate and coordinate themselves with our shared world experience. The radical simplifications of revisionary theories also turn out to be enormously valuable within this horizon, provided that – in the wake of their triumphs – they do not give in to the "greedy" (Dennett 1995, p. 92) temptation to go too quickly to the bottom of the phenomenon they are trying to explain.

Against the background of this non-imperialistic, fallibilistic, truly empiricist attitude, a non-naive version of phenomenological realism looms up. One of its sources is no less than Aristotle, whose renowned definition of reality – "what appears (*dokei*) to all, this we call Being" (*Nicomachean Ethics*, 1172b36) – looks still admirable as far as

---

[5] See Taylor (1971, pp. 180–1): "The fact is that many of the great paradigms of scientific progress can be used to teach more than one lesson. Does the revolution in physics in seventeenth-century tell in favour of mechanism because it was mechanist, or does it show rather how the hold of a powerful traditional conceptual scheme (Aristotelian in the seventeenth-century; mechanist in ours) on the scientific community can impede progress? We shall have to await the outcome of present disputes to see who has been cast in the role of Galileo and who in that of his obtuse Aristotelian critics".

concision is concerned. Such a non-emphatic realism tries to reconcile the subjective and objective dimensions of experience, reminiscent of the fact that, as Thomas Nagel aptly noted, an inflated claim to objectivity always runs the risk of turning over into an extreme form of idealism. After all, to quote Taylor (1989, p. 57) once again, "what better measure of reality do we have in human affairs than those terms which on critical reflection and after correction of the errors we can detect make the best sense of our lives"?

In this sense, even our boldest efforts to understand the "nature" of the self cannot go beyond the limits of intelligibility, which underlie the rule of "saving the phenomena". We simply cannot jump outside the relational field that makes the self both possible and actual. But, then, does this mean that future neuroscientific discoveries cannot possibly undermine our phenomenological sense of self? Have we no reason to be concerned at all?

This would seem odd at a first glance. It reminds us of a well-known paradox conjured up by Michael Walzer (1990) at the height of the Liberal–Communitarian Debate. Why bother about the liberal unencumbered self? "If the sociological argument of liberal theory is right, if society is actually decomposed without residue, into the problematic coexistence of individuals, then we might well assume that liberal politics is the best way to deal with the problems of decomposition. ... If we really are a community of strangers, how can we do anything else but put justice first?" (Walzer 1990, p. 146). But, on the contrary, if the communitarian portrait of human beings is correct, "how are we to understand this extraordinary disjunction between communal experience and liberal ideology, between personal conviction and public rhetoric, and between social bondedness and political isolation?" (Walzer 1990, p. 147). Either we are unencumbered selves – then we can do nothing to promote our favorite view of the social life – or we are "thick" selves – then we have nothing to worry about. (In its general lines, of course, this kind of argument goes back at least to Epicurus' consoling thoughts about the fear of death.)

But, of course, we would be very surprised if this kind of argument worked. Much more is needed in order to exorcize such long-standing anxieties over the consistency of what we most care about – ourselves. In particular, we need a reliable view of what exactly is at stake here. And this demands something more than a quick rejoinder or a witty remark. Besides, modernity is by definition a culture of crisis. Out-of-balanceness is its natural condition. The modern individual is at her best when she finds herself in a precariously balanced situation (the above mentioned ``crisis'') where she is required to exercise a faculty of judgment relieved from the weight of tradition and is free to figure out and endorse her own standards of evaluation (``critique''). After all, it is the future – something indeterminate, which is not yet – that a restless identity, such as the modern one, is oriented to, while seeking to shape itself into the desired mold. Things being so, it does seem hopeless to aim at a perfectly stable condition.

Yet, modern men cannot feed only on restlessness. There actually are specifically modern antidotes to modern anxieties. One has only to think of influential new ideas such as progress, autonomy, or self-determination. These are powerful ideals that served and still serve today as orienting and motivating forces for a lot of people. Manipulation – especially self-manipulation and self-control – is obviously another of these powerful ideals. It is hard to picture something more reassuring and empowering than the thought that we are able to put reality in perspective, take an objectifying stand towards it and manipulate it in order to control it better. And what when the manipulable thing is your main subject of concern? What when it is your very self that you are promised to be able to control and manipulate? That sounds exhilarating, indeed. But exactly therein is the problem and the main danger of the present situation. First of all, because manipulating and controlling is not the same as knowing what we are manipulating or controlling. For we can control the enabling conditions of a phenomenon without ever knowing what the phenomenon really is and how worthy it is. Thus, when someone such as M. J. Farah (2005, p. 38) rhetorically asks: ``Is there anything about people that is not a feature of their bodies?'', she is actually raising two different questions. (1) Is there anything in our mental and physical life that does not entail a form of embodiment? (The answer to this question is very probably no.) And (2) do we know everything or enough about a phenomenon when we have learnt how to manipulate it or control it? (The most probable answer to this question is another ringing no.) After all, we can also manipulate a person's identity by preventing her from making a full use of her lived body or by concealing or revealing a crucial piece of information about her personal history (let us think only of an adopted child who lately comes to discover her true origins). We do not need to mess up or tinker with her brain. To the extent that it is an activity based upon a web of relations, the self is a fragile thing that can be injured in many different ways since it entails a wide range of enabling conditions (bodily, social, cognitive, spiritual, etc.). But it does not overlap with any of them. That´s why a shared view of the self is urgently needed. And this kind of view, in all probability, calls for ``an ontology with more than one level´´, where – as Taylor (1971, p. 186) has rightly claimed – acknowledging that ``some principles govern the behaviour of all things´´ does not prevent us from supposing that ``others apply only to some; and yet the latter cannot be shown as special cases of the former´´.

However, one thing that we surely cannot fully control is our ``belief environment´´ (Dennett 2006), that is to say the horizon of meaning against which our practical self-understanding takes place. But, then, is scientific progress likely to damage or radically undermine the cognitive and moral framework (or the social, anthropological, metaphysical imaginaries) within which our lives are shaped? My personal hunch is that it is an exaggeration – and not a particularly useful or innocent one – to paint the situation in such dark colors. Modern science is not a belief system that opposes *en bloc* another belief system in order to totally replace it. It is, rather, a generator of beliefs that works its way into a thick and dynamic web of mostly non-thematized, and generally underdetermined, convictions, opinions, and certainties, causing wholly unforeseeable changes and fluctuations. To this extent, it might be said that the different world views – materialist, idealist, religious, etc. – share a single common space and, when they clash, they never collide head-on, but, as it were, erode each other by acting on the joints by which the beliefs are connected. Accordingly, it should be clear why a military imaginary cannot supply a suitable framework for understanding this kind of cultural conflicts. The problem, of course, is not that the clash between different belief conglomerates does not provoke violent reactions in their self-appointed spokesmen – just the opposite – but that no conflict is able to fully unravel the web or tangle of beliefs. As a matter of fact, the polarization of the debate is less an inescapable feature of the situation, than a psychological device to motivate the contenders.

To sum up, science cannot directly undermine our sense of self, but it can indirectly affect our self-understanding by providing us with pieces of information that may radically upset our current reflective equilibrium. But the only alternative to a disrupted balance, is another more steady balance. We cannot get out of the appearances as far as the self is concerned. The only way to get out is by acting on the enabling (bodily, social, intellectual) conditions in such a way as to make a sense of self utterly impossible. But it is hard even to imagine what this outcome would look like. The fact that we are and we are going to be more and more able to physically manipulate the self's enabling conditions does not mean that the self is a sort of substance that we can isolate, objectify, and manipulate. Personal identity is first of all a matter of bodily, social and normative relations and ought to be understood as an ordered whole, but not as a too tightly and hierarchically organized system. For such a homogeneous view of the self does not permit us to properly grasp its dynamic, articulate, active, heterogeneous and inherently conflictual nature. We are not to understand the self as a kind of monocratic, vertical, bureaucratic government, but rather as a horizontal mixed government with a strong deliberative leaning. Our Self is more like a public realm where self-rule is first of all made possible by the agents´ responsiveness to the space of reasons and by their tacit respect of the constitutive rules (or ``point´´) of its defining practices. As a matter of fact, when it is not understood in terms of sameness, identity can also mean discontinuity (and not only continuity), mis-cognition (and not only recognition), articulacy (and not only unity), impersonality (and not only personality). In a nutshell, the self is a necessary pre-condition for having a world, which also makes it indispensable for scientists of any sort (including hyper-reductionist ones).

REFERENCES

Chalmers, D. J. 1996. *The Conscious Mind. In Search of a Fundamental Theory.* Oxford: Oxford University Press.

Costa, P. 2005. Natura e identità umana. In Costa, P. & Michelini, F. (eds.) *Natura Senza Fine. Il Naturalismo Moderno e le sue Forme.* Bologna: EDB, pp. 119–50.

Costa, P. 2007. *Un´Idea di Umanità. Etica e Natura dopo Darwin.* Bologna: EDB.

Dennett, D. 1995. *Darwin´s Dangerous Idea. Evolution and the Meanings of Life.* New York: Simon & Schuster.

Dennett, D. 2006. How to protect human dignity from science. *Draft for the Bioethics Commission,* August 16. Available at http://ase.tufts.edu/cogstud/papers/dignityscience3.pdf.

Farah, M. J. 2005. Neuroethics: the practical and the philosophical. *Trends in Cognitive Sciences* **9**: 34–40.

Gauchet, M. 2004. *La Condition Historique. Entretiens avec François Azouvi et Sylvain Piron,* 2nd edn. Paris: Gallimard.

Larmore, C. 1998. Person und Anerkennung. *Deutsche Zeitschrift für Philosophie* **46**: 459–64.

Larmore, C. 2004. *Les Pratiques du Moi.* Paris: Presses Universitaires de France.

Larmore, C. 2006. The thinking thing. *The New Republic,* June 19, pp. 37–41.

Merleau-Ponty, M. 1945. *Phénoménologie de la Perception.* Paris: Gallimard.

Midgley, M. 1994. *The Ethical Primate. Humans, Freedom and Morality.* London: Routledge.

Nagel, T. 1986. *The View from Nowhere.* Oxford: Clarendon Press.

Nussbaum, M. 1986. *The Fragility of Goodness. Luck and Ethics in Greek Tragedy and Philosophy.* Cambridge: Cambridge University Press.

Nussbaum, M. 2001. *Upheavals of Thought. The Intelligence of Emotions.* Cambridge: Cambridge University Press.

Olafson, F. A. 1995. *Naturalism and the Human Condition.* London: Routledge.

Parfit, D. 1987. *Reasons and Persons,* 3rd edn. Oxford: Clarendon Press.

Quine, W. V. O. 1966. *The Ways of Paradox and Other Essays.* New York: Random House.

Ricoeur, P. 1990. *Soi-même comme un Autre.* Paris: Éditions du Seuil.

Searle, J. 2007. *Freedom and Neurobiology. Reflections on Free Will, Language, and Political Power.* New York: Columbia University Press.

Seigel, J. 2005. *The Idea of the Self. Thought and Experience in Western Europe since the Seventeenth Century.* Cambridge: Cambridge University Press.

Stroud, B. 1996. The charm of naturalism. *Proceedings and Addresses of the American Philosophical Association* **70**: 43–55. [Now in *Naturalism in Question,* ed. M. De Caro & D. Macarthur. Cambridge, MA: Harvard University Press, 2004, pp. 21–35.]

Taylor, C. 1971. How is mechanism conceivable? In *Human Agency and Language: Philosophical Papers I.* Cambridge: Cambridge University Press, pp. 164–86.

Taylor, C. 1973. Peaceful coexistence in psychology. In *Human Agency and Language: Philosophical Papers I.* Cambridge: Cambridge University Press, pp. 117–38.

Taylor, C. 1976. Responsibility for self. In Rorty, A. O. (ed.) *The Identities of Persons.* Berkeley, CA and Los Angeles, CA: University of California Press, pp. 281–99.

Taylor, C. 1989. *Sources of the Self. The Making of the Modern Identity.* Cambridge, MA: Harvard University Press.

Trilling, L. 1972. *Sincerity and Authenticity.* Cambridge, MA: Harvard University Press.

Walzer, M. 1990. The Communitarian Critique of Liberalism. *Political Theory* **18**: 6–23. [Now in *Politics and Passion. Toward a More Egalitarian Liberalism.* New Haven and London: Yale University Press, 2004, pp. 141–63.]

Williams, B. 1995. Making sense of humanity. In *Making Sense of Humanity and Other Philosophical Papers.* Cambridge: Cambridge University Press, pp. 79–89.

Wollheim, R. 1980. On persons and their lives. In Rorty, A. O. (ed.) *Explaining Emotions.* Berkeley, CA and Los Angeles, CA: University of California Press, pp. 299–321.

Wollheim, R. 1984. *The Thread of Life.* New Haven, CT, and London: Yale University Press.

Wrathall, M. A. 2005. Motives, reasons, and causes. In Carmen, T. & Hansen M. B. N. (eds.) *The Cambridge Companion to Merleau-Ponty.* Cambridge: Cambridge University Press, pp. 111–28.

6

Religious issues and the question of moral autonomy

A. AUTIERO & L. GALVAGNI

AUTONOMY: A BRIEF HISTORY OF THE CONCEPT

No other concept has played such a decisive role in the history of ethical thought as that of autonomy. It reached maturation in modern moral philosophy, within a theory of the ethical subject, but in fact autonomy has a much longer history. Its origins can be traced to the culture of classical antiquity, which made use of the concept in a paradigm of thought distinct from that existing today. The approach was primarily of a political character in that the concept of autonomy served to characterize the nature and identity of sociopolitical entities (e.g. cities), which, albeit maintaining their relationship to the state (Athens) and recognizing its primacy, claimed their independence and the right to enact their own laws (Thucydides and Herodotus).

Later, in the European context of the seventeenth century wars of religion, the concept of autonomy returned in the form of a legal–political notion. It affirmed the ability of every individual to exercise his right to freedom of religion and conscience. Moreover, the social aspect of autonomy was claimed as a condition for the existence and development of single spheres of individual and collective life, within the community of states. As the modern idea of state developed in Europe, the concept of autonomy accompanied the history of emancipation and the liberation of individual life from the arrogant and destructive supremacy of dictatorial notions in politics as in social life.

Scientific and Philosophical Perspectives in Neuroethics, ed. J. J. Giordano & B. Gordijn. Published by Cambridge University Press. © Cambridge University Press 2010.

This second approach prepared the way for the third, typical of modernity and substantiated in an originally ethical conception. This approach was manifest in the philosophical and anthropological reflections of I. Kant, according to whom the autonomy of the subject is the substance of morality. The ethical subject is constituted as such only to the extent that he is able to develop within himself the heteronomous and extrinsic forces of moral obligation and build awareness of his condition as a free agent; able to undertake self-obligations in fulfilment of the exigencies of the moral good. Evidently here, it is decisive to recognize rational capacity as the factor that makes autonomy possible. The latter therefore stands in strict relationship to the self-awareness, self-consciousness, and openness to rationality of the ethical subject.

There was no lack of reaction to, or rejection of, the strongly anthropological and ethical focus of this modern concept of autonomy, because it too markedly evinced the danger of anti-religiosity inherent in the concept. It was viewed as causing alienation from the transcendental reference and withdrawal of the ethical subject into himself. This suspicion imbued a large part of theological tradition, as expressed especially in Catholic moral philosophy, and it emphasized the emancipatory dimensions of the concept of autonomy. In reality, however, the modern concept of autonomy was well received even within religious thought. Indeed, a re-reading of the genuine tradition of theology, particularly of the medieval reflections of Thomas Aquinas, would reveal close compatibility between modernity's concept of autonomy and the vision of the human species as an active and intelligent participant in divine wisdom and providence. Here, there are many points that should be developed and enhanced.

Perhaps it can be said that the entire history of the concept of autonomy is embedded in strongly abstract, substantialist, and metaphysical terms. Today, the implication of the concept resides in systems that regulate action, more than in metaphysical approaches that define the essence of humanity. Above all, reflection in applied ethics – particularly that conducted to understand and solve dilemmas in bioethics – shows that the idea of autonomy is used to respond to more moderate demands. It seems increasingly to be a *functional–practical* concept regulating the choice of the actions to adopt or eschew.

This shift of emphasis places the theme of autonomy in a context of greater plasticity and concreteness, where the dimension of a person's being-in-the-world, his participation in shaping his personal and relational history, acquires a greater importance, expressed in his

bodily condition. Embodiment therefore becomes the locus of autonomy in the human sphere. Exploring this connection is important to
remedy the abstractness of the concept, but also to use it appropriately,
and to respond to the expectations that it brings to the current ethical
debate.

EMBODIMENT, CONSCIOUSNESS, AND SENSE OF SELF (HERETOFORE REFERRED TO AS INTERIORITY)

Following discoveries of neurosciences and cognitive sciences, questions that have traditionally preoccupied philosophy and religions
have returned to the fore: for instance, the problem of the soul, the
issue of free will, moral autonomy, and the question of the existence of
interiority. The strong emphasis placed by neurosciences and cognitive
sciences on the question of the structure and function of the brain, as
well as interpretation and expression of the mind, has also led to a
reformulation of the problem of human identity. According to some,
these discoveries have made it possible to come closer to the root of
human subjectivity and therefore to re-examine the moral dynamics of
freedom and the will. Scenarios, currently only hypothetical, such as
the ability to ``read´´ the thoughts of the human mind, or to decode
what a person is thinking, induce us to wonder whether it will ever be
possible to make the human being ``transparent´´, and, if this does
become possible, whether it would be opportune and/or morally sound
to do so (see Chapters 12 and 13, this volume).

The problem of conscience and reflexivity has been reformu-
lated within this debate. Attention has returned to the conditions of
reason and knowledge, and to their relationship with the dimensions
of desires, beliefs, and intentions. Analysis of the dynamics governing
the manifestation of feelings, emotions, and attitudes has resumed.
Less space and, perhaps, less thorough debate have concerned
examination of the interactions between mind and interiority,
between mind and freedom, and between reason and spirituality.
However, there is increasing interest among theologians in the
neurosciences and the issues that they raise, so much so that one
speaks of neurotheology (see, for example, Hick 2006; Runehov 2007;
Russell *et al.* 2002).

If neurobiology furnishes a possible theoretical corpus from
which to draw answers and interpretations in regard to the dimensions
of identity and interiority, what is the position of embodiment in
relation to these scenarios? And, again, what is it that enables us to

define the human being as such, understood both as a single individual and in anthropological terms? In a 1969 essay on the theme of brain death and its recent redefinition in light of transplant surgery (Jonas 1969, 1974) the philosopher Hans Jonas argued that the new criterion selected for declaration of death – namely brain death – was unsatisfactory because the practical interest of the transplants vitiated the theoretical perspective. For Jonas, this definition disguised a resumption of mind/body dualism in the new formula of a brain/body dualism: cerebral functions, in fact, had come to be considered the decisive discriminants in definition of the human person. Jonas proposed that it should once again be the human organism as a whole that defined the identity of the individual.

> The body is as uniquely the body of this brain and no other, as the brain is uniquely the brain of this body and no other. What is under the brain´s central control, the bodily total, is as individual, as much ``myself´´, as singular to my identity (fingerprints!), as non-interchangeable, as the controlling (and reciprocally controlled) brain itself. My identity is the identity of the whole organism, even if the higher functions of personhood are seated in the brain. How else could a man love a woman and not merely her brains? How else could we lose ourselves in the aspects of a face? Be touched by the delicacy of a frame? It´s this person´s, and no one else´s. Therefore, the body of the comatose, so long as – even with the help of the art – it still breathes, pulses, and functions otherwise, must still be considered a residual continuance of the subject that loved and was loved, and as such is still entitled to some of the sacrosanctity accorded to that subject by the laws of God and men. That sacrosanctity decrees that it must not be used as a mere means.
>
> Jonas (1974), p. 139.

This observation by Jonas yields interesting insights in regard to the debate aroused by the neurosciences. In fact, an ill-concealed dualism seemingly reappears today, and it does so frequently, with the strong bias of the neurosciences and cognitive sciences towards the brain, to the detriment of a more global interpretation of the human organism. It is of interest to examine the re-reading of the organism in its bodily dimension and the re-evaluating of embodiment and the lived body as determinants of personal and existential identity. Important insights in this regard can be drawn from phenomenological reflection on the body and embodiment. The phenomenological approach stresses the centrality of the body, which is the ``cognitive geometral´´ (Merleau-Ponty 1962) through which human beings make contact with reality, gain experience of the world, interrelate with each other, and interact.

It is the body, perceived and lived, which mediates definition of the identity; it is through the body that the conditions arise for the onset of subjectivity, for its capacity for expression, and for its manifestation in autonomy. And autonomy itself can be defined in its bodiliness (Mackenzie 2001). The lived experience of embodiment, the conscious reprocessing of experiences performed by all of us, also constitutes the basis of the symbiotic relationship between the body and the self: what happens to my body also happens to me. The lived body is also sometimes defined as bodily consciousness, given that it is the conscience that mediates the relationship with the world and processes experiences. The conscience has traditionally been considered the locus of human reflection upon conditions and experiences; it is measured with time, through memory, reflection, and intentionality; and understood as interaction with the world and also as future capacity.

The conscience, which in the moral tradition has often been identified as the locus *par excellence* of moral capacity and choice, is where we converse with ourselves. It is consequently considered the ``seat´´ of our liberty, of our existential possibility to judge and to choose; and for this reason it is identified as the seat of an essential moral capacity. But the conscience is always prospective and contextual. It grasps only a certain part of reality, and it processes only some of the infinite experiences possible. Once again, it is the body that mediates this relationship, and therefore also defines our affective states and our emotional experiences. The shared basis of rationality and the emotions is our body, our corporeity.

This central role played by the body, in definition of our identity, also enables us to understand the possible relational basis of autonomy. We form ourselves through bodily relationships, and we grow and mature through forms of interaction and exchange represented by physical, affective, linguistic, and symbolic relationships. Our personality, and with it our moral autonomy, also grows and evolves in these different forms. Paradoxically, but only apparently so, our ability to make choices reflecting our vision of the world and life develops through relationships and constant comparisons with other persons and other identities. These relationships are primarily ones of exchange, real or symbolic, and always mediated by the body.

SITUATED FREEDOM

Considered in terms of embodiment, the concept of autonomy loses its tendency toward abstractness and recovers substantive legitimacy as a regulative idea of action. This involves renewal of the connection between the idea of autonomy and the conception of freedom as established by Kant and the tradition of early modernity. Attesting to this is Kant's statement in the *Grundlegung zur Metaphysik der Sitten* (AA, 4, 446) that ``the concept of freedom is the key that explains the autonomy of the will.'' Moreover, the endeavor that prepared the modern tradition for the rise of the concept of autonomy can only be fully understood in light of the affirmation of the idea of freedom as a substantial and distinctive characteristic of man. The program of modernity and the Age of Enlightenment did nothing other than investigate the conditions in which freedom is possible, interrogating the relationship between conditioning and freedom, between constraints applied by the sensible world and the spaces of freedom produced by the intelligible world. Located in this typically modern dialectic was the theme of freedom as a given condition and as a task to be undertaken; both granted for humans but also constructed by them. Kant's critique of determinism and Christian Wolff's (1679–1754) *Schulphilosophie* restored a necessary balance between human's participation in the sensible world (*Sinnenwelt*), and therefore their subjection to natural causality, and their participation in the intelligible world (*Verstandeswelt*), where there is the greatest valorization of the law of freedom and therefore the largest opening for the autonomy of will.

But what is meant by this law of freedom? Of what freedom can one speak? Two types of criticism have been brought against the modern idea of freedom, or at any rate against how it has been construed in some quarters. The first criticism starts from awareness that the theme of freedom has been separated from that of truth. Particular testimony to this criticism is provided by a certain tradition of Catholic theological thought as expressed in Pope John Paul II's encyclical *Veritatis Splendor* (1993), which at section 32 states that today the theme of freedom assumes such magnitude and extent that liberty is often glorified. But its connection with the truth is neglected, and this, according to the encyclical, empties the notion of freedom of meaning.

The second criticism arises above all from the recent debate in the neurosciences, and it resumes some aspects of previous traditions that considered the weight of determinism in the notion of freedom. The accusation of abstractness in the conception of freedom was correct in a certain sense and requires a substantial change of direction. But the tradition of modernity already comprised interesting and fertile approaches indicative of the balance to achieve. In his practical philosophy, Hegel developed a concept of *konkrete Freiheit* (concrete freedom) as the pivot of the liberal–bourgeois thought and an integration of Kant's critical thought. One element in this tradition was Hegel's concept of *Anerkennung* (recognition), as a logical–practical device for a heuristic of the situatedness of concrete subjects in their history and as an operational basis for the concept of freedom. According to Hegel and the tradition following him, the encounter among subjects takes place within a concrete framework of conditions and conditionings that make freedom a concrete *topos* of definition of what is human. Hence it was modernity itself that made it possible to supersede the abstractness of freedom and which incorporated into its understanding a paradigm of conversion to the concrete. A more recent development in this direction has been the ethical–political approach taken by Martha C. Nussbaum, whose humanistic project for a ``materialism of freedom´´ seeks no more than to induce consideration of persons in their concreteness and indigence, in their aspirations and real possibilities. The approach of ``capability´´ to be developed in every individual, recognized in his/her dignity as a free being, opposes the abstractness of universalistic systems that espouse a vague idea of justice and equality by stressing the particularity of concrete subjects. But it also opposes the functional and utilitarian vision by highlighting the ``substantial´´, and not only instrumental, nature of the idea of the good life and therefore also of freedom. With this reflexive and situated equilibrium, freedom does not disappear from the domain of morality; rather, it acquires concrete features that inspire theoretical reflection in applied ethics, acting as a heuristic criterion for normative choices on matters concerning both individual and public ethics.

WHAT AUTONOMIES AND WHAT FREEDOMS? AUTONOMY AND NEUROSCIENCES ON A PRACTICAL LEVEL

The interpretation furnished by the neurosciences of the human condition frequently under-emphasizes dimensions such as autonomy, interiority, and openness to transcendence, while favoring parameters such as heteronomy and exteriority. Or it tends to exclude the possibility of transcendent referents. The imbalance thus created also radically changes the perception of what may be important in defining the human condition. Although it is a complex undertaking to furnish an interpretation that considers the meanings and values of lived experiences in the knowledge process and in the maturation of our awareness, this unbalanced interpretation neglects or only gives little space to the dimensions that characterize human life from an existential point of view. It is therefore important to reinstate these components in the interpretation thus provided of the human being.

On an existential level understood in both mental and more specifically moral terms, there is a trajectory in the maturation and growth of liberty that seems to involve a progressive shift from the level of norms to that of values. There exists a form of maturation of the subject which, starting from the heteronomous phase of respect for the norms, becomes an understanding of, and an autonomous adherence (which is personal and existential) to, the values subsumed by those norms. It is thus possible to develop and manifest deliberate adherence to the value of which the norm is the bearer (Gius & Coin 1999; Gius 2004). It is at this level that there arises our capacity for interiority, whereby we also define our deepest-lying identity.

But what is the connection among maturation, affective life, and the experience of values? Moral autonomy in its essence seemingly derives from some sort of personal maturation, from a process in which we learn to integrate the rationality of choices and the possible impersonality of norms with the emotional and affective components ever-present in our vision of the world and life, and which guide us. This capacity for interiority and imagination possessed by human beings, and the uniqueness of each individual, are well expressed by our behaviors and attitudes, as well as via the medium of language and the multiple meanings that it can communicate.

Hannah Arendt wrote in *The Life of the Mind*:

> ... all mental activities withdraw from the world of appearances, but this withdrawal is not toward an interior of either the self or the soul. Thought with its accompanying conceptual language, since it occurs in and is spoken by a being at home in a world of appearances, stands in need of metaphors in order to bridge the gap between a world given to sense experience and a realm where such immediate apprehension of evidence can ever exist. But our soul-experience are body-bound to such an extent that to speak of an `inner life´ of the soul is as unmetaphorical as to speak of an inner sense thanks to which we have clear sensations of the functioning of our inner organs. It is obvious that a mindless creature cannot possess anything like an experience of personal identity (...) The language of the soul in its mere expressive stage, prior to its transformation and transfiguration through thought, is not metaphorical; it does not depart from the senses and uses no analogies when it talks in terms of physical sensations.
>
> Arendt 1971

There are areas in which what Hannah Arendt indicates as ``language of the soul´´ is most evident. One of them is undoubtedly the use of images and metaphors. Accounts of illness make intense use of metaphors and images – precisely where and when bodily and moral autonomy seems most compromised. In this case their function is not solely rhetorical or decorative, for they convey experiences that would otherwise be difficult to recount, almost as if they were a concentrate of experiences that can only be expressed in language. In the knowledge process, moreover, the oral and logical expression generally termed ``conceptual´´ is a second level with respect to the imaginative–analogic expression that constitutes its primary level.

Where the experience of the body is most intense, it reshapes our modes of expression into more incisive ones better suited to expressing the complexity of the moment and conditions being experienced. The sense of time, itself, is changed. The metaphors or images used are therefore important because they synthesize past experience and memory, present vision and initiative, and future choice or intention (Ricoeur 1975, 1983-5). In this sense metaphor is characterized as a moment of innovation and initiative.

If we assume with Ricoeur that our identity is narrative (Ricoeur 1992), we can understand how autonomy can also pass through those accounts, the remnants of stories, that persist when rational capacity is seriously compromised by illness, mental aging, or pain; or also when it is still not fully expressed, as with children.

When illness devastates the body, afflicts the mind, and reduces autonomy, our identity does not diminish. The profound mental and/or physical changes undergone by persons in these circumstances induce them to redefine their identities. Even in the image and the condition of a destroyed body, a meaning can be found: a provisional identity which, however, is essential at that time because it enables the sufferer to modulate a new perspective and a new interpretation of his/her life-condition. It is necessary to try to assemble these various stories, these fragments, even when a cure seems impossible. There are numerous scenarios in which this task can be performed. In the case of degenerative neurological diseases, Alzheimer´s disease for example, it is necessary to understand what still remains of the person´s moral autonomy, and to what extent they can express themselves in non-traditional ways.

This requires us to understand how the person´s autonomy is re-shaped in these situations. People find a new language with which to express their moral values when they are no longer able to formulate the moral reasons that determine their choices and their behavior. Listening to different needs and new desires is a way to show respect for those persons, their interiority, and their partially new identity.

In the case of degenerative neurological diseases, the restriction of autonomy is evident. It is first of all restriction of bodily autonomy, because those who suffer from such diseases are unable to walk on their own, to keep their balance, to remain standing for some time, or to cover long distances. The use of a walking stick, and to a greater extent, a walker or a wheelchair, enables them to regain some of their lost autonomy. These instruments sometimes become akin to parts of the body, and they can be perceived and experienced as real extensions of the person's autonomy (Toombs 2001). The great uncertainty experienced in these cases also induces sufferers from degenerative neurological illnesses to change their vision and to re-define their life perspective. It is not surprising that the metaphors and images used by such sufferers forcefully express the change in their embodiment and their different kind of autonomy.

What changes, what life alterations, what bodily experiences make us understand that we still have autonomy? While the body slows down, time may expand, and this is not necessarily experienced negatively. Time becomes different because it can change our perceptions, and experiences. That which counts, for instance, is the experience of the moment, the day that is granted, which becomes remarkable because it gives the possibility of living a little longer. Even just one day, even another unexpected year, becomes significant, and leads to re-defining what constitutes our identity. We can perceive the passage of time precisely because it changes our consciousness and changes the traversing flow.

Change in bodily condition re-defines our perceptions and influences our intentionality. The horizon is different, and so too is the way in which it is perceived. In addition, the language that expresses our moral values may be different and may enable us to express our position when we are no longer able to express our moral reasons. In this expanded space of time, there frequently return images and languages that speak to us of other dimensions, those that we generally call spiritual or interior. And perhaps this happens in the new space of a somewhat different body, where we become able to listen to our experience and to grasp its limits, thus opening ourselves to other dimensions.

And what happens to the autonomy of people when they have lost consciousness and are living without any possibility of restoring it?

What do these uninhabited bodies represent? What are the signs of their identity, at this time and in these conditions?

We can observe that our human being is defined by many different components: our identity is formed from the complex manifestations of the body, the mind, the conscience, and from their interactions, which change according to the influences of individual development, character and personality, education, culture, and environment. The whole of these different elements – their synthesis, so to speak – also contributes to forming our interiority, which represents the privileged ``space´´ of our possibility and capacity to express ourselves as human beings. This dimension of interiority is also expressed by the image, the dense metaphor, of the heart (De Monticelli 2003). It is within interiority that we cultivate our ability to still be surprised, to intuit processes and aspects that we would not see otherwise, to modulate our desires, and to let our being´s most profound needs speak. It is to these interiorities that we must listen when it is no longer possible to use the most usual forms of communication and relationality.

Autonomy – with its inevitable relational and mutual dimension – and the language of the body can still express our desires and our expectations, which, precisely when they are at their most fragile, must be listened to once again.

REFERENCES

Arendt, H. 1971. *The Life of the Mind*. London: Secker & Warburg.
De Monticelli, R. 2003. *L´ordine del Cuore. Teoria ed Etica del Sentire*. Milan: Garzanti.
Gius, E. 2004. *Teoria della Conoscenza e Valori. Prospettive Psicologiche*. Milan: Giuffrè.
Gius, E. & Coin, R. 1999. *I Dilemmi dello Psicoterapeuta: il Soggetto tra Norme e Valori*. Milan: Cortina.
Hick, J. 2006. *The New Frontier of Religion and Science: Religious Experience, Neuroscience and the Transcendent*. New York: Palgrave Macmillan.
Jonas, H. 1969. Philosophical reflections on experimenting with human subjects. *Daedalus* **98**(2): 219–47.
Jonas, H. 1974. Against the stream: comments on the definition and redefinition of death. In Jonas, H. (ed.) *Philosophical Essays: From Ancient Creed to Technological Man*. Englewood Cliffs, NJ: Prentice-Hall, pp. 132–40.
Joseph, R. (ed.) 2003. *Neurotheology: Brain, Science, Spirituality, Religious Experience*. San Jose, CA: University Press.
Mackenzie, C. 2001. On bodily autonomy. In S. K. Toombs (ed.) *Handbook of Phenomenology and Medicine*. Amsterdam: Kluwer, pp. 417–39.
Merleau-Ponty, M. 1962. *Phenomenology of Perception*. London: Routledge.
Ricoeur, P. 1975. *La Metaphore Vive*. Paris: Editions du Seuil.
Ricoeur, P. 1983–5. *Temps et Recit*. Paris: Editions du Seuil.
Ricoeur, P. 1992. *Soi-même comme un Autre*. Paris: Editions du Seuil.

Runehov, A. L. C. 2007. *Sacred or Neural? The Potential of Neuroscience to Explain Religious Experience*. Göttingen: Vandenhoeck & Ruprecht.

Russell, R. J., Murphy, N., Meyering, T. C. & Abib, M. A. (eds.) 2002. *Neuroscience and the Person. Scientific Perspectives on Divine Action*. Vatican City/Berkeley, CA: Vatican Observatory, Center for Theology and the Natural Sciences.

Toombs, S. K. 2001. Reflections on bodily change: the lived experience of disability. In S. K. Toombs (ed.) *Handbook of Phenomenology and Medicine*. Dordrecht: Kluwer, pp. 247–61.

7

Toward a cognitive neurobiology
of the moral virtues

P. M. CHURCHLAND

In the ten years since this chapter was originally written – for an issue of the journal *Topoi* devoted to the topic of moral reasoning – the hopes expressed in its opening paragraph have been fulfilled beyond even my own fond expectations. Since then, brain imaging has revealed a number of neuroanatomical locations that seem disproportionately active during moral reasoning and various forms of social interaction. At a lower level, neuroethology and neurophysiology have jointly identified several distinct neurotransmitter chemicals that play a major role in long-term pair-bonding, in the establishment of mutual trust and cooperation between individuals, and in the commitment of personal resources to the joint parenting of shared offspring, both in animals and in humans. Beyond this, the role of our so-called ``mirror neurons´´ in comprehending the behavior and the emotions of one´s fellow creatures, and in grounding one´s capacity for social mimicry, has revealed a major brain mechanism for simultaneously sustaining both social perception and social behavior. And these brain-focussed disciplines have recently been joined by the social sciences from above and by evolutionary biology from below, yielding a multi-level and multidisciplinary portrait of our precious capacity for moral cognition. This capacity for morality, it now seems clear, is not unique to the human species; many other creatures display it as well. But none does so as thoroughly and intricately as we humans. It binds us together, and gives us collective (and individual!) wings, to a degree that is downright startling. But it is

Reprinted with kind permission from Springer Science & Business Media: *Topoi*, ``Toward a cognitive neurobiology of the moral virtues´´, **17**:2, 1998, 83–96, Paul M. Churchland.

Scientific and Philosophical Perspectives in Neuroethics, ed. J. J. Giordano & B. Gordijn. Published by Cambridge University Press. © Cambridge University Press 2010.

146

not a matter of *mere* biology or neuroscience. As even Aristotle stressed, moral character is still very much a matter of gradual *learning*, and of learning within the context of an already-established *moral environment*. The concerns of the following chapter, therefore, still lie at the focus of our desire to understand the nature of moral cognition. And the lessons it urges are no less salient now than they were ten years ago.

INTRODUCTION

These are the early days of what I hope will be a long and fruitful intellectual tradition, a tradition fueled by the systematic interaction and mutual information of cognitive neurobiology on the one hand and moral theory on the other. More specifically, it is the traditional sub-area we call *metaethics,* including moral epistemology and moral psychology, that will be most dramatically informed by the unfolding developments in cognitive neurobiology. And it is metaethics again that will exert a reciprocal influence on future neurobiological research: more specifically, into the nature of moral perception, the nature of practical and social reasoning, and the development and occasional corruption of moral character.

This last point about reciprocity highlights a further point. What we are contemplating here is no imperialistic takeover of the moral by the neural. Rather, we should anticipate a mutual flowering of *both* our high-level conceptions in the domain of moral knowledge *and* our lower-level conceptions in the domain of normal and pathological neurology. For each level has much to teach the other, as this chapter will try to show.

Nor need we resist this interaction of distinct traditions on grounds that it threatens to deduce normative conclusions from purely factual premises, for it threatens no such thing. To see this clearly, consider the following parallel. Cognitive neurobiology is also in the process of throwing major illumination on the philosophy of *science* – by way of revealing the several forms of neural representation that underlie scientific cognition, and the several forms of neural activity that underlie learning and conceptual change (see, for example, Churchland 1989a, chapters 9–11). And yet, substantive science itself will still have to be done by scientists, according to the various methods by which we make scientific progress. An adequate theory of the brain, plainly, would not constitute a theory of stellar evolution or a theory of the underlying structure of the periodic table. It would constitute, at most, only a theory of how we generate, embody, and manipulate such worthy cognitive achievements.

Equally, and for the same reasons, substantive moral and political theory will still have to be done by moral and political thinkers, according to the various methods by which we make moral and political progress. An adequate theory of the brain, plainly, will not constitute a theory of Distributive Justice or a body of Criminal Law. It would still constitute, at most, only a theory of how we generate, embody, and manipulate such cognitive achievements.

These reassurances might seem to rob the contemplated program of its interest, at least to moral philosophers, but we shall quickly see that this is not the case. For we are about to contemplate a systematic and unified account, sketched in neural-network terms, of the following phenomena: moral knowledge, moral learning, moral perception, moral ambiguity, moral conflict, moral argument, moral virtues, moral character, moral pathology, moral correction, moral diversity, moral progress, moral realism, and moral unification.

This collective sketch will serve at least to outline the program, and even at this early stage it will provide a platform from which to address the credentials of one prominent strand in pre-neural metaethics, the program of so-called "Virtue Ethics", as embodied in both an ancient writer (Aristotle), and three modern writers (Johnson, Flanagan, and MacIntyre).

THE RECONSTRUCTION OF MORAL COGNITIVE PHENOMENA IN COGNITIVE NEUROBIOLOGICAL TERMS

This chapter builds on work now a decade or so in place, work concerning the capacity of recent neural-network models (of micro-level brain activity) to reconstruct, in an explanatory way, the salient features of molar-level cognitive activity. That research began in the mid-1980s by addressing the problems of perceptual recognition, motor-behavior generation, and other basic phenomena involving the gradual learning of sundry cognitive *skills* by artificial "neural" networks, as modeled within large digital computers (Gorman & Sejnowski 1988; Lehky & Sejnowski 1988; Rosenberg & Sejnowski, 1987; Lockery *et al.* 1991; Cottrell 1991; Elman 1992). From there, it has moved both downward in its focus, to try to address in more faithful detail the empirical structure of biological brains (Churchland & Sejnowski, 1992), and upward in its focus, to address the structure and dynamics of such higher-level cognitive phenomena as are displayed, for example, in the human pursuit of the various theoretical sciences (Churchland 1989a).

For philosophers, perhaps the quickest and easiest introduction to these general ideas is the highly pictorial account in Churchland (1995), to which I direct the unprepared reader. My aim here is not to recapitulate that groundwork, but to build on it. Even so, that background account will no doubt slowly emerge, from the many examples to follow, even for the reader new to these ideas, so I shall simply proceed and hope for the best.

The model here being followed is my earlier attempt to reconstruct the epistemology of the *natural* sciences in neural-network terms (Churchland 1989a). My own philosophical interests have always been centered around issues in epistemology and the philosophy of science, and so it was natural, in the mid-1980s, that I should first apply the emerging framework of cognitive neurobiology to the issues with which I was most familiar. But it soon became obvious to me that the emerging framework had an unexpected generality, and that its explanatory power, if genuine at all, would illuminate a much broader range of cognitive phenomena than had so far been addressed. I therefore proposed to extend its application into other cognitive areas such as mathematical knowledge, musical knowledge, and moral knowledge. (Some first forays appear in chapters 6 and 10 of Churchland 1995.) These further domains of cognitive activity provide, if nothing else, a series of stiff *tests* for the assumptions and explanatory ambitions of neural-network theory. Accordingly, the present paper presumes to draw out the central theoretical claims, within the domain of metaethics, to which a neural-network model of cognition commits us. It is for the reader, and especially for professional moral philosophers themselves, to judge whether the overall portrait that results is both explanatorily instructive and faithful to moral reality.

Moral knowledge

Broadly speaking, to teach or train any neural network to embody a specific cognitive capacity is gradually to impose a specific *function* onto its input–output behavior. The network thus acquires the ability to respond, in various but systematic ways, to a wide variety of potential sensory inputs. In a simple, three-layer feedforward network with fixed synaptic connections (Figure 7.1a), the output behavior at the third layer of neurons is completely determined by the activity at the sensory input layer. In a (biologically more realistic) *recurrent* network (Figure 7.1b), the output behavior is jointly determined by sensory input *and* the prior dynamical state of the entire network. The purely

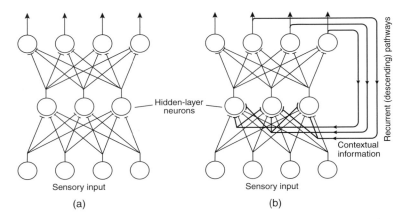

Figure 7.1 (a) A simple feedforward network. (b) A simple recurrent network. For a quick grip on the functional significance of such models, think of the lower or input layer of neurons as the sensory neurons, and think of the upper or output layer of neurons as the motor or muscle-driving neurons.

feedforward case yields a cognitive capacity that is sensitive to spatial patterns but blind to temporal patterns or to temporal context; the recurrent network yields a capacity that is sensitive to, and responsive to, the changing cognitive contexts in which its sensory inputs are variously received. In both cases, the acquired cognitive capacity actually resides in the specific configuration of the many synaptic *connections* between the neuronal layers, and learning that cognitive capacity is a matter of slowly adjusting the size or ``weight´´ of each connection so that, collectively, they come to embody the input–output function desired. On this, more in a moment.

Evidently, a trained network has acquired a specific skill. That is, it has learned how to respond, with appropriate patterns of neural activity across its output layer, to various inputs at its sensory layer. Accordingly, and as with all other kinds of knowledge, my first characterization of moral knowledge portrays it as a *set of skills*. To begin with, a morally knowledgeable adult has clearly acquired a sophisticated family of *perceptual* or *recognitional* skills, which skills allow him a running comprehension of his own social and moral circumstances, and the social and moral circumstances of the others in his community. Equally clearly, a morally knowledgeable adult has acquired a complex set of *behavioral* and *manipulational* skills, which skills make possible his successful social and moral interaction with the others in his community.

According to the model of cognition here being explored, the skills at issue are embodied in a vast configuration of appropriately weighted synaptic connections. To be sure, it is not intuitively obvious how a thousand, or a billion, or a trillion such connections can constitute a specific cognitive skill, but we begin to gain an intuitive grasp of how they can do so when we turn our attention to the collective behavior of the neurons at the layer to which those carefully configured connections happen to attach.

Consider, for example, the second layer of the feedforward network in Figure 7.1(a). That neuronal population, like any other discrete neuronal population, represents the various states of the world with a corresponding variety of *activation patterns* across that entire population. That is to say, just as a pattern of brightness levels across the 200,000 pixels of your familiar TV screen can represent a certain two-dimensional scene, so can the pattern of activation levels across a neuronal population represent specific aspects of the external world, although the ``semantics´´ of that representational relation will only rarely be so obviously ``pictorial´´. If the neuronal representation is auditory, for example, or olfactory, or gustatory, then obviously the representation will be something other than a 2-D ``picture´´. What is important for our purposes is that the abstract *space* of *possible* representational patterns, across a given neuronal population, slowly acquires, in the course of training the synapses, a specific structure – a structure that assigns a family of dramatically preferential abstract *locations,* within that space, in response to a preferred family of distinct stimuli at the network's sensory layer. This is how the mature network manages to categorize all possible inputs, either as rough instances of one-or-other of its learned family of prototypical *categories,* or, failing that, as instances of unintelligible noise. Before training, *all* inputs produce noise at the second layer. After training, however, that second layer has become preferentially sensitized to a comparatively tiny subset of the vast range of possible input patterns (most of which are never encountered). Those ``hot-button´´ input patterns, whenever they occur, are subsequently assimilated to the second layer's acquired set of *prototypical categories.*

Consider an artificial network (Figure 7.2a) trained to discriminate human faces from non-faces, male faces from female faces, and a handful of named individuals as presented in a variety of distinct photographs. As a result of that training, the abstract space of *possible* activation patterns across its second neuronal layer has become *partitioned* (Figure 7.2b), first into a pair of complementary subvolumes for

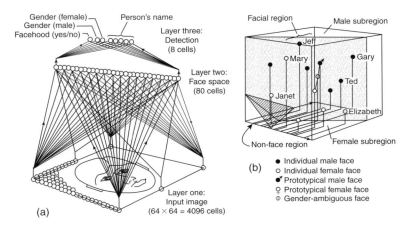

Figure 7.2 (a) A feedforward neural network for recognizing human faces and distinguishing gender. (b) The hierarchy of categorial partitions, acquired during training, across the space of possible neuronal activation patterns at the network´s middle or ``hidden´´ layer.

neuronal activation patterns that represent sundry faces and non-faces respectively. The former subvolume has become further partitioned into two mutually exclusive subvolumes for male faces and female faces, respectively. And within each of these two subvolumes, there are proprietary ``hot-spots´´ for each of the named individuals that the network learned to recognize during training.

Following this simple model, the suggestion here advanced is that our capacity for *moral* discrimination also resides in an intricately configured matrix of synaptic connections, which connections also partition an abstract conceptual space, at some proprietary neuronal layer of the human brain, into a hierarchical set of categories, categories such as ``morally significant´´ vs. ``morally non-significant´´ actions; and within the former category, ``morally bad´´ vs. ``morally praiseworthy´´ actions; and within the former subcategory, sundry specific categories such as ``lying´´, ``cheating´´, ``betraying´´, ``stealing´´, ``tormenting´´, ``murdering´´, and so forth (Figure 7.3).

That abstract space of possible neuronal-activation patterns is a simple model for our own conceptual space for moral representation, and it displays an intricate structure of similarity and dissimilarity relations: relations that cluster similar vices close together and similar virtues close together; relations that separate highly dissimilar action categories into spatially distant sectors of the space. This high-dimensional similarity space (of course, Figure 7.3 ignores all but three of its

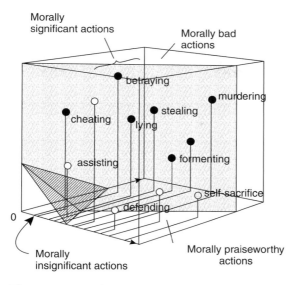

Figure 7.3 A (conjectural) "activation space" for moral discrimination.

many neuronal axes) displays a structured family of categorical "hotspots" or "prototype positions", to which actual sensory inputs are assimilated with varying degrees of closeness.

An abstract space of *motor neuron* activation patterns will serve a parallel function for the generation of actual social behavior, a neuronal layer that presumably enjoys close functional connections with the sensory neurons just described. All told, these structured spaces constitute our acquired knowledge of *the structure of social space,* and *how to navigate it effectively.*

Moral learning

Moral learning consists in the gradual generation of these internal perceptual and behavioral prototypes, a process that requires repeated exposure to, or practice of, various *examples* of the perceptual or motor categories at issue. In artificial neural networks, such learning consists in the repeated adjustment of the weights of their myriad synaptic connections, adjustments that are guided by the naive network's initial performance *failures,* as measured by a distinct "teacher" program. In living creatures, learning also consists in the repeated adjustment of one's myriad synaptic connections, a process that is also driven by one's ongoing experience with failure. Our artificial "learning technologies" are currently a poor and pale reflection of what goes on in real brains, but in both cases – the artificial networks and living brains – those gradual synaptic readjustments lead to an appropriately structured high-dimensional similarity space, a space partitioned into a hierarchical family of categorical subspaces, which subspaces contain a central hot-spot that represents a *prototypical* instance of its proprietary category.

Such learning typically takes time, often large amounts of time. And as the network models have also illustrated, such learning often needs to be structured, in the sense that the simplest of the relevant perceptual and behavioral skills need to be learned first, with the more sophisticated skills being learned later, and only after the elementary ones are in place. Moreover, such learning can display some familiar pathologies, those that derive from a narrow or otherwise skewed population of training examples. In such cases, the categorical framework duly acquired by the network fails to represent the full range and true structure of the social/moral domain it needs to represent, and performance failures are the inevitable result.

These remarks barely introduce the topic of moral learning, but we need to move on. The topic will be re-addressed below, when we discuss moral progress.

Moral perception

This most fundamental of our moral skills consists in the *activation*, at some appropriate layer of neurons at least half a dozen synaptic connections away from the sensory periphery, of a specific pattern of neuronal excitation levels that is sufficiently close to some already learned moral *prototype* pattern. That nth-layer activation pattern is jointly caused by the current activation pattern across one or more of the brain's sensory or input layers, and by the series of carefully trained synaptic connections that intervene. Moral perception is thus of a piece with perception generally, and its profile displays features long familiar to perceptual psychologists.

For example, one's spontaneous judgments about the social and moral configuration of one's current environment are strongly sensitive to contextual features, to collateral information, and to one's current interests and focus of attention. Moral perception is thus subject to ``priming effects´´ and ``masking effects´´. As well, moral perception displays the familiar tendency of cognitive creatures to ``jump to conclusions´´ in their perceptual interpretations of partial or degraded perceptual inputs. Like artificial networks, we humans have a strong tendency automatically to assimilate our current perceptual circumstances to the nearest of the available moral prototypes that our prior training has created in us.

Moral ambiguity

A situation is morally ambiguous when it is problematic by reason of its tendency to activate *more than one* moral prototype, prototypes that invite two incompatible or mutually exclusive subsequent courses of action. In fact, and to some degree, ambiguity is a chronic feature of our moral experience, partly because the social world is indefinitely complex and various, and partly because the interests and collateral information each of us brings to the business of interpreting the social world differ from person to person and from occasion to occasion. The recurrent or descending pathways within the brain (illustrated, in stick-figure form, in Figure 7.1b) provide a continuing stream of such background information (or misinformation) to the ongoing process of perceptual interpretation and prototype activation. Different ``perceptual takes´´, on one and the same situation, are thus inevitable. Which leads us to our next topic.

Moral conflict

The activation of distinct moral prototypes can happen in two or more distinct individuals confronting the same situation, and even in a single individual, as when some contextual feature is alternatively magnified or minimized and one´s overall perceptual take flips back and forth between two distinct activation patterns in the neighborhood of two distinct prototypes. In such a case, the single individual is morally conflicted (``Shall I *protect* a friend´s feelings by keeping silent on someone´s trivial but hurtful slur, or shall I be forthright and *truthful* in my disclosures to a friend?´´).

Interpersonal conflicts about the moral status of some circumstance reflect the same sorts of divergent interpretations, driven this time by interpersonal divergences in the respective collateral information, attentional focus, hopes and fears, and other contextual elements that each perceiver brings to the ambiguous situation. Occasional moral conflicts are thus possible, indeed they are inevitable, even between individuals who had identical moral training and who share identical moral categories.

There is, finally, the extreme case where moral judgment diverges because the two conflicting individuals have fundamentally different moral conceptual frameworks, reflecting major differences in the acquired structure of their respective activation spaces. Here, even communication becomes difficult, and so does the process by which moral conflicts are typically resolved.

Moral argument

On the picture here being explored, the standard conception of moral argument as the formal deduction of moral conclusions from shared moral premises starts to look procrustean in the extreme. Instead, the administration and resolution of moral conflicts emerges as a much more dialectical process whereby the individuals in conflict take turns highlighting or making salient certain aspects of the situation at issue, and take turns urging various similarities between the situation at issue and various shared prototypes, in hopes of producing, within their adversary, an activation pattern that is closer to the prototype being defended (``It´s a mindless clutch of cells, for heaven´s sake! The woman is not obliged to preserve or defend it.´´) and/or farther from the prototype being attacked (``No, it´s a miniature person! Yes, she is obliged.´´). It is a matter of nudging your interlocutor´s current neuronal activation-point *out* of the attractor-category that has captured it, and *into* a distinct attractor-category. It is a matter of trying to change the probability, or the robustness, or the proximity to a shared neural prototype-pattern, of your opponent´s neural behavior.

In the less tractable case where the opponents fail to share a common family of moral prototypes, moral argument must take a different form. I postpone discussion of this deeper form of conflict until the section on moral progress, below.

Moral virtues

These are the various skills of social *perception,* social *reflection, imagination, and reasoning,* and social *navigation and manipulation* that normal social learning produces. In childhood, one must come to appreciate the high-dimensional background structure of social space – its offices, its practices, its prohibitions, its commerce – and one must learn to recognize its local configuration swiftly and reliably. One must also learn to recognize one´s own current position within it, and the often quite different positions of others. One must learn to anticipate the normal unfolding of this ongoing commerce, to recognize and help repair its occasional pathologies, and to navigate its fluid structure while avoiding social disasters, both large and small. All of this requires skill in divining the social perceptions and personal interests of others, and skill in manipulating and negotiating our collective behavior.

Being skills, such virtues are inevitably acquired rather slowly, as anyone who has raised children will know. Nor need their continued development ever cease, at least in individuals with the continued opportunities and the intelligence necessary to refine them. The acquired structures within one's neuronal activation spaces – both perceptual and motor – can continue to be sculpted by ongoing experience and can thus pursue an ever deeper insight into, and an effectively controlling grasp of, one's enclosing social reality. Being skills, they are also differently acquired by distinct individuals, and they are differentially acquired within a single individual. Each brain is slightly different from every other in its initial physical structure, and each brain's learning history is unique in its myriad details. No two of us are identical in the profile of skills we acquire, which raises our next topic.

Moral character

A person's unique moral character is just the individual profile of his or her perceptual, reflective, and behavioral skills in the social domain. From what has already been said, it will be evident that moral character is distinguished more by its rich diversity across individuals than by its monotony. Given the difficulty in clearly specifying any canonical profile as being uniquely ideal, this is probably a good thing. Beyond the unending complexity of social space, the existence of a diversity of moral characters simply reflects a healthy tendency to explore that space and to explore the most effective styles of navigating it. By this, I do not mean to give comfort to moral nihilists. That would be to deny the reality of social learning. What I am underwriting here is the idea that long-term moral learning across the human race is positively served by tolerating a Gaussian distribution of well-informed ``experiments´´ rather than by insisting on a narrow and impossible orthodoxy.

This view of the assembled moral virtues as a slowly acquired network of skills also contains an implicit critique of a popular piece of romantic nonsense, namely, the idea of the ``sudden convert´´ to morality, as typified by the ``tearful face of the repentant sinner´´ and the post-baptismal ``born-again´´ charismatic Christian. Moral character is not something – is not *remotely* something – that can be acquired in a day by an Act of Will or by a single Major Insight.

The idea that it can be so acquired is a falsifying reflection of one or other of two familiar conceptions of moral character, herewith discredited. The first identifies moral character with the acceptance of a canonical set of behavior-guiding rules. The second identifies moral character with a canonical set of desires, such as the desire to maximize the general happiness, and so on. Perhaps one can embrace a set of rules in one cathartic act, and perhaps one can permanently privilege some set of desires by a major act of will. But neither act can result in what is truly needed: namely, an intricate set of finely-honed perceptual, reflective, and sociomotor skills. These take several decades to acquire. Epiphanies of moral commitment can mark, at most, the initiation of such a process. Initiations are welcome, of course, but we do not give children a high-school diploma for showing up for school on the first day of the first grade. For the same reasons, ``born-again´´ moral characters should probably wait a similar period of time before celebrating their moral achievement or pressing their moral authority.

Moral pathology

This is a large topic, since, if there are many different ways to succeed in being a morally mature creature, there are even more ways in which one might fail. But as a first pass, moral pathology consists in the partial absence, or subsequent corruption, of the normal constellation of perceptual, reflective, and behavioral skills under discussion. In terms of the cognitive theory that underlies the present approach, it consists in the failure to achieve, or subsequently to activate normally, a suitable hierarchy of moral prototypes within one's neuronal activation space. And at the lowest level, this consists in a failure, either early or late, to achieve and maintain the proper configuration of the brain's 10^{14} synaptic weights, the configuration that sustains the desired hierarchy of prototypes and makes possible their appropriate activation.

The terms ``normally´´, ``suitable´´, ``proper´´, and ``appropriate´´ all appear in this quick characterization, and they will all owe their sense to a inextricable mix of *functional* understanding within cognitive neurobiology and genuine *moral* understanding as brought to bear by common sense and the civil and criminal law. The point here urged is that we can come to understand how displays of moral incompetence, both major and minor, are often the reflection of specific functional failures, both large and small, within the brain. This is not a specula-tive remark. Thanks to the increasing availability of brain-scanning technologies such as positron emission tomography (PET) and mag-netic resonance imaging (MRI), neurologists are becoming familiar with a variety of highly specific forms of brain damage that display themselves in signature forms of cognitive failure in moral perception, moral reasoning, and social behavior (Damasio *et al.* 1991; Damasio 1994; Bechara *et al.* 1994; Adolphs *et al.* 1996).

Two quick examples will illustrate the point. The neurologists Antonio and Hanna Damasio have a patient, known in the literature as ``Boswell'', who is independently famous for his inability to lay down any new long-term memories because of bilateral lesions to his medial temporal lobe, including his hippocampus. Since his illness, his ``remembered past'' is a moving window that reaches back no more than forty seconds. More importantly, for our purposes, it later emerged that he also displays a curious inability to ``see evil'' in pic-tures of various emotionally-charged and potentially violent scenes. In particular, he is unable to pick up on the various negative emotions as expressed in people's *faces,* and he will blithely confabulate innocent explanations of the socially and morally problematic scenes shown him. There is nothing wrong with Boswell's eyes or visual system, however. His cognitive deficit lies roughly a dozen synaptic steps and a dozen neuronal layers behind his retinas.

As the MRI scans revealed, Boswell's herpes-simplex encephalitis had also damaged the lower half of both of his temporal lobes, which includes the area called ``IT'' (infero-temporal) known for its critical role in discriminating individual human faces and in coding facial expressions. He can no longer recognize the identity of faces well known to him before the illness (movie stars and presidents, for example), and his moral perception has been selectively impaired in the manner described.

A second patient, EVR, had a normal life as a respected account-ant, devoted father, and faithful husband. In his mid-40s, a ventromedial frontal brain tumor was successfully removed, and subsequent tests revealed no change in his original IQ of 140. But within six months he had lost his job for rampant irresponsibility, made a series of damaging financial decisions, was divorced by his frustrated wife, briefly married and then was left by a prostitute, and had generally become incapable of the normal prudence that guides complex planning and intricate social interactions. Subsequent MRI scans confirmed that the surgical removal of the tumor had lesioned the ventromedial frontal cortex (the seat of complex planning) and its connections to the amygdala (a primitive limbic area that apparently embodies fear and anxiety).

The functional consequence of this break in the wiring was to *isolate* EVR´s practical reasonings from the ``visceral´´ somatic and emotional reactions that normally accompany the rational evaluation of practical alternatives. In normals, those ``somatic markers´´ (as the Damasios have dubbed them) constitute an important dimension of socially relevant information and a key factor in inhibiting one´s decisions. In EVR, they have been cut out of the loop, resulting in the sorts of behavior described above.

These two failures, of moral perception and moral behaviour, respectively, resulted from sudden illness and consequent damage to specific brain areas, which is what brought them to the attention of the medical profession and led to their detailed examination. But these and many other neural deficits can also appear slowly, as a result of developmental misadventures and other chronic predations – childhood infections, low-level toxins, abnormal metabolism, abnormal brain chemistry, abnormal nutrition, maternal drug use during pregnancy, and so forth. There is no suggestion, let me emphasize, that all failures of moral character can be put down to structural deficits in the brain. A proper moral education – that is, a long stretch of intricate socialization – remains a necessary condition for acquiring a well-formed moral character, and no doubt the great majority of failures, especially the minor ones, can be put down entirely to sundry inadequacies in that process.

Even so, the educational process is thoroughly entwined with the developmental process and deeply dependent on the existence of normal brain structures to embody the desired matrix of skills. At least some failures of moral character, therefore, and especially the most serious failures, are likely to involve some confounding disability or marginality at the level of brain structure and/or physiological activity. If we wish to be able wisely to address such major failures of moral character, in the law and within the correctional system, we would therefore do well to understand the many dimensions of neural failure that can collectively give rise to them. We can´t fix what we don´t understand.

Moral correction

Consider first the structurally and physiologically *normal* brain whose formative social environment fails to provide a normal moral education. The child´s experience may lack the daily examples of normal moral behavior in others, it may lack opportunities to participate in normal social practices, it may fail to see others deal successfully and routinely with their inevitable social conflicts, and it may lack the normal background of elder sibling and parental correction of its perceptions and its behavior. For the problematic young adult that results, moral correction will obviously consist in the attempt somehow to make up a missed or substandard education.

That can be very difficult. The cognitive plasticity and eagerness to imitate found in children is much reduced in a young adult. And a young adult cannot easily find the kind of tolerant community of innocent peers and wise elders that most children are fortunate to grow up in. Thus, not one but two important windows of opportunity have been missed.

The problem is compounded by the fact that children in the impoverished social environments described do not simply fail to learn. Rather, they may learn quite well, but *what* they learn is a thoroughly twisted set of social and moral prototypes and an accompanying family of skills which – while crudely functional within the impoverished environment that shaped them, perhaps – are positively dysfunctional within the more coherent structure of society at large. This means that the young adult has some substantial unlearning to do. Given the massive cognitive ``inertia´´ characteristic even of normal humans, this makes the corrective slope even steeper, especially when young adult offenders are incarcerated in a closely knit prison community of similarly twisted social agents.

This chapter was not supposed to urge any substantive social or moral policies, but those who do trade in such matters may find relevant the following purely factual issues. The US budget for state and federal prisons is said to be somewhat larger than its budget for *all* of higher education, for its elite research universities, its massive state universities, its myriad liberal arts colleges, and all of its technical colleges and two-year junior colleges combined. It is at least conceivable that this enormous penal-system budget might be more wisely spent on prophylactic policies aimed at raising the quality of the social environment of disadvantaged children, rather than on policies that struggle, against much greater odds, to repair the damage once it is done.

A convulsive shift, of course, is not an option. Whatever else our prisons do or do not do, they keep at least some of the dangerously incompetent social agents and the outright predators off our streets and out of our social commerce. But the plasticity of the young over the old poses a constant invitation to shift our corrective resources childwards, as due prudence dictates. This policy suggestion hopes to reduce the absolute input to our correctional institutions. An equally important issue is how, in advance of such ``utopian´´ advances, to increase the rate at which they are emptied, to which topic I now turn.

A final point, in this regard, about normals. The cognitive plasticity of the young – that is, their unparalleled capacity for learning – is owed to neurochemical and physiological factors that fade with age. (The local production and diffusion of nitric oxide within the brain is one theory of how some synaptic connections are made selectively subject to modification, and there are others.)

Suppose that we were to learn how to *recreate* in young adults, temporarily and by neuropharmacological means, that perfectly normal regime of neural plasticity and learning aptitude found in children. In conjunction with some more effective programs of re-socialization than we currently command (without them, the pharmacology will be a waste of time), this might re-launch the ``disadvantaged normals´´ into something much closer to a normal social trajectory and out of prison for good.

There remain, alas, the genuine abnormals, for whom moral correction is first a matter of trying to repair or compensate for some structural or physiological defect(s) in brain function. Even if these people are hopeless, it will serve social policy to identify them reliably, if only to keep them permanently incarcerated or otherwise out of the social mainstream. But some, at least, will not be hopeless. Where the deficit is biochemical in nature – giving rise to chronically inappropriate emotional profiles, for example – neuropharmacological intervention, in the now familiar form of chronic subdural implants, perhaps, will return some victims to something like a normal neural economy and a normal emotional profile. That will be benefit enough, but they will then also be candidates for the re-socialization techniques imagined earlier for disadvantaged normals.

This discussion presumes far more neurological understanding than we currently possess, and is plain speculative as a result. But it does serve to illustrate some directions in which we might well wish to move, once our early understanding here has matured. In any case, I shall close this discussion by re-emphasizing the universal importance of gradual socialization by long interaction with a moral order already in place. We will never create moral character by medical intervention alone. There are too many trillions of synaptic connections to be appropriately weighted and only long experience can hope to do that superlatively intricate job. The whole point of exploring the technologies mentioned above will be to maximize everyone´s chances of engaging in and profiting from that traditional and irreplaceable process.

Moral diversity

I here refer not to the high-dimensional bell-curve diversity of moral characters within a given culture at a given time, but to the non-identity, across two cultures separated in space and/or in time, of the overall *system* of moral prototypes and prized skills common to most normal members of each. Such major differences in moral consciousness typically reflect differences in substantive economic circumstances between the two cultures, in the peculiar threats to social order with which they have to deal, in the technologies they command, the metaphysical beliefs they happen to hold, and other accidents of history.

Such diversity, when discovered, is often seen as grounds for a blanket scepticism about the objectivity or reality of moral knowledge. That was certainly its effect on me in my later childhood, a reaction reinforced by the astonishingly low level of moral argument I would regularly hear from my more religious schoolchums, and even from the local pulpits. But that is no longer my reaction, for throughout history there have been comparable differences, between distinct cultures, where *scientific* knowledge was concerned, and comparable block-headedness in purely ``factual´´ reasoning (think of ``New Age medicine´´, for example, or ``UFOlogy´´). But this very real diversity and equally lamentable sloppiness does not underwrite a blanket skepticism about the possibility of scientific knowledge.

It merely shows that it is not easy to come by, and that its achievement requires a long-term process of careful and honest evaluation of a wide variety of complex experiments over a substantial range of human experience. Which points to our next topic.

Moral progress

If it exists – and there is some dispute about this – moral progress consists in the slow change and development, over historical periods, of the moral prototypes we teach our children and forcibly impose on derelict adults, a developmental process that is gradually instructed by our collective *experience* of a collective life lived under those perception-shaping and behavior-guiding prototypes.

From the neurocomputational perspective, this process looks different only in its ontological focus – the *social* world as opposed to the *natural* world – from what we are pleased to call *scientific progress*. In the natural sciences as well, achieving adult competence is a matter of acquiring a complex family of perceptual, reflective, and behavioral skills in the relevant field. And there, too, such skills are embodied in an acquired set of structural, dynamical, and manipulational proto-types. The occasional deflationary voice to the contrary, our scientific progress over the centuries is a dramatic and encouraging reality, and it results in part from the myriad instructions (often painful) of an ongoing experimental and technological life lived under those same perception-shaping and behavior-guiding scientific prototypes.

Our conceptual development in the moral domain, I suggest, differs only in detail from our development in the scientific domain. We even have institutions whose job it is continually to fine-tune and occasionally to reshape our conceptions of proper conduct, permissible practice, and proscribed behavior. Civic, state, and federal legislative bodies spring immediately to mind, as does the civil service, and so do the several levels of the judiciary and their ever-evolving bodies of case-law and decision-guiding legal precedents. As with our institutions for empirical science, these socially-focused institutions typically outlive the people who pass through their offices, often by centuries and sometimes by many centuries. And as with the payoff from our sci-entific institutions, the payoff here is the accumulation of unpreced-ented levels of recorded (social) experience, the equilibrating benefits of collective decision making, and the resulting achievement of levels of moral understanding that are unachievable by a single individual in a single lifetime.

To this overarching parallel it may be objected that science addresses the ultimate nature of a fixed, stable, and independent reality, while our social, legislative, and legal institutions address a plastic reality that is deeply dependent on the organizing activity of humans. But this presumptive contrast disappears almost entirely when one sees the acquisition of both scientific and moral wisdom as the acquisition of sets of *skills*. Both address a presumptively implastic part of their respective domains: the basic laws of nature in the former case, and basic human nature in the latter. And both address a pro-foundly *plastic* part of their respective domains: the articulation, manipulation, and technological exploitation of the natural world in the case of working science, and the articulation, manipulation, and practical exploitation of human nature in the case of working morals and politics. A prosperous city represents simultaneous success in both dimensions of human cognitive activity. And the resulting artificial technologies, both natural and social, each make possible a deeper insight into the basic character of the natural universe and of human nature, respectively.

Moral unity/systematicity

This parallel with natural science has a further dimension. Just as progress in science occasionally leads to welcome unifications within our understanding – as when all planetary motions come to be seen as special cases of projectile motion, and all optical phenomena come to be seen as special cases of electromagnetic waves – so also does progress in moral theory bring occasional attempts at conceptual unification, as when our assembled obligations and prohibitions are all presented (by Hobbes) as elements of a *social contract,* or (by Kant) as the local instantiations of a *categorical imperative,* or (by Rawls) as the reflection of *rules rationally chosen from behind a veil of personal ignorance.* These familiar suggestions, and others, are competing attempts to unify and systematize our scattered moral intuitions or antecedent moral understanding, and they bring with them (or hope to bring with them) the same sorts of virtues displayed by intertheoretic reductions in science, namely, greater simplicity in our assembled conceptions, greater consistency in their application, and an enhanced capacity (born of increased generality) for dealing with novel kinds of social and moral problems.

As with earlier aspects of moral cognition, this sort of large-scale cognitive achievement is also comprehensible in neurocomputational terms, and it seems to involve the very same sorts of neurodynamical changes that are (presumptively) involved when theoretical insights occur within the natural sciences. Specifically, a wide range of perceptual phenomena – which (let us suppose) used to activate a large handful of distinct moral prototypes, m_1, m_2, m_3, ..., m_n – come to be processed under a new regime of recurrent manipulation (recall the recurrent neuronal pathways of Figure 7.1b) that results in them all activating an unexpected moral prototype M, a prototype whose typical deployment has hitherto been in other perceptual domains entirely, a prototype that now emerges as a *superordinate* prototype of which the scattered lesser prototypes, m_1, m_2, m_3, ..., m_n can now be seen, retrospectively, as so many subordinate instances.

The preceding is a neural-network description of what happens when, for example, our scattered knowledge in some area becomes *axiomatized.* But axiomatization, in the linguaformal guise typically displayed in textbooks, is but one minor instance of this much more general process, a process that embraces the many forms of non-discursive knowledge as well, a process that embraces science and ethics alike.

Reflections on some recent ``virtue ethics´´

As most philosophers will perceive, the general portrait of moral knowledge that emerges from neural-network models of cognition is a portrait already under active examination within moral philosophy, quite independently of any connections it might have with cognitive neurobiology. Its original champion is Aristotle and its current research community includes figures as intellectually diverse as Mark Johnson (1993), Owen Flanagan (1991), and Alasdair MacIntyre (1981), all of whom came to this general perspective for reasons entirely of their own. For the many reasons outlined in the body of this paper, I am compelled (and honored) to count myself among them. But I am not entirely comfortable in this group, for two of the philosophers just mentioned take a view, on the matter of moral progress, very different from that just outlined. Flanagan (1996) has expressed frank doubts that human moral consciousness ever makes much genuine ``progress´´, and he suggests that its occasional changes are better seen as just a directionless meander made in local response to our changing economic and social environment.

MacIntyre (1981) voices a different but comparably skeptical view, wherein he hankers after the lost innocence of pre-Enlightenment human communities, which were much more tightly knit by a close fabric of shared social practices, which practices provided the sort of highly interactive and mutually dependent environment needed for the many moral virtues to develop and flourish. He positively laments the emergence of the post-Enlightenment, liberal, secular, and comparatively anonymous and independent social lives led by modern industrial humans, since the rich soil necessary for moral learning, he says, has thereby been impoverished. The familiar moral virtues must now be acquired, polished, and exercised in what is, comparatively, a social vacuum. If anything, in the past few centuries we have suffered a moral *regress.*

I disagree with both authors, and will close by outlining why. I begin with MacIntyre, and I begin by conceding his critique of the (British) Enlightenment´s cartoon-like conception of *Homo economicus,* a hedonic calculator almost completely free of any interest in or resources for evaluating the very desires that drive his calculations. I likewise concede his critique of the (Continental) Enlightenment's conception of *pure reason* as the key to identifying a unique set of behavior-guiding rules. And my concessions here are not reluctant. I agree wholeheartedly with MacIntyre that neither conception throws much light on the nature of moral virtue.

But as crude as these moral or meta-moral ideas were, they were still a step up from the even more cartoonlike conceptions of *Homo sheepicus* and *Homo infanticus* relentlessly advanced by the pre-Enlightenment Christian Church. Portraying humanity as sheep guided by a supernatural Shepherd, or as children beholden to a supernatural Father, was an even darker self-deception and was even less likely to serve as a means by which to climb the ladder of moral understanding.

I could be wrong in this blunt assessment, and if I am, so be it. For the claim of the preceding paragraph does *not* embody the truly important argument for moral progress at the hands of the Enlightenment. That argument lies elsewhere. It lies in the permanent opening of a tradition of cautious *tolerance* for a diversity of local communities each bonded by their own fabric of social practices; it lies in the establishment of lasting institutions for the principled *evaluation* of diverse modes of social organization, and for the institutionalized *criticism* of some and the systematic *emulation* of others. It lies, in sum, in the fact that the Enlightenment broke the hold of a calcified moral dictatorship and replaced it with a tradition that was finally prepared to learn from its deliberately broad experience and its inevitable mistakes in first-order moral policy.

Once again, I am appealing to a salient parallel. The virtue of the Enlightenment, in the moral sphere, was precisely the same virtue displayed in the scientific sphere, namely, the legitimation of responsible theoretical diversity and the establishment of lasting institutions for its critical evaluation and positive exploitation. It is this long-term process, rather than any particular moral theory or moral practice that might fleetingly engage its attention, that marks the primary achievement of the Enlightenment.

MacIntyre began his Introduction to *After Virtue* with a thought-provoking science fiction scenario about the loss of an intricate practical tradition that alone gives life to its corresponding family of theoretical terms, and the relative barrenness of their continued use in the absence of that sustaining tradition. This embodies the essentials of his critique of our moral history since the Enlightenment. But we can easily construct, for critical evaluation, a parallel critique of our *scientific* history since the same period, and that parallel, I suggest, throws some welcome light on MacIntyre's rather conservative perspective.

Consider the heyday of Aristotelian Science, from the fourth century BC to the seventeenth century AD (even longer than the Christian domination of the moral sphere), and consider the close-knit and unifying set of intellectual and technological practices that it sustained. There is the medical tradition running from Rome's Galen to the four Humors of the late medieval doctors. There is the astronomical/astrological tradition that extends through Alexandria's Ptolemy to Prague's Johannes Kepler, who was still casting horoscopes for the wealthy despite his apostate theorizing. There is the intricate set of industrial practices maintained by the alchemists from the Alexandrian Greeks to seventeenth century Europe, which tradition simply owned the vital practices of metallurgy and metal-working, and of dyemaking and medicinal manufacture as well. These three traditions, and others that space bids me pass over, were closely linked by daily practice as well as by conceptual ancestry, and they formed a consistent and coherent environment in which the practical and technological virtues of late antiquity could flourish. As they did. MacIntyre's first condition is met.

So is his second, for this close-knit ``paradise'' is well and truly lost, having been displaced by a hornet's nest of distinct sciences, sciences as diverse as astrophysics, molecular biology, anthropology, electrical engineering, solid-state physics, immunology, and thermodynamic meteorology. Modern science now addresses and advances on so many fronts that the research practice of individual scientists and the technological practice of individual engineers is increasingly isolated from all but the most immediate members of their local cognitive communities. And the cognitive virtues they display are similarly fragmented. They may even find it difficult to talk to each other.

You see where I am going. There may well be problems – real problems – arising from the unprecedented flourishing of the many modern sciences, but losing an earlier and somehow more healthy ``golden age'' is certainly not one of them. Though real, those problems are simply the price that humanity pays for growing up, and we already attempt to address them by way of interdisciplinary curricula, interdisciplinary conferences and anthologies, and by the never-ending search for explanatory unifications and intertheoretic reductions.

I propose, for MacIntyre's reflection, a parallel claim for our moral, political, and legal institutions since the Enlightenment.

Undoubtedly there are problems emerging from the unprecedented flourishing of the many modern industrial societies and their sub-societies, but losing touch with a prior golden age is not obviously one of them. The very real problems posed by moral and political diversity are simply the price that humanity pays for growing up. And as in the case of the scattered sciences, we already attempt to address them by constant legislative tinkering, by the reality-driven evolution of pre-cedents in the judicial record, by tolerating the occasional political ``divorce´´ (e.g. Yugoslavia, the Soviet Union, the Scottish Parliament), and by the never-ending search for legal, political, and economic uni-fications. Next to the discovery of fire and the polydoctrinal example of ancient Greece, the Enlightenment may be the best thing that ever happened to us.

The doctrinal analog of MacIntyre´s implicit Communitarianism in moral theory is a hyperbolic form of Kuhnian conservatism in the philosophy of science, a conservativism that values the (very real) virtues of any given ``normal science´´ tradition (such as Ptolemaic astronomy, classical thermodynamics, or Newtonian mechanics) over the com-paratively fragile institutions of collective evaluation, comparison, and criticism that might slowly force their hidden vices into the sunlight and pave the way for their rightful overthrow at the hands of even more promising modes of cognitive organization. One can certainly see Kuhn´s basic ``communitarian´´ point: stable scientific practices make many valuable things possible. But tolerant institutions for the evalu-ation and modification of those practices make even *more* valuable things possible – most obviously, new and more stable practices.

This particular defense of the Enlightenment also lays the foundation for my response to Flanagan´s quite different form of skepticism. As I view matters from the neural-network perspective explained earlier in this essay, I can find no difference in the pre-sumptive brain mechanisms and cognitive processes that underwrite moral cognition and scientific cognition. Nor can I find any significant differences in the respective social institutions that administer our unfolding scientific and moral consciousness, respectively. In both cases, learning from experience is the perfectly normal outcome of both the neural and the social machinery. That means that moral progress is no less possible and no less likely than scientific progress. And since none of us, at this moment, is being shown the instruments of torture in the Vatican´s basement, I suggest it is actual as well.

There remains the residual issue of whether the *sciences* make genuine progress, but that issue I leave for another time. The take-home claims of the present essay are that (1) whatever their ultimate status, moral and scientific cognition are on an *equal* footing, since they use the same neural mechanisms, show the same dynamical profile, and respond in both the short and the long term to similar empirical pressures; and (2) in both moral and scientific learning, the fundamental cognitive achievement is the acquisition of *skills,* as embodied in the finely tuned configuration of the brain's 10^{14} synaptic connections.

REFERENCES

Adolphs, R., Tranel, D., Bechara, A., Damasio, H. & Damasio, A. R. 1996. Neuropsychological approaches to reasoning and decision making. In A. R. Damasio *et al.* (eds.), *The Neurobiology of Decision-Making.* Berlin: Springer-Verlag, pp. 157–80.

Bechara, A., Damasio, A., Damasio, H. & Anderson, S. W. 1994. Insensitivity to future consequences following damage to human prefrontal cortex. *Cognition* **50**: 7–15.

Churchland, P. M. 1989a. *A Neurocomputational Perspective: The Nature of Mind and the Structure of Science.* Cambridge MA: The MIT Press.

Churchland, P. M. 1989b. On the nature of theories: a neurocomputational perspective. In W. Savage (ed.) *Scientific Theories: Minnesota Studies in the Philosophy of Science*, Vol. 14. Minneapolis, MN: University of Minnesota Press, pp. 59–101.

Churchland, P. M. 1989c. On the nature of explanation: a PDP approach. In Churchland, P. M. (ed.) *A Neurocomputational Perspective: The Nature of Mind and the Structure of Science.* Cambridge, MA: The MIT Press, Chapter 10. (Reprinted in J. Misiek (ed.) 1995. *Rationality,* Vol. 175 of *Boston Studies in the Philosophy of Science.* Dordrecht: Kluwer.)

Churchland, P. M. 1989d. Learning and conceptual change. In Churchland, P. M. (ed.) *A Neurocomputational Perspective: The Nature of Mind and the structure of science.* Cambridge, MA: The MIT Press, Chapter 11.

Churchland, P. M. 1995. *The Engine of Reason, The Seat of the Soul: A Philosophical Journey into the Brain.* Cambridge, MA: The MIT Press.

Cottrell, G. 1991. Extracting features from faces using compression networks: face, identity, emotions and gender recognition using holons. In Touretzky, D., Elman, J., Sejnowski, T. & Hinton, G. (eds.) *Connectionist Models: Proceedings of the 1990 Summer School.* San Mateo, CA: Morgan Kaufmann, pp. 328–37.

Damasio, A. R. 1994. *Descartes' Error.* New York: Putnam & Sons.

Damasio, A. R., Tranel, D. & Damasio, H. 1991. Somatic markers and the guidance of behavior. In Levin, H. *et al.* (eds.) *Frontal Lobe Function and Dysfunction.* New York: Oxford University Press, pp. 217–29.

Elman, J. L. 1992. Grammatical structure and distributed representations. In Davis, S. (ed.) *Connectionism: Theory and Practice. Vancouver Studies in Cognitive Science*, vol. 3. Oxford: Oxford University Press.

Flanagan, O. 1991. *Varieties of Moral Personality: Ethics and Psychological Realism.* Cambridge, MA: Harvard University Press.

Flanagan, O. 1996. The moral network. In McCauley, B. (ed.) *The Churchlands and Their Critics.* Cambridge, MA: Blackwell, pp. 192–215.

Gorman, R.P. & Sejnowski, T.J. 1988. Analysis of hidden units in a layered network trained to classify sonar targets. *Neural Networks* **1**: 75–89.

Johnson, M. 1993. *Moral Imagination*. Chicago, IL: Chicago University Press.

Lehky, S. & Sejnowski, T.J. 1988. Network model of shape from shading: neuronal function arises from both receptive and projective fields. *Nature* **333**: 452–54.

Lehky, S. & Sejnowski, T.J. 1990. Neural network model of visual cortex for determing surface curvature from images of shaded surfaces. *Proceedings of the Royal Society of London* **B240**: 251–78.

Lockery, S.R., Fang, Y. & Sejnowski, T.J. 1991. A dynamical neural network model of sensorimotor transformation in the leech. *Neural Computation* **2**: 274–82.

MacIntyre, A. 1981. *After Virtue*. Notre Dame, CA: University of Notre Dame Press.

Rosenberg, C.R. & Sejnowski, T.J. 1987, Parallel networks that learn to pronounce English text. *Complex Systems* **1**: 145–68.

Saver, J.L. & Damasio, A.R. 1991. Preserved access and processing of social knowledge in a patient with acquired sociopathy due to ventromedial frontal damage. *Neuropsychologia* **29**: 1241–9.

8

From a neurophilosophy of pain to a neuroethics of pain care

J. J. GIORDANO

Every sentient being knows what is meant by pain, but the true significance of pain eludes the most sapient. For philosophers, pain is a problem of metaphysics ... for clinicians a symptom to be understood and an ill to be relieved.

C. F. Illingworth (1941)

THE NEUROSCIENCE AND NEUROPHENOMENOLOGY OF PAIN

The problem of pain

If the profession and practices of pain therapeutics are to be focally dedicated to right and good care of those in pain, then it is imperative to (1) pursue knowledge of the mechanisms and effects of the disorder that has rendered them to be patients, and (2) recognize and acknowledge that the uniqueness of pain as sensation and experience is inextricably bound to these neural event(s) (Giordano 2006). In this chapter I argue that these facts establish the progressive epistemological basis for a neurophilosophy of pain that both informs and sustains the direction for ongoing research, and gives rise to a neuroethics of pain care.

Some forty-seven years ago, British scientist and novelist C. P. Snow described what he believed was a deeply entrenched, widening rift between the ``two cultures´´ of modern society: the sciences and the humanities (Snow 1959). Yet, one of the most significant

Scientific and Philosophical Perspectives in Neuroethics, ed. J. J. Giordano & B. Gordijn. Published by Cambridge University Press. © Cambridge University Press 2010.

accomplishments of contemporary neuroscience has been to make ardent strides toward what biologist E. O. Wilson calls consilience: "... a jumping together of knowledge by the linking of facts and fact-based theory across disciplines to create a common groundwork for explanation". (Wilson 1998). Wilson speaks to the unity of purpose for both philosophy and science, and addresses how such intellectual fusion (albeit from divergent perspectives) has reconciled particular dialectics and expanded the perspectives both within and between fields. I agree with Wilson, and believe that the relation of science and the humanities is not new, novel, nor insanable. Philosophical questions have classically provided the impetus and initiative direction for much of scientific study, and reciprocally, scientific discovery has afforded information that has not simply answered, but frequently furthered philosophical inquiry. Recent advances in the ever-growing disciplines that are nested within the rubric of neuroscience (and/or perhaps more accurately, neurophilosophy) reflect an intellectual inertia that has allowed a broader, more comprehensive and philosophical approach to studying the brain, mind, and pain. Science and philosophy become ever more consilient as we continue to ponder the question of "what is pain?"

The apparent simplicity of this question veils the fact that there is not a singular answer, for pain is inveterately complicated. It is a physiological event, subtended by distinct systems in the peripheral and central nervous systems in response to insult or injury, or as an independent, distinct pathology. At the same time, it is a psychological event, evoked by the co-activation of neural systems that are involved in cognition, emotion, and behaviors (Chapman 2005; see also Varela *et al.* 1991). This neuropsychological foundation instills pain as an event of phenomenal conscious processes, reflecting alteration of the perceived internal dimensionality of the lived-body that is construed as the "self". Attempts at explaining the neural event of pain cannot ignore the experiential dimension(s), and any description of the phenomenal embodiment of pain must account for the role of brain–mind in consciousness.

Thus, any meaningful definition of pain must infer both scientific explanation and subjective understanding. But in many ways our approach(es) to the study of pain are bounded by "the hermeneutic circle": to understand the parts requires an understanding of the whole, yet the whole cannot be understood without knowledge of its constituent parts (Palmer 1969). In addition, knowledge of pain is limited by problems of understanding and explanation: what is sub-jectively understood cannot be directly explained, and what can be explained does not directly reflect that which is subjectively under-stood (Jaspers 1963).[1] Pain is subjective, and while we may have knowledge of the neural mechanisms and systems that are involved in pain transmission, third-person assessment does not allow apprehen-sion of what pain ``feels like´´, and hence the discernment, differenti-ation, and diagnosis of particular pain syndromes is reliant, in a large part, upon the meaningful combination of objective data with some type(s) of first-person information obtained from the patient.

The heuristic value of the neuroscience of pain

Through contributions from various disciplines (e.g. biology, chemistry, psychology, physics, philosophy) and advances in genomic, molecular, physiologic, and imaging technologies, contemporary neuroscience has resolved prior peripheralist–centralist and cell-reticularist arguments, and shown pain to involve mechanisms of both the peripheral and central nervous systems functioning as a complex, networked hierarchy (Giordano 2008a).[2] Older, somewhat esoteric, temporal classifications of pain have given way to more detailed etiologic and nosologic taxon-omies that reflect the involvement of heterogeneous molecular and anatomical substrates (Woolf & Max 1994).[3] I posit that pain may be considered as something of a spectrum disorder, with differential expression reflecting dynamical, complex-systems effects that interact from the genomic to the populational levels. The elucidation of genetic elements capable of establishing definable endo- and exo-phenotypes that may subserve particular pain syndromes strengthens this hypoth-esis (Mogil et al. 2000; see also Mogil 1999). Furthermore, it may be that such geno- and phenotypes variably exist,[4] may be related to the (co-)

---

[1] For further discussion and distinction of the concepts of understanding (*Verstehen*) and explanation (*Erklarung*), see also Appel (1988).

[2] Excellent discussion of these reconciliations within an expanded conceptualization of pain can be found in Harcastle (1999).

[3] For an overview of older classification schemes of pain, see Merskey & Bogduk (1994).

[4] Perhaps as balanced polymorphisms within populations and communities, as constituents of larger ``families´´ of genetic polymorphisms that are capable of co-expressing sensitivities to pain and/or molecular pathologies that contribute to types of pain and other CNS dysfunction(s) as spectrum disorders. See Turk et al. (1987); Lander & Schnork (1994); Tisch & Merikangas (1996).

morbidity of other CNS and non-neural characteristics and disorders, and explain, to some extent, particular (individual, familial, and/or community) patterns of susceptibility to chronic pain and co-terminal syndromes (e.g. depression, anxiety, etc.).

These variations may establish bases for potential changes in neural function and (micro and macro)structure that (1) fortify the algesic neuraxis; (2) de-construct non-linear, adaptive pain-modulating networks; (3) incur progressive, aberrant linearity within pain-transmitting pathways; and (4) ultimately produce alteration(s) at higher loci to more broadly affect hierarchical network processes within multiple substrates of the core neural structures of conscious process(es).(Giordano 2005; see also Katchalsky *et al.* 1974; Posner & Dehaene 1994; Kelso 1995). Thus, the neural events of persistent pain can induce changes at intermediate levels of the cognitive neuraxis to affect the experience of self and the lived body (i.e. *consciousness of* the body in pain), as well as incur more pervasive changes at lower and higher levels of cognitive function to affect apperception and awareness (i.e. the *state of consciousness* that contributes to the feeling(s) of ``being''). In this way, the pathology of pain can alter the brain to affect ``mind''.[5]

There is evidence from recent imaging studies to support the neuroanatomical basis of such a conceptualization (Peyron *et al.* 2000; Casey & Bushnell 2000; Flor & Bushnell 2005–17).[6] But, while it is tempting to turn to technology to depict ``how'' pain affects the brain, and ``where'' such effects occur, it is erroneous to assume that a given anatomical structure creates a particular function, as this reflects what Bennett and Hacker have called the ``mereological fallacy'' of attributing the function of the whole (i.e. the brain–mind, as well as the embodied conscious ``self'') to a specific part (i.e. a given anatomical locus or structure) (Bennett & Hackett 2003). More appropriately, while various neuroanatomic regions may contribute to the assemblage that is the functional network (of local and distant neuronal and glial effects) of the brain–mind, it is the focussed engagement of a particular

---

[5] The concept of consciousness as the parallel and/or serial processing of neural inputs within a hierarchical core of neural assemblies is addressed by Prinz (2004); see also Jackendoff (1987).

[6] Although it should be noted that neuroimaging is not without criticisms, not least of which are (1) improper discriminability of signal: noise ratios through disproportionate establishment of the selective Gaussian kernel that does not allow for depiction of ``real'' neuronal network activation, and (2) the more general concern of assigning attributes to the consequential. For detailed discussion of these concerns and criticisms, see Chapters 11 and 12, this volume.

neural work space or dynamical core that actually produces the sensations, cognitions, emotions, and behaviors of any event, including pain (Baars 2002; Edelman 2004; see also Llinas 1998). Thus, no single site or locus produces ``pain´´ per se, but rather the ``feeling of pain´´ reflects the vectored activity within some myriad combination of microcircuits within somewhat larger regional anatomic components of a networked ``whole´´ (namely, the body–brain–mind), and thus the experience of pain (as any other) is potentially (and most likely) unique to each individual. Given this uniqueness, the adage that ``. . . no two pains are exactly alike´´, while trite, actually bespeaks a profound truth with regard to pain as acute event, as a self-sustaining, neuropatholo-gical process, and ultimately as manifest subjective illness.

Maldynia: neuropathology expressed as the subjective illness of pain

The term *maldynia* was proposed by Lippe to reflect the ``abnormality´´ of neuropathic pain (1998). But the concept of abnormality in this condition is relative, for as the algesic system undergoes plastic change (s), these then become ``normalized´´ as distinctly new parameters and patterns of function (Slater & Woolf 2005). If we regard pain as a spectrum disorder, then at the extreme of such a spectrum, pre-dis-positional factors would sustain the pathologic process(es) of pain to engage (and perhaps alter) the neuraxis and express illness. In this light, I have proposed that maldynia be reconsidered to be the multi-dimensional constellation of symptoms and signs that represent the syndrome of persistent pain as phenomenal illness (Giordano 2005, 2008c). Clearly, multiple biological and psychosocial factors contribute to, and are affected by maldynic pain. Given that (1) maldynia induces functional and structural changes in the neurological axis from per-iphery to brain; (2) there are distinct regions in the brain that are responsible for the conditions and awareness of this network as a discriminable internal dimensionality; and (3) maldynia-induced changes in these brain regions are capable of evoking alteration of the sensed internal state that is consciousness, I posit that maldynia is a disorder of the body–brain that (directly or indirectly) affects the expressed embodied ``mind´´. In this way, maldynia is both the conscious *state of* pain, and a consciousness *of* pain as a condition of the internal domain of the lived body and first-person identifiable ``self´´.

This approach grounds maldynia to hierarchical neural event(s) evoked by successively engaged mechanisms of pain. It also allows for, and in fact may instigate philosophical speculation upon, whether pain is a state, and/or is a conscious representation of that state. This is attractive because it (1) establishes a physiological and anatomical basis of pain, and (2) validates the experience of pain as a neurobiological event, thereby making it resonant with the epistemology of much of contemporary medicine. Still, any neurobiological consideration of pain will confront the ``hard question´´, namely the epistemological gap(s) involved in explaining the process(es) by which mind is evoked from brain. In addition, bodies, brains, minds, and ``selves´´ are engaged by and expressed within various sociocultural environments. Thus, a naturalistic orientation to the problem, event, and experience of pain must account for biopsychosocial dimensions. This prompts the question of whether the illness of pain can be knowable through solely objective means (Giordano 2005, 2006a, 2008c). Given that the neurobiological substrates of pain are in some way foundational to consciousness, and consciousness is transparent only in the first person, then it is obvious that some form of contextual, inter-subjective knowledge must be necessary to truly afford the clinician an understanding of the unique nature of pain and suffering of an ``other´´ – at least at this point in time, given the capacities and limitations of extant neurotechnology.

The value of integrative pain research

Comprehending the complexity of maldynic pain involves both scientific and humanistic inquiry and is fundamental to the provision of technically right and morally good care (Giordano 2006). Research sustains the knowledge base that both informs clinical therapeutics and initiates policy. I have previously argued, and re-iterate here, that *what* we learn about pain should direct *how* we study pain, and *how* pain studies are conducted may provide critical insight(s) to new types and domains of knowledge (Giordano 2004, 2006c). Thus, if we re-conceptualize pain as a spectrum disorder that exists along a continuum of disease and illness affecting body, brain, and mind, we must recognize that neurobiological functions can affect and be affected by both internal and external environments, and any study of the body–brain–mind must acknowledge the manifestation(s) of such effects, ``. . . from synapses to social groups´´ (Rees 2004), and be committed to methods that allow such inquiry. These methods must be valid, reliable, elucidative, applicable, and time- and cost-effective, as (1) research serves and fulfills a public good, and (2) supportive resources are not without limits and therefore should not be frivolously utilized. Scientific philosophy dictates paradigmatic self-evaluation, self-criticism, and self-revision so as to be anti-dogmatic (Bechtel 1988). It is important to assess whether current research methods and protocols effectively address the problem of pain in light of our contemporary knowledge of the relationship(s) between body, brain, and mind, and selves, others, and the environment.

Such knowledge provides the epistemic grounding, and compels a more thorough consideration of the philosophical and practical basis of pain and pain care, for it provides a mechanistic and phenomenal explanation of pain. This knowledge is both heuristic and allows a hermeneutic approach – relating explanatory constructs to the understood experience. This epistemic foundation undergirds the anthropologic and ethical dimensions of pain care: if we appreciate the fact of pain as neural mechanism, sensation, psychological event(s), and phenomenal experience, then we must objectively acknowledge its intrinsic, subjective harm, and be dedicated to effective compassionate care as a core moral obligation.

THE LIMITATIONS OF NEUROSCIENCE

... Nature is only showing us the tail of the lion, but I have no doubt that the lion belongs to it even though, because of its large size, it cannot totally reveal itself all at once ...

Albert Einstein (2000)

Implications for a neurophilosophy of pain

An enhanced understanding of neuroscience together with a broadened concept of ``mind´´ has instigated pragmatic and ethical concerns about the experience of pain (Giordano 2008c). Clearly, such concerns must account for both the neural process of pain, and its proximate and more durable effects – as neural event and cognitive and emotional experience – that occur in painient beings existing within particular environments, communities, and cultures (Morris 1998). The newly popular phrase of ``... see one brain, see *one* brain´´ would thereby suggest the improbability, if not impossibility, of the colloquialism ``... I feel your pain´´ as it is likely that the sensation and experience of pain are individually variant, subjective, and in reality, knowable only to the one who suffers. In essence, we cannot ``feel´´ another´s pain any more than we can know what it is like to be another being (Nagel 1979). Rather, we can only recognize or know others´ experiences in relation to our own subjectivity (Dilthey 1990; Grondin 1995). We do this through (1) objectifying others' experiences by applying intellectual knowledge of common processes that are equivalent or similar in ourselves and others (i.e. phenomenological relativism), (2) perception of some set of knowable reactions, responses, and/or semiotics, and/or (3) the direct explanation of subjective experience(s) by others. This makes pain assessment pragmatically and morally difficult in those situations in which linguistic and/or communicative barriers exist, such as between cultures; when dealing with patients who are profoundly mentally impaired, demented, or obtunded; when dealing with animals; and/or when considering the possibility of pain and suffering in non-organic, ``artificially intelligent'' entities.

Knowledge of the development, structure, and function of the systems that mediate pain and analgesia is vital, but it is equally important to recognize the boundaries of objective information, and what this infers about the uncertainty of others' subjective experience. The imperative to evaluate and treat pain and suffering has been a major incentive for the development of new medical techniques and technologies (Giordano 2008d). Perhaps neurotechnology will one day allow the completely objective assessment of pain (and its experience). To date, however, this has not been the case, and even if this were possible, we still must confront the limitations, burdens, and risks – along with the benefits – of any technologic advance, and the information it may deliver (Jonas 1985).

Current neuroscience informs that the relationships of body, brain, mind, and self are not linear or wholly deterministic, and this expanding epistemologic framework may be the basis of a new (neuro) philosophy of pain that more clearly defines what pain is, and what such definitions of pain mean with regard to our conduct toward both human and non-human others. An iterative understanding of the structure and function of various organisms' nervous systems (and of the human organism at various stages and states of existence) allows – or perhaps more accurately dictates – consideration that particular organisms can, and likely do feel pain (Niebroj *et al.* 2008). Given that pain cannot be directly assessed solely through objective means, in the absence of subjective reports and descriptions, the fact that an organism has the *capacity* to feel pain must both satisfice our belief *that* they experience pain, and guide our treatment of such (potential for) pain and suffering with some strong measure of precaution. This would base pain care upon a naturalistic (neuro)philosophy that is built upon the most current epistemic capital, and acknowledges the experience of pain as one of the most elemental qualities of anthropological and ethical concern.

For now, perhaps, this may be enough to compel an overarching obligation to treat pain. Yet, if the core incentive of neuroscientific inquiry is not simply knowledge ``for knowledge's sake,'' but the acquisition of knowledge that can be applied toward the achievement of an identifiable, humanitarian purpose, then moral consideration is required to determine not just ``why'' but ``how'' care for those in pain must be rendered so as to enact individual and social good (Niebroj et al. 2008).

TOWARD A NEUROETHICS OF PAIN CARE

Purpose and potential

> ``... analysis makes for unity, but not necessarily goodness ...''
>
> Sigmund Freud (1966)

This speaks to the need for an ethics that both reflects, and is directly relevant to the current neuroscience of pain, acknowledgment, and appreciation of the sentient being in pain, effects of cultural value(s), and the nature of healing; in other words, a neuroethics of pain care that is consistent with both of its major ``traditions'', so as to consider (1) the neural bases for and of moral decision-making, and (2) the moral basis and ethics of neuroscientific research, applications, and related practice(s). We have posited that there is a certain deontic framework that defines the profession of pain medicine, which is built upon and shaped by the facts of pain, realities of medicine, and its practical and moral claims (Maricich & Giordano 2007). But such rules cannot, and do not, provide the answers for each and every dilemma in all situations.

A number of ethical issues arise at the intersection of neuroscience, pain, medicine, and society. For example, the principle of respect for autonomy has played a central role in much of contemporary bioethical thought, based upon varying constructs of the ``self'' (Miller 2004). In the strictest sense, autonomy can be understood to be (1) a particular kind of potentiality of being, (2) the ability of such a being to make independent decisions and actions, and (3) the negative right of refusal (Kant 1963). Autonomy in the first sense (i.e. a being as an autonomous moral subject) is in some ways related to the manifestations of a being's independent decisions, and actions (Niebroj et al. 2008).

But who (or what) is a moral subject? What of those circumstances in which the level of neural function makes a being unable to act autonomously? This often occurs because of individuals' immaturity (e.g. neonates, young children), not being fully conscious, or being mentally impaired. Very often, these individuals also cannot express their sentience or pain. Because of this, should we not regard pain in the very young, the very old, and the very sick? And what of non-human pain? Probably, like never before, an understanding of animal nervous systems has allowed a consideration of the possibility of pain equivalence in animals, if not of animal minds more broadly, and this latter possibility has initiated dispute about previously held notions of consciousness, mentation, autonomy, and moral value (Sorabji 1993; Radner & Radner 1996; Ryder 1989).

If this neuroscientifically informed epistemology is to be applicable to, and engage, the philosophical domains of anthropology and ethics, we must also recognize that our relationships to any and all other (human and even non-human) beings are not uniform (Kant 1998). While we are learning more about the relative capacities of other brains and other minds, asymmetries still exist in our relationships with others based upon their ability to exert autonomous action, level of dependence, and vulnerabilities, and there has been a renewed call to acknowledge this relational asymmetry and tend to those who are vulnerable (Ving 1993). In this way, the moral imperative to treat pain and alleviate suffering is not directed at pain as an object, but rather can be seen as a regard for the impact and effects of pain upon a sentient being who is the subject of our respect (Schweitzer 1936; Ryder 2001). Clearly, the heightened vulnerability of the pre-nate, neonate, young, infirm, obtunded/vegetative, and aged (as well as non-human sentient beings) strengthens our responsibility for their care.

Such respect reflects a reverence for the experience and value of life in both oneself and others (Woodruff 2002) and has been seen as a fundamental characteristic of medicine (Giordano & Pedroni 2007). In upholding a regard for the ``power of nature, enigma of life, health, pain, [and] suffering'' it provides a basis to appreciate both what has the potential to harm, as well as what is good, and thereby ``directs . . . good intentions and actions'' (Schweitzer 1936). It is this latter dimension of reverence that guides beneficence (Giordano 2006c).

When enacted within pain care – as a medical profession – such beneficence entails striving toward the ends of providing right and ``good'' treatment to patients (Pellegrino 1999; Giordano 2006b). I argue that if pain medicine – as a practice – is to be authentic, it requires knowledge of (1) the brain–mind, (2) the pathology of pain, (3) available treatments that could possibly mitigate the harm(s) incurred by pain, and (4) the being who is the pain patient, so as to discern (a) the nature and extent of such harms, (b) the relative and appropriate ``goodness´´ of potential interventions, in order to (c) determine what care can and should be provided (Giordano & Schatman 2008).

Still, defining what is ``good´´ in a pluralized population can be problematic, and becomes ever more so given the imperative to establish a framework for ethically sound, globalized pain care (UNESCO 2008). The diversity of patients´ and physicians´ values, various exigencies, and general uncertainties that are the reality of the medical relationship and clinical encounter are such that rarely (if ever) do circumstances allow for consideration – or use – of a simple definition of the good, or any given principle with ``all things being equal´´ (Clouser & Gert 1999). Such discord is often directly related to the scope of the social sphere in which health care is provided. Characteristically, the larger the recipient population, the greater the potential and likelihood for the diversity of circumstance(s), values, and dissonance in such values (Herskovits 1973).

Neuroethical questions and issues in pain care

> ... man was not born to solve the problems of the universe, but to put his finger on the problem and then keep within the limits of the comprehensible ...
>
> Johann Wolfgang von Goethe (1966)

Considering the nature of the ``good´´ of pain care in neurocentric contexts gives rise to several fundamental questions. For example, is there some threshold of pain and suffering that can or should be validated in order to incur and/or justify clinical intervention? At what point does the treatment of pain and suffering become ``excessive´´ and would such intervention be considered ``enhancement´´? Can neuroscience contribute this metric or rule? To what level(s) might we take diagnostics and therapeutics? Given the capacities and limitations of neuroimaging (e.g. fMR, fNIR, PET, SPECT, mEEG, etc.) what can we realistically expect this technology to yield in pain medicine, and how can we employ these methods so as to avoid (1) the mereological fallacy (Bennett & Hacker 2003), (2) the error of attributing antecedents to the consequential (Uttal 2003; Illes 2003; see also Chapter 12, this volume), and/or (3) being seduced into the lure of what Ludwig Wittgenstein referred to as ``picture thinking´´ (Wittgenstein 1958, 1961)?

Similarly, we must be cautious when employing neurogenetic information to diagnose the pre-disposition or likelihood of pain syndromes, so as to (1) avoid over-simplification of genotype–phenotype–disorder relationships; (2) assume full responsibility to use this information equitably and with appropriate confidentiality in order to prevent social, economic, and/or vocational stigmatization, and disproportionate under-allocation of insurance benefits; and (3) address the problems that arise when diagnosing disorders that cannot be cured.

In addition, we must confront the crucial questions of neural stem cell research (Kass 2004), and the use of stem cells in pain medicine. However, the stem cell debate is but one of the contentious issues that surround the possible trajectories of neural transplantation (Freed 1999; see also Chapter 9, this volume). While human–human and animal–human (i.e. xenograft) transplantation techniques and technologies may offer considerable promise for generating and remodeling new neural pathways, we must ask what extent of new tissue is required to affect the entirety of the neural network (that might constitute operational definitions of mind and self). The use of exogenous material to restore or repair neural function is not limited to living tissue, and we must also examine the benefits, difficulties, and problems that arise from the direct interface of technology and human neural systems (e.g. transcranial magnetic stimulation, implanted bioelectric devices, nano-neurotechnology), and the iterative ``cyborgization´´ of the human body. While such notions of cyborgization have traditionally been viewed as the stuff of science fiction, Francis Fukuyama (2002) and Chris Gray (2001) note that biologically relevant machines have already become the norm throughout many domains of society, and Moore´s theorem (namely the advancement of technologies that are based upon the multiplication of computer-based applications and derivatives) predicts this machine interfacing to progress with fluidity and rapidity. These developments are influenced by a number of social forces, including various political and economic climates, often providing both the inertia, and steering imperatives for patterns of use and/or misuse. How shall we regulate which developments should be utilized and which should not? Just because we might be able to obliterate pain, should we, or might we regard some forms of pain as a means toward ``existential gain´´, and if so, what forms, for whom, and who decides? In other words, how might and should we determine what pains are to be treated and which are not? And what of justice; how, and to whom shall these new and novel developments in pain treatment be provided? For sure, each and all of these questions contribute to the problematic nature of pain care (Giordano 2008b), give rise to variable social possibilities, and could incur both utopian and dystopian manifestations (Gordijn 2005).

CONCLUSION

Proceeding with prudence

... virtue in itself is not enough; there must also be the power to translate it into action.

Aristotle (1944)

It may be that neuroethics provides a viable meta-construct for pain care – providing illustration of the facts and possibilities, as well as grounding moral decisions to a naturalistic regard for neural mechanisms involved in moral cogitation, sentience, self-reflection, and the experience of pain. This neuroethics would need to acknowledge the uniquity of the individual, and must take into accord the process(es) by which cognition and emotions contribute to pain, and to moral constructs and actions.

As applied to pain care it would need to address at least three core questions: First, how does pain affect the experience and existence of the painient? Second, is this effect significant enough to warrant some form of (mitigating) action or intervention? Third, how can and should such pain be treated? While the first and second question may have ``evolved´´ from an objective appreciation of neuroscience and contemporary re-appraisal of consciousness, sentience, and painience in humans and non-humans, the third speaks to the need to utilize this information in ways that allow for accurate evaluation of the potential goods, burdens or harms that might be incurred by treating or non-treating pain in particular ways.

Obviously, no single dimension of knowledge or skill can or will afford universal answers or abilities. I have previously opined, and re-state here, that an agent-based ethics that is critically reliant upon the virtue of practical wisdom may be most functionally viable (Giordano & Schatman 2008; Giordano 2007), not because other ethical systems are invalid, but rather because it comports well with our current understanding of neural mechanisms of decision-making and social interaction (Casebeer 2003). If nothing else, practical wisdom must strive to be ``operationally beneficent´´, taking into accord relational asymmetry, and an appreciation for the phenomenal experience of others.

Frankena's conceptualization of multi-leveled beneficence (ranging from the obligatory to the supererogatory, and from the individual to social) (Frankena 1982), coupled to Pellegrino and Thomasma's description of how the acts of medicine affect the multidimensional flourishing of each patient as a moral agent (Pellegrino & Thomasma 1987), allows for a broader, more useful understanding of ``good'', and how it could and should be enacted (within both pain medicine and societies). This beneficence (1) encompasses non-harm through a reverent regard for each sentient and painient individual, and thereby (2) affords respect for each individual's agency, autonomy, intrinsic worth, and environmental and sociocultural nestedness.

Such consideration would compel the prudent use of the most current scientific knowledge together with an enhanced humanitarian regard for the one in pain so as to guide the need for, and provision of safe, effective, and equitable pain care. Ultimately, pain care – like other forms of medicine – is a science of probabilities that in many ways remains a hermeneutic exercise. Just as any single type of knowledge cannot completely serve these functions, the use of a single ethical approach could be equally constraining. Thus, a neuroethics of pain care may need to ``paint from a broader palette'' requiring a more integrative approach that allows – if not obligates – alignment of facts, social values, and moral attitudes in an ongoing process of re-investigation, analysis, and revision of what we know and don't know about brains, minds, and selves, and how we regard and treat the painient. In its naturalizing quality, a neuroethics of pain care may achieve a relatively balanced equilibrium, as it would tend to reflect the relatedness of science, philosophy, and ethics, such that science depends upon philosophy to provide perdurable questions of ethical import, and ethics depends upon the sciences for information about how – and upon which – moral judgments can best be made (Baggini & Fosl 2007).

To be sure, the questions and issues that have arisen in the study and treatment of pain do not have readily facile answers. Nor is it likely that the questions or answers will get any simpler or easier as we forge ahead at the frontiers of neurotechnology, and extend the boundaries of understanding. In light of this, it becomes evident that both neuroethics and pain medicine must rely upon new scientific information and knowledge, meet the challenges posed by advances in scientific understanding and technology, and work to address the ever-widening and -deepening questions, issues, and imperatives that these developments are likely to generate.

ACKNOWLEDGMENTS

This work was funded in part by a grant from the Laurance S. Rockefeller Trust.

REFERENCES

Appel, K. O. 1988. *Understanding and Explanation* (Warnke, G., transl.). Cambridge, MA: MIT Press.

Aristotle. 1944. *Politics. Aristotle in 23 volumes*, Vol. 21, transl. H. Rackham. Cambridge, MA: Harvard University Press; London: William Heinemann Ltd.

Baars, B. 2002. Conscious access hypothesis. *Trends in Cognitive Sciences* **6**(1): 47–62.

Baggini, J. & Fosl, P. 2007. *The Ethics Toolkit: A Compendium of Ethical Concepts and Methods*. Oxford: Blackwell, pp. 90–191.

Bechtel, W. 1988. *Philosophy of Science: An Overview of Cognitive Science*. New York: Lawrence Erlbaum Associates.

Bennett, M. R. & Hacker, P. M. S. 2003. *Philosophical Foundations of Neuroscience*. Malden, MA: Blackwell.

Casebeer, W. 2003. Moral cognition and its neural constituents. *Nature Reviews Neurosciences* **4**: 841–6.

Casey, K. L. & Bushnell, M. C. 2000. *Pain Imaging*. Seattle, WA: IASP Press.

Chapman, C. R. 2005. Psychological aspects of pain: a conscious studies perspective. In Pappagallo, M. (ed.) *The Neurological Basis of Pain*. New York: McGraw-Hill, pp. 157–67.

Clouser, K. D. & Gert, B. 1999. Concerning principlism and its defenders: reply to Beauchamp and Veatch. In Kopelman, L. (ed.) *Building Bioethics*. London: Kluwer, pp. 183–99.

Dilthey, W. 1990. *Gesammelte Schriften*, vol. 5. Stuttgart: B. & B. G. Teubner Verlagsgessellschaft.

Edelman, G. 2004. *Wider Than the Sky*. New Haven, CT: Yale University Press.

Einstein, A. 2000. In Calaprice A. (ed.) *The Expanded Quotable Einstein*. Princeton, NJ: Princeton University Press, p. 232.

Flor, H. & Bushnell, M. C. 2005. Central imaging of pain. In Hunt, S. & Koltzenburg, M. (eds.) *The Neurobiology of Pain*. Oxford: Oxford University Press, pp. 311–32.

Frankena, W. 1982. Beneficence in an ethics of virtue. In Shelp, E. (ed.) *Beneficence and Health Care*. Dordrecht: Reidel, pp. 63–81.

Freed, W. 1999. *Neural Transplantation: An Introduction*. Cambridge, MA: MIT Press.

Freud, S. 1966. In Auden, W. H. & Kronenberger, L. (eds.) *The Viking Book of Aphorisms*. New York: Dorset Press, p. 340.

Fukuyama, F. 2002. *Our Post-Human Future: Consequences of the Biotechnology Revolution*. New York: Farrar; Straus and Giroux.

Giordano, J. 2004. Pain research: can paradigmatic expansion bridge the demands of medicine, scientific philosophy and ethics? *Pain Physician* **7**: 407–10.

Giordano, J. 2005. The neurobiology of nociceptive and anti-nociceptive systems. *Pain Physician* **8**: 277–91.

Giordano, J. 2005. Toward a core philosophy and virtue-based ethics of pain medicine. *Pain Practitioner* **15**(2): 59–66.

Giordano, J. 2006. On knowing: the use of knowledge and intellectual virtues in practical pain management. *Practical Pain Management* **6**(3): 65–7.

Giordano, J. 2006a. Competence and commitment to care. *Pain Practitioner* **16**(2): 10–16.

Giordano, J. 2006b. Moral agency in pain medicine: Philosophy, practice and virtue. *Pain Physician* **9**: 71–6.

Giordano, J. 2006c. Good as gold? The randomized controlled trial – paradigmatic revision and responsibility in pain research. *American Journal of Pain Management* **16**(2): 66–9.

Giordano, J. 2006d. Agents, intentions and actions: moral virtue in pain medicine. *Practical Pain Management* **6**: 76–80.

Giordano, J. 2007. Pain, the patient and the physician: philosophy and virtue ethics in pain medicine. In Schatman, M. (ed.) *Ethical Issues in Chronic Pain Management*. New York: Informa, pp. 1–18.

Giordano, J. 2008a. Complementarity, brain-mind, and pain. *Forschende Komplementarmedizin* **15**: 2–6.

Giordano, J. 2008b. Ethics in and of pain medicine: constructs, content, and contexts of application. *Pain Physician* **11**: 1–5.

Giordano, J. 2008c. Maldynia: chronic pain as illness, and the need for complementarity in pain care. *Forschende Komplementarmedizin* **15**: 277–81.

Giordano, J. 2008d. Technology in pain medicine: research, practice, and the influence of the market. *Practical Pain Management* **8**(3): 56–8.

Giordano, J. & Pedroni, J. 2007. The legacy of Albert Schweitzer's virtue ethics within a contemporary philosophy of medicine. In Ives, D. & Valone, D. (eds) *Reverence for Life Revisited: The Legacy of Albert Schweitzer*. Newcastle: Cambridge Scholars' Press.

Giordano, J. & Schatman, M. 2008. A crisis in chronic pain care – an ethical analysis. Part two: Proposed structure and function of an ethics of pain medicine. *Pain Physician* **11**: 589–95.

Goethe, J.W. 1966. In Auden, W.H. & Kronenberger, L. (eds.) *The Viking Book of Aphorisms*. New York: Dorset Press, p. 339.

Gordijn, B. 2005. Nanoethics: from utopian dreams and apocalyptic nightmares towards a more balanced view. *Science and Engineering Ethics* **11**(4): 521–33.

Gray, C. 2001. *Cyborg Citizen: Politics in the Posthuman Age*. New York: Routledge.

Grondin, J. 1995. *Sources of Hermeneutics*. Albany, NY: State University of New York Press.

Harcastle, V.G. 1999. *The Myth of Pain*. Cambridge, MA: MIT Press.

Herskovits, M. 1973. *Cultural Relativism: Perspectives in Cultural Pluralism*. New York: Vintage Books.

Illes, J. 2003. Neuroethics in a new era of neuroimaging. *American Journal of Neuroradiology* **24**: 1739–41.

Illingworth, C.F. 1941. *Lectures on Peptic Ulcer*. New York: MacMillan.

Jackendoff, R. 1987. *Consciousness and the Computational Mind*. Cambridge, MA: MIT Press.

Jaspers, K. 1963. *Allegemeine Psychopathologie*. Berlin: Springer.

Jonas, H. 1985. *The Imperative of Responsibility: In Search of an Ethics for the Technological Age*. Chicago, IL: University of Chicago Press.

Kant, I. 1963. *Lectures on Ethics*. Translated by L. Infield. New York: Harper and Row.

Kant, I. 1998. *Groundwork for the Metaphysics of Morals*, Gregor, M. (ed.) Cambridge: Cambridge University Press.

Kass, L. 1961. *Monitoring stem cell research. Report of the President's Council on Bioethics*. Washington, D.C.: US Government Printing Office.

Katchalsky, A. K., Rowland, V. & Blumenthal, R. 1974. Dynamic patterns of brain cell assemblies. *Neuroscience Research Program Bulletin* **12**: 152.

Kelso, J. A. S. 1995. *Dynamic Patterns*. Cambridge, MA: MIT Press.

Lander, E. S. & Schnork, N. J. 1994. Genetic dissection of complex traits. *Science* **265**: 2037–48.

Lippe, P. M. 1998. An apologia in defense of pain medicine. *Clinical Journal of Pain* **14**(3): 189–90.

Llinas, R. 1998. The neuronal basis of consciousness. *Philosophical Transactions of the Royal Society of London* **353**: 1841–9.

Maricich, Y. & Giordano, J. 2007. Pain, suffering and the ethics of pain medicine: is a deontic foundation sufficient? *American Journal of Pain Management* **17**: 130–8.

Merskey, H. & Bogduk, N. 1994. *Classification of Chronic Pain*, 2nd edn. Seattle, WA: IASP Press.

Miller, B. 2004. Autonomy. In Post, S. G. (ed.) *Encyclopedia of Bioethics*, 3rd edn, vol. 1. New York: Thompson, pp. 246–51.

Mogil, J. S. 1999. The genetic mediation of individual differences in sensitivity to pain and its inhibition. *Proceedings of the National Academy of Sciences, USA* **96**: 7744–75.

Mogil, J. S., Yu, L. & Basbaum, A. I. 2000. Pain genes? Natural variation and transgenic mutants. *Annual Review Neuroscience* **23**: 777–811.

Morris, D. B. 1998. *Illness and Culture in the Postmodern Age*. Berkeley, CA: University of California Press.

Nagel, T. 1979. *Mortal Questions*. Cambridge: Cambridge University Press.

Niebroj, L., Jadamus-Niebroj, D. & Giordano, J. 2008. Toward a moral grounding of pain medicine: consideration of neuroscience, reverence, beneficence, and autonomy. *Pain Physician* **11**: 7–12.

Palmer, R. E. 1969. *Hermeneutics*. Evanston, IL: Northwestern University Press.

Pellegrino, E. 1999. The goals and ends of medicine: how are they to be defined? In Hanson, M. & Callahan, D. (eds.) *The Goals of Medicine, the Forgotten Issues in Health Care Reform*. Washington, D.C.: Georgetown University Press, pp. 55–68.

Pellegrino, E. & Thomasma, D. 1987. *For the Patient's Good: The Restoration of Beneficence in Health Care*. New York: Oxford University Press.

Peyron, R., Laurent, B. & Garcia-Larrea, L. 2000. Functional imaging of brain responses to pain: a review and meta-analysis. *Neurophysiologie Clinique* **30**; 263–88.

Posner, M. I. & Dehaene, S. 1994. Attentional networks. *Trends in Neurosciences* **17**: 75–9.

Prinz, J. A. 2004. Neurofunctional theory of consciousness. In Brook, A. & Adkins, K. (eds.) *Philosophy and Neuroscience*. Cambridge: Cambridge University Press.

Radner, D. & Radner, M. 1996. *Animal Consciousness*. New York: Prometheus Books.

Rees, J. 2004. Fundamentals of clinical discovery. *Perspectives in Biology and Medicine* **47**(4): 597–607.

Ryder, R. 1989. *Animal Revolution: Changing Attitudes towards Speciesism*. Oxford: Blackwell.

Ryder, R. 2001. *Painism: A Modern Morality*. London: Centaur Press.

Schweitzer, A. 1936. The ethics of reverence for life. *Christendom* **1**: 225–39.

Slater, M. W. & Woolf, C. J. 2005. Cellular and molecular mechanisms of central sensitization. In Hunt, S. & Koltzenburg, M. (eds.) *The Neurobiology of Pain*. Oxford: Oxford University Press, 95–114.

Snow, C. P. 1959. *The Two Cultures. The Rede Lectures.* Cambridge: Cambridge University Press.

Sorabji, R. 1993. *Animal Minds and Human Morals: Origin of the Western Debate.* Ithaca, NY: Cornell University Press.

Tisch, N. & Merikangas, K. 1996. The future of genetic studies of complex human diseases. *Science* **273**: 1516–17.

Turk, D. C., Flor, H. & Rudy, T. E. 1987. Pain and families: etiology, maintenance and psychosocial impact. *Pain* **30**: 3–27.

UNESCO. 2008. Universal Declaration on Bioethics and Human Rights. http:// unesdoc.unesco.org/images. Accessed 14 July 2008.

Uttal, W. 2003. *The New Phrenology: The Limits of Localizing Cognitive Processes in the Brain.* Cambridge, MA: MIT Press.

Varela, F., Thompson, E. & Rosch, E. 1991. *The Embodied Mind.* Cambridge, MA: MIT Press.

Ving, V. 1993. The coming technological singularity: how to survive in the post-human era. *Whole Earth Review* Winter. Available online at http://www-rohan.sdsu.edu/faculty/vinge/misc/singularity.html.

Wilson, E. O. 1998. *Consilience: The Unity of Knowledge.* New York: Random House.

Wittgenstein, L. 1958. *The Blue and Brown Books: Preliminary Studies for the 'Philosophical Investigations'.* New York: Harper and Row.

Wittgenstein, L. 1961. *Tractatus Logico-Philosophicus*, D. Pears & B. McGuinness (transl.) London: Routledge.

Woodruff, P. 2002. *Reverence.* New York: Oxford University Press.

Woolf, C. J. & Max, M. B. 2001. Mechanism-based pain diagnosis: issues for analgesic drug development. *Anesthesiology* **95**: 241–9.

9

Transplantation and xenotransplantation
Ethics of cell therapy in the brain revisited

G. J. BOER

INTRODUCTION

Although adult-to-adult organ transplantation has developed in the past 50 years in the surgical arenas, neurosurgeons have had no options to take out damaged brain areas and to implant new tissue from adult donors. Adult neurons do not survive isolation and transplantation. The neurosurgeon, moreover, cannot take out malfunctioning brain tissue or cells without severely damaging the nervous system in its still intact parts. However, the possibility of neural tissue repair by implantation rather than by transplantation became an option, with observations in animal research that has shown that immature nerve cells not only survive and mature following implantation in the adult nervous system, but also integrate and become functionally active in existing networks. Implantation of neurons to supplement lost neurons in cases of neurodegenerative diseases and neurotrauma thus became a challenging perspective for the neurosurgeon.

Parkinson´s disease (PD) was the test bed disease for this approach, as it is primarily characterized by a defined loss of neurons in the substantia nigra serving a dopaminergic input in the striatum of the central nervous system (CNS). Grafting fetal substantia nigra dopaminergic cells into the striatum of substantia nigra-lesioned rats reversed the motor disturbances, and similar studies in non-human primate models were successful as well. These results prompted clinical trials with human

Scientific and Philosophical Perspectives in Neuroethics, ed. J. J. Giordano & B. Gordijn. Published by Cambridge University Press. © Cambridge University Press 2010.

fetal dopaminergic neurons implanted into the striatum of PD patients. The grafted neurons indeed survived and became active cells as shown by functional brain scans. However, although amelioration of the motor behavioral syndrome was reported in many studies, functional results were variable and unwanted side effects were seen in some patients. The treatment has therefore not developed into a reproducibly efficacious therapy for PD. On the other hand the feasibility of neural grafting or neurotransplantation[1] in the human brain has been demonstrated, and this fostered further studies on neurotransplantation in other neurological disorders, such as Huntington´s disease (HD), Alzheimer´s disease (AD), multiple systemic atrophy (MSA), multiple sclerosis (MS), epilepsy, stroke, and spinal cord injury.

Clinical neurotransplantation has triggered ethical debate on the use of human fetal tissue from elective abortion. Several national and international health and governmental organizations as well as science organizations have discussed this issue in the past and have contributed guidance for the retrieval and use of human fetal tissues, either in formal guidelines or by national legislation. Currently, however, it is clear that whenever cell implants for the brain becomes a therapy, the supply and logistics of viable tissue from abortion clinics will not be nearly sufficient to retrieve enough material for the large numbers of patients with neurodegenerative diseases or brain trauma. Research has therefore moved into the putative use of stem cells. The proliferation characteristics and differentiation multipotency of these cells into large and perhaps endless numbers of any cell type (thus not only brain cells) make them candidates for growing transplants in the laboratory. This has revived the ethical debate especially in light of the use of embryonic stem cells (ESCs) isolated from in vitro human blastocysts.

Not only does the retrieval and use of human embryonic and fetal tissues give rise to ethical debate, but neurotransplantation in human brain also raises other issues, such as the risk/benefit in clinical trials, the proper design of the clinical trial, and the informed consent of patients with a neurological (and frequently also mental) disorder. Concerning the risks, separate from the risk of the surgery process itself and the biological safety of the implant, one has to realize that neurotransplantation is an intracranial intervention in

---

[1] Despite the fact that cells or tissue fragments are inserted without taking out the cells or tissue, and thus no genuine replacement is carried out, the field uses the term ``neurotransplantation´´.

an organ that is related to personality. Characteristics such as thinking, feeling, perception, will, learning, and memory all reside in the brain. The question can be raised as to whether the new cells, in addition to repairing the affected nervous system, also reorganizes other neuronal networks, since cell implantation by injection will never bring back the pre-disease or -injury structural organization of the brain.

In this chapter, the above issues will be discussed in view of new developments in the field. Neurotransplantation nowadays entails more than just the implantation of immature nerve cells to repair the brain. Treatments to supplement loss of glial cells and treatments with neural and non-neural cells – encapsulated and/or of animal origin – to support neuroregeneration or to prevent or retard neurodegeneration are under investigation as well. So the debate on the ethical issues must also consider the differences of approach, cell type, and cell origin in each of the various scenarios of neurotransplantation.

VARIOUS TYPES OF CELL IMPLANT FOR THE BRAIN

Immature neurons for grafting in the brain can be obtained directly from the aborted remains of human embryos or fetuses. The developmental age of the embryo or fetus at the time of tissue retrieval determines which neuronal group of cells is at a developmental stage for optimal survival, as different groups of nerve cells arise in different periods of encephalogenesis. Cells isolated for grafting should be a nerve cell but not yet have grown too many processes and synaptic contacts. Substantia nigra cells, for instance, derived from 6–8 week old human embryos, survived much better than cells from fetuses of 10–11 weeks (Brundin *et al.* 1986). Thus, not all neuronal cell types can be obtained at the optimal developmental stage for graft survival, as some are either too mature or not yet developed in the common period of (legal) elective abortion.

The problem of obtaining sufficient amounts of immature neurons of a specific phenotype may potentially be solved by the laboratory ``production´´ of immature nerve cells from stem cells. These cells can clone themselves indefinitely and can grow and differentiate into any cell type for transplants, as mediated by external factors. Stem cells with the potential to differentiate into neuronal cells can be collected as (i) ESCs from the blastocyst (pre-implantation embryo), (ii) embryonic germ cells from post-implantation embryos, or

(iii) somatic stem cells (SSCs) from organs in late embryonic, fetal, neonatal, and even adult stages, including brain and umbilical cord blood. ESCs are easy to culture and are truly pluripotent, whereas SSCs perform less well in the laboratory. The presence of SSCs in adult organs (often also called adult stem cells) in principle introduces the possibility for neural autografts: the patient as his/her own donor. However, not all organ-derived stem cells have equal potential for growth into neural transplants. In addition, brain-committed cell lines, for instance LBS neurons (Layton BioScience neurons) originating from a human teratocarcinoma, can be used to grow transplants of immature nerve cells (Borlongan *et al.* 1998). Finally, as neurons of non-human mammals can match the functional capabilities of human cells (Isacson & Deacon 1997), implants of porcine fetal brain origin are also applicable to humans and this has already been explored, albeit with very limited functional response, in human PD patients (Larsson & Widner 2000).

However, cell therapeutic approaches other than supplementation of nerve cells are needed when a brain anomaly results from an indirect effect on neurons, such as the loss of oligodendrocytes in MS. Implantation of glial precursor cells is then indicated. Finally, the feasibility of cell implantation in the brain has also opened avenues to implant cells that release compounds to substitute the function of lost neurons (*molecular* versus *cellular* replacement) or to release protein compounds that can stop, prevent, or counteract the degeneration or malfunction of diseased neurons (molecular treatment). Such cells do not need to be neural but can also be fibroblasts genetically modified to overexpress a therapeutic factor. The latter has been explored using autologous nerve growth factor-releasing cells in a phase I trial with Alzheimer's disease patients as a means to reactivate cholinergic neurons of the nucleus basalis of Meynert in an attempt to fight the dementia (Tuszynski *et al.*, 2005). A molecular treatment is also possible through genetically modified cells encapsulated by a semipermeable membrane before implantation. This method allows the cells to be removed with the capsule and prevents autoimmune responses against the donor cells and therefore allows the use of non-human cells as removable biological drug-delivery devices (Bachoud-Lévi *et al.* 2000; Bloch *et al.* 2004).

In summary, either immature neuronal or glial cells are implanted to supplement or compensate for cell death or cell dysfunction in the nervous system (neural grafting), or cells – either immature or mature, neural or non-neural, human or non-human, encapsulated or not – are placed in the nervous system to treat neuronal dysfunction or ameliorate neurodegeneration. Thus for a molecular cell therapy donor, cells need not always come from immature human donors, i.e. aborted tissue remains.

GUIDANCE FOR THE RETRIEVAL OF HUMAN TISSUES AND CELLS

Various types of neurotransplantation for neural disease thus require different types of cellular implant, and therefore a variety of methods of retrieval, direct use or in vitro expansion and differentiation can be distinguished.

Primary cells

Experimental cell supplementation surgery in the human brain primarily uses human embryonic and fetal tissues as available, maximally efficacious, and safe sources for grafting. Guidance for the retrieval and use of the remains of human abortions has been developed to solve the related ethical issues, although for parts of society the use of human abortion tissues (as well as abortion itself) remains a moral obstacle. However, given the fact that in many countries elective abortion is legal, one cannot simply forbid the use of the remains for therapeutic use in the CNS or in any other organ. Even if induced abortion is regarded as unethical, it does not necessarily make the user compliant in the action of ending the life of an unborn (De Wert et al. 2002). It is peculiar to notice that the grafting of embryonic neurons in a common disease such as PD has re-opened the discussion of ethical acceptability, whereas research on pre-viable and non-viable embryos and fetuses has been carried out for decades by embryologists and physiologists (Falkner & Tanner 1978; O'Rahilly & Müller 1987). In part, this may be due to the notion that the use of embryonic and fetal cells would become of therapeutic value for large groups of patients and that this might induce a great demand, which in turn would encourage induced abortions that would otherwise not have occurred. Any sound ethical guidance must therefore address the relationship between the occurrence and practice of the elective abortion and the particular needs for cell or tissue transplantation (Boer 1994, 1999).

Many national and international organizations, national institutes of ethics, as well as scientists in the field, have provided ethical guidelines for the subsequent use of body remains for experimental and clinical research (DHSS 1972; CNESVS 1992; BMA 1988; Boer 1994; see also review by De Wert *et al.*, 2002). Despite marked differences, all aim to solve the above-mentioned ethical problem by trying to achieve complete separation between the decision about abortion (whether, how, and when) and the possible donation of the remains (the so-called *separation principle*) (Boer 1999; De Wert 2002). It would then be similar to the generally accepted use of organs or tissue from deceased babies, children or adults for research or clinical use. The separation principle proposes that the possible donation of the abortion tissues should not be considered before a final decision has been made on ending pregnancy. Of course, informed consent should then be obtained from the woman for the donation. The main additional requirements are that the timing and method should not compromise efficient medical handling in the interest of the woman and the conceptus, and that no remuneration, self-donation, or person-appointed donation is involved. Adhering to this principle has a strategic function, as it visualizes that abortion and the use of the remains are separate practices, thereby circumventing any of the accusations of complicity or moral taint as discussed above.

Concerning consent for donation two points may be added. First, one could argue that when the application of embryonic or fetal cells and tissues becomes a well-known and established therapy for common diseases, this knowledge will make the decision on elective abortion easier. One can doubt whether this will be an important aspect for a woman who has to make a difficult, complex, and emotional judgment about her situation. Moreover, in practice, a planned implantation surgery is often cancelled for the simple reason that not enough donor tissue was available. Second, there are practical arguments to seek consent for donation from the woman only and not from the man, despite the equal positions of men and women (in Western societies) (Boer 1994). Some women do not want to involve a spouse or partner in the process of terminating the pregnancy, (or the inseminator is unknown at the time of abortion). In the case of a mutual parental relationship, the partner's view will in any event, be taken into account by the woman.

Stem cells

The discoveries on the potential of stem cells to grow transplants generated discussion on the ethical guidance for the retrieval of donor material, because ESCs are still better source material compared to

SSCs or any other stemcell-like tissue(s). The retrieval of SSCs from human embryos and fetuses can be guided by the same rules as formulated above for the retrieval of primary immature cells. SSCs from adults can be obtained under current guidance and legislation of organ and tissue donation. No ethical objections for retrieval are present in these cases as long as the profit of subsequent treatment or amelioration of the severe disease symptoms of the subject outweighs the possible burden for the donor (which may be the patient him/herself). However, the use of ESCs, (the pluripotent stem cells with superior proliferation capacities and differentiation potentials) raises additional issues. ESCs are isolated from the inner cell mass of *pre-implantation embryos* (blastocysts) either available as spares from an in vitro fertilization (IVF) program or created in vitro as a means-to-the-end. Ethically speaking – although the blastocyst has biologically the same status – the donor situation in the latter cases is quite different and needs separate evaluation.

Owing to the burden of the necessary hormonal treatment, current practice in IVF protocols is that the collection of egg cells and subsequent fertilization is performed once. After some days of growth and quality control in blastocysts are then implanted in the uterus vitro, or deep frozen for a second trial or subsequent pregnancies. Surplus blastocysts (also called rest, residual, spare, or supernumerary embryos) often remain, and pragmatism leads to destruction at some point in time. If the use of the remains of an aborted post-implantation embryo can be ethically justified, thawing the ``surplus´´ blastocysts to collect valuable stem cells cannot be rejected. The protection of the *in vitro* human blastocyst, a liquid-filled tissue sphere with undifferentiated cells (Singer 1990), should not be held in higher esteem than that of an intrauterine human embryo in which organogenesis into a visible human-being-to-be has taken shape. So, the decision to destroy the blastocyst opens the case for donation. Ethical guidance would then be similar to the donation of embryonic or fetal remains after elective abortion. In both cases conception is not intended to prepare cells for research or experimental implantation, and it should be morally acceptable to use this tissue rather than destroy it. The IVF couple should provide informed consent, the separation principle can be maintained, and no elongated in vitro growth of the intact blastocyst towards post-implantation developmental stages comparable with that beyond 14 days post-conception, i.e. the intrauterine pre-implantation period, should be applied (FIGO, 2003). Theoretically, ESCs from a single human blastocyst would be sufficient to treat large cohorts of patients (Thomson *et al.* 1998). However, the precise conditions to achieve and harness cell lines for neural cell supplementation are far from established (Rosser *et al.* 2007; Rao 2008) and therefore research using human pre-implantation embryos remains necessary.

A different issue is the creation of human blastocysts solely for the above purpose, either by the same IVF technique but with donated egg cells and sperm, or by *therapeutic cloning*, whereby a donated egg cell is used to transplant the adult cell nucleus (somatic cell nuclear transfer, SCNT) (Cibelli *et al.* 2001). The latter approach can be used to grow a blastocyst whose ESCs immunologically match the graft recipient in order to avoid tissue rejection and long-term immune suppression (Wolf *et al.* 1998). The use of specially created blastocysts for stem cell production can be seen as exploitation of human life as it creates life solely for the purpose of sacrificing it. Blastocysts have been created to serve the quality of IVF, and, hence, the quality of life for persons conceived in this way (McLaren 1996). However, for restorative cell surgery, non-reproductive creation of the human blastocyst must indeed be regarded as the instrumental use of a human-being-to-be. The question is whether this a priori has to be ethically condemned, especially since no definitive guidelines exist for the most efficacious and safe way to grow cell implants for putative cellular therapy for severely physically and/or mentally handicapping neuro-diseases (such as, for example, PD, AD, MS, and brain stroke). SCNT with animal egg cells is not an alternative, as biologically speaking, the blastocyst has human DNA and should therefore be regarded as human.

This alternative source for human ESCs (as well as the other alternatives, i.e. SSCs, especially those of the bone marrow, and adult somatic cells dedifferentiated to somatic stem cells (Lewitzky & Yamanaka 2007), still have to prove their definitive value and safety for the production of defined cell types for therapy. One has to ethically weigh the respect for human dignity by ex vivo creating and destroying a human blastocyst against the burden of severe or untreatable brain anomalies (or as some patient organizations have put it: ``place the severely ill patient next to the respect for … human cells´´). It will be difficult, however, to reach a universal consensus, as societal and religious views on human value and respect for life at the early stages of a fertilized egg (day 0), morula (4–5 days), and blastocyst (5–10 days after fertilization) may simply differ too much (De Wert *et al.* 2002; Matthiesen 2002).

Currently, research on the in vitro growth of neurografts (and other organotypic grafts) can be performed using IVF residual embryos, and there is presently no need to create human blastocysts to collect ESCs for in vitro differentiation purposes (McLaren 2001; Outka 2002). As well, clinical therapies are evolving for neurodegenerative and traumatic brain disorders based on viral vector-mediated gene transfer for factors that replace neuronal function, or stop degeneration and/or stimulate regeneration (Korecka *et al.* 2007). However, it is difficult to claim that isolating primary neural cells or SSCs from human abortion remains or ESCs from ``surplus'' or created pre-implantation embryos is violating the ethical *principles of proportionality* and *subsidiarity* as these approaches serve an important goal in the interest of human health. Autologous hESCs may still be a better source to grow neural grafts (except for cases of hereditary brain disorders like HD).

Animal cells

In view of the limited availability of human embryonic or fetal tissue, xenogenic tissue is seen as an alternative. Xenografting makes use of the chimeric plasticity of undifferentiated or immature mammalian nerve cells (Isacson & Breakefield 1997). For instance, human neuro-progenitor cells transplanted in the germinal ventricular zones of the postnatal developing rat brain readily assume the ontogenic characteristics of rat cells (Flax *et al.* 1998). Pig fetal mesencephalic grafts placed in the rat model for PD exhibit allograft-like morphology and remarkable axonal target specificity, and restore motor function (Galpern *et al.* 1996). For human application, scientific, practical, and ethical reasons make the pig a top source for graft material (Dunning *et al.* 1994). A pig's brain size is comparable to that of a human, and there is extensive experience in breeding these animals for organ transplants (Nuffield Council on Bioethics 1996). The welfare of the source animals, the dangers of infections and long-term immunosuppressive treatment, and psychological acceptance by the recipient all were considered not to rule out xenografting. Animal protectionists, however, remain generally opposed to the use of specially bred animals as a source of transplants, since the special breeding conditions – necessary to control the pathogen status of the source animals – would introduce yet another violation of animal integrity and a new type of factory farming. Ethically speaking, there should be no difference between breeding animals for food or breeding them to harvest cells or organs for transplantation (Daar 1997), provided that suffering can be kept to a minimum. One might even say that breeding for transplants serves a higher goal than food production.

For both PD and HD, pilot pig xenografts were applied in small patient groups, but essentially this was a failure because of limited graft survival (Fink *et al.* 2000; Larsson & Widner 2000).

RISK/BENEFIT ASPECTS

Ideally, cell therapy for brain disorders should completely reverse signs and symptoms in a safe way without side effects and without negatively affecting the mental state of the patient.

Surgical safety

Neurotransplantation is a surgical intervention that involves injection microliter quantities of cells or tissue fragments into stereotactically precisely defined target areas of a *c.* 1.5 liter volume of human brain mass. The safety of this surgery compares with other intracranial interventions such as the placement of electrodes for deep brain stimulation. One important additional requirement, however, is quality and the microbiological safety of the implanted cells. Current practice with the use of tissues isolated for neurografting is the rapid serology testing for HIV 1 and 2, hepatitis B and C, *Treponema pallidum*, and HTLV-I and II (nowadays this is legally required in the EU; EC Directive 2004). When neurografts are grown from stem cells, control for the presence of pathogens is easier and can (and in fact does) form part of the ``good laboratory practice'' (GLP) of the cell line production facility. Cell lines derived from human ESCs appear to be sensitive for mutations (Maitra *et al.* 2005), which makes periodic monitoring for genetic and epigenetic alterations necessary to maintain quality. A major problem, however, is the probability of tumor formation in stemcell-based therapy. ESCs injected in an undifferentiated state and not given proper trophic guidance can form a tumor in virtually any location (Asano *et al.* 2006). Experimental application in the human brain should therefore not be started until this effect is better understood and controlled. As there is no evidence to date that cancer is caused by bonemarrow-derived SSCs, these can be used as an autograft and are not ethically controversial, so current stem cell therapies focus more on the use of SSCs. However, as claimed above, ESC may ultimately prove to be more viable because of their genuinely pluripotent character.

Physiological safety

It is clear that any restorative intervention in an injured brain will never totally bring about the "prior structural and organizational situation." Any therapeutic effect will therefore be reached with neural circuits that deviate and differ in structure and capacities from the pre-disease situation, because plasticity phenomena may have taken place during the progress or course of the disease. Slight changes in the cellular make-up or molecular functioning of the brain *will* have physiological and behavioral consequences. Thus, any and all surgical brain interventions will have side effects! Side effects must be accepted, but are they identifiable? And if so, of course, they should be outweighed by clinical improvement.

The report that, PD patients who received an intrastriatal human fetal mesencephalic graft, dyskinesias occurred more frequently than in sham-controlled subjects (Olanow *et al.* 2003; Hagell *et al.* 2002) indicates one such side effect. The new dopaminergic neurons, integrated in the host striatum and improving the motor control, apparently act within a neuronal network that deviates from the normal non-PD situation. The effect was only recognized after a long history of dopaminergic cell grafting in PD patients, indicating that negative symptoms are sometimes hidden. It also re-emphasized that animal models are never completely predictive of the results in the human and that unexpected side effects may show up in the clinical trial. Such an observation clearly may compel the clinical neuroscientist to design new strategies for improved experimentation in humans, if at all feasible.

Psychological safety

Changes in personality can occur in any brain disease, and are either directly or indirectly related to the disease: directly when particular nervous functions are affected; indirectly because the physical, psychological, and social situation of patients suffering from brain (and other) diseases is altered by the burden of the symptoms, limited potential, fear, depression, stress, uncertainties about the future, and a possible loss of self-respect and self-confidence. If the burden of the symptoms can be eliminated or alleviated by restorative interventions, many of these psychological aspects will improve. The patient feels better and healthier. These are welcome effects, and not unwanted side effects. In this respect brain interventions are no different from a pharmaceutical therapy that aims to treat the origin of a disease. Possible negative consequences of the latter treatments, however, are largely reversible when medication is stopped. The question therefore remains whether neural reconstruction by cell therapy can or will also affect the psyche in an unwanted but hidden or subtle way.

The answer appears to be that so far psychologic risks of cell implants are limited or hardly recognizable. Personality and identity are not linked to a single defined brain structure or set of structures. Identity as a reflection of declarative information on self, others, time, and environment involves much of the entire brain and its networks in a dynamic fashion (the brain is not static but continuously changing and adapting its neuronal cell function, sensitivity and cellular connectivity). Neurotransplantation adds only small neural cell masses to the recipient brain; it does not and cannot replace large parts of the nervous system as in organ transplantation (see introduction). However, small changes in the nervous system can indeed produce personality changes, as indicated from functional neuroteratology or behavioral teratology studies, neurografting studies in intact animals, and human neurological, anomalies themselves (Boer 2006; Merkel *et al.* 2007). In other words personality changes can be acquired by subtle changes, small injuries, or reorganizations in the nervous system, and surgical interventions may introduce changes in addition to the ones that are caused by pathology. Psychological, alterations may also present as side effects. In experimental restorative neurosurgery with fetal dopaminergic neurons in PD, personality changes were rarely more than subtle (Sass *et al.* 1995; Diederich & Goetz 2000; McRae *et al.* 2003) and thus would not counter the gain of therapeutic effects.

Transfer of psychological elements

Transfer of personality has been put forward as a possible unwanted side effect of neurotransplanting human fetal brain tissue (HMSO 1989; Linke 1993). Personality, as stated above, is not located in a single neuronal cell type or in a small brain area, but comes to expression from the activity of the neuronal networks of the brain and the body. The maturational fate and functional integration of implanted fetal neurons will, be directed by the adult conditions, which are totally different from those in the fetal brain. Thus, transfer of personality through the implantation of (minced or suspended) immature fetal donor tissue to an adult host brain is erroneously been posed as a possible drawback in neurotransplantation. Having said this, it is also clear that pig neural xenografts, which integrate and function to repair the injured brain of other non-mammalian species (Isacson *et al.* 1995; Galpern *et al.* 1996), do not have that danger either. For pig neurografts, animal-to-human transmissible diseases (Barker *et al.* 2000) or zoonosis (Bach *et al.* 1998), as well as the disadvantages of lifelong immune suppression therapy, are to be considered, not the risks of acquiring pig-like behavior.

NEUROTRANSPLANTATION CLINICAL TRIALS: WHEN AND HOW?

The history of cellular intervention in human brain disorders started with the autologous implantation of adrenal medulla tissue fragments in the striatum of the PD patient. The adrenal medulla can produce dopamine, and in rat models striatal implantation reversed motor symptoms. The first presentation of these studies in 1987 provoked the question of whether this was enough evidence to justify a clinical trial. It pointed out the difficulty of determining whether animal studies justify experimentation in the human. If the answer is yes, then the question arises of how to perform the clinical study in a safe and ethically responsible way, as cell implantation is an irreversible intervention.

Role of animal experimentation

One of the fundamental requirements in clinical research is that a sufficient body of relevant animal studies must be reported before trials on human beings can be performed. This can be ethically controversial, but is generally regarded as necessary to ensure the safety of the procedures and the possibility of beneficial effects (Sladek & Shoulson 1988). The factors to be considered are (i) the risk/benefit ratio for patients, (ii) the need for treatment in light of the severity of the disease, (iii) the time and money required, and (iv) the effects of trials on the experimental animals involved, in particular non-human primates. Animal ``models'' for brain diseases, however, will never completely match the symptomatology and prognoses of human patients. In addition, many risks can be evaluated in animal experiments, but the above mentioned possible psychologic side effects are not easily measurable in animals, if at all. Thus, the final efficacy of any brain intervention will require trials in human beings that also carry some risk of negative effects. The brain is a very heterogeneous organ and both the type and site of intervention will differ in every disease, and thus evaluations on when to initiate and justify a clinical trial will also vary.

The Norwegian/Swedish team that performed the first stereotactic neurotransplantation of autologous adrenal medulla tissue argued that the frustrating lack of treatment for advanced PD patients had weighed heavily in considerations before medico-ethics committees (Backlund et al. 1985)[2]. Cell implantation surgery appeared safe, but only after very positive results presented by Madrazo et al. (1987), in which hundreds of patients world wide were subjected to this autotransplant surgery. In the end, however, one had to conclude that cell survival and recovery effects were both negative, which then also became clear in the monkey PD model. This history illustrates the difficulty of determining what level of prior animal experimentation is required to establish the efficacy of a new clinical treatment. It also illustrates that a move towards the first clinical trial is often prompted by the absence of existing effective treatment (Boer 1996, 1999, 2006). A basic requirement, however, is that any brain disorder elected for cell transfer therapy must have a defined target for the intervention, determined by the results of animal experiments. A new trial without such a background cannot be accepted because of unknown risks for human brain functions.

Clinical trial design

When a human brain disorder finally becomes eligible for experimental cell therapy, strategies on how to control efficacy and safety need to be defined. A cell implantation trial in the nervous system is not comparable to a pharmacological clinical trial, for which a gold standard exists of a double-blind placebo-controlled randomized evaluation (CPMP 1990). Drug treatment can be stopped, but cell implantation cannot be undone, only destroyed, and not without consequences for the intact neighboring tissue[3] (perhaps only minimally in the case of implants of encapsulated cells for a molecular treatment). Moreover, a placebo treatment would mean the insertion

---

[2] Extensively discussed at the Eric K. Fernstrom Foundation Symposium on ``Neural grafting in the human CNS'', Lund, Sweden, 18–22 June 1984.

[3] Before implantation, cells can be equipped with the thymidine kinase (HSV-tk) gene, rendering them susceptible to the cytotoxic effects of ganciclovir, which will subsequently kill the cells that were implanted. An inflammatory response to remove the debris is the consequence.

of non-therapeutic nonsense cells in the brain of a patient, which would be impracticable and surely unethical. Owing to the invasiveness of cell-based therapeutic trials in the brain, placebo surgery is problematic and poses more of a risk than in other organs, since self-repair is virtually absent in nervous tissues.

Human experiments that are methodologically bound to give non-interpretable results are unethical, but so are unnecessary control treatments in human beings. A clinical trial, however, must show that a particular treatment correlates with a hypothesized outcome (Kenny 1979). Comparison of pre- versus post-treatment measurements in an individual human subject can easily be biased by artifacts (Kraemer 2004), and therefore regarded as inferior, or at the least less superior in comparison with research using placebo controls. In experimental neurotransplantation, or for that matter in any experimental neuro-surgery, one needs to establish what control can be or should be included to obtain meaningful results. General guidelines for medical interventions given by the WHA Declaration of Helsinki (2000), and by the Council of Europe Convention on Human Rights and Biomedicine (1997) do not provide answers. Double-blind sham-controlled surgery, i.e. surgery without intracranial needle insertions for placement of cells, has been advocated (Freeman *et al.* 1999) and applied (Freed *et al.* 2001; Olanow *et al.* 2003) as control treatment. Sham-controlled or imitation surgery trials, however, control only for the placebo effects on the expectations of the surgery and not for the result of the cellular or molecular intervention itself. Moreover, the plea for controls involving treatments up to the stage of drilling a hole in the skull can be, and has been, challenged both on the basis of the outcome of the open studies, on ethical arguments (Macklin 1999; Dekkers & Boer 2001; London & Kadane 2002; Clark 2002), and by proposing alternative study designs (Boer & Widner 2002).

Sham surgery as control: yes or no?

The plea for sham surgery in clinical neurotransplantation research published by Freeman *et al.* (1999) was based on the observation that (i) up to that time, open trials of neural grafing in PD patients had always been performed under different conditions of donor tissue treatment, graft placement, surgical approach, and pre- and post-grafting treatment and symptom evaluation, (ii) surgical outcome was therefore variable from center to center; and (iii) the reported efficacy in some centers could be criticized, as investigator bias and placebo effects on the patient side might have had a role. Freeman *et al.* (1999) subsequently listed three criteria that must be met before randomized double blind sham-controlled trials could be carried out: (i) the study should address an important research question that cannot be answered with an alternative design that poses a lower risk to the subjects, (ii) there must be preliminary but not conclusive evidence that the intervention is effective; and (iii) the treatment should be sufficiently developed so that it is unlikely that it will become obsolete before the study has been completed. For neurotransplantation in PD – the case discussed by Freeman *et al.* (1999) – the latter two criteria pose no problems (Dekkers & Boer 2001) as it was at that time generally acceptable to assume that the treatment could be effective, though still to be improved and perfected, and that adverse effects had not been prominent (Brundin *et al.* 2000; Dunnett *et al.* 2001). The discussion therefore centers upon the first one, which is a general point for all clinical trials of experimental restorative neurosurgery. The justification for control of investigator bias or placebo effects are only defensible when risks of participation in the control arm are ``reasonable'' in relation to the possible benefits (Dekkers & Boer 2001). Frank *et al.* (2005) recently reviewed side effects reported in the double-blind sham surgery-controlled trials for PD, and concluded that (i) surgery was generally safe and well tolerated, (ii) placebo effects were not attributed to the surgery, and (iii) harm occurred more frequently in subjects with the ``true'' intervention. In general the risks of surgery, were not zero, however, and they must be regarded as major compared with a placebo drug treatment (Boer & Widner 2002). Of mention are the medical risks of local or general anesthesia (6–8 h), of the surgery itself, the immune suppression therapy (at least 6 months cyclosporin), and the risks related to the significant irradiation dose for the repeated PET scans needed in an evaluation period. These procedures were thus enforced on control PD patients at a moment when (i) the neurografting technique remains suboptimal in terms of neuronal survival and striatal reinnervation, (ii) a significant number of PD patients worldwide had adrenal medulla cell implants without evidence of long-lasting therapeutic effect, and (iii) compelling evidence had been presented that the clinical course of the engrafted PD patients parallels the development of the dopaminergic graft measured with the surrogate marker F-dopa uptake in PET scans (Lindvall 1999; Dunnett *et al.* 2001). This all is evidence that imitation surgery can be predicted to have no effects in PD patients. The actual data indeed showed no improvements of symptoms over 1–2 years post-surgical evaluation period in the sham-treated PD group (Freed *et al.* 2001; Olanow *et al.* 2003).

Macklin (1999), London and Kadane (2002), and Clark (2002) criticized the sham approach from a different perspective, mainly based on the moral claims that researchers used individuals as means to an end for the study, and the problem of valid informed consent in view of the risks. Patients desperate about their disease state easily agree to participate in clinical studies and sometimes eagerly desire participation, because they believe, often erroneously, that the study will benefit them. Such an unrealistic expectation of benefit undermines the validity of the consent given by the patient in a hypothetical research trial. Kim *et al.* (2006) found that PD patients willing to participate did not differ in their perception of personal benefit as a precondition for volunteering from patients not willing to participate. However, those willing to participate tended to perceive lower probability of risk, were more tolerant of greater risks, and were more optimistic about science and progress for society. In the sham-controlled studies described above, sham patients after being told that they would not be enrolled in the grafting surgery arm after one year because of higher-than-anticipated incidence of adverse events, were not relieved to have undergone apparently safer sham surgery, but were sometimes even outraged about the situation. They said they might not have participated in the study if they had known they would have to wait so long for the ``real´´ surgery. Therapeutic misconception is not easy to avoid when the study results are disclosed. Thus, the argument referring to obtaining the proper informed consent (Macklin 1999) is indeed one of the major obstacles for the introduction of imitation surgery in experimental cell therapy (Dekkers & Boer 2001).

Sham surgery in itself is defensible, as the first open neural grafting trials in PD using dopaminergic adrenal medulla tissue for implantation took place in a balanced, and ethically acceptable fashion (Boer 2006). Progress in brain tissue repair by cell therapy will be terminated if one cannot accept surgery studies with some risks! There is no absolute requirement for direct benefit for research subjects when aspirational benefit, i.e. benefit for the patient group in future studies, can be ascertained. (Dekkers & Boer, 2001; Albin 2002). As argued above, controlling new experimental therapy is of the utmost importance, as an experimental study should not be performed when interpretable data cannot be compiled. Although one cannot a priori exclude the need to include control-treated patients, a basic question should be: might there be an alternative method that can control or nearly control for investigator bias and placebo effect, thereby sparing subjects the invasive imitation brain surgery?

Core assessment protocol

Shortly after the first clinical trials of cell therapy in PD patients, it became obvious that there was a critical need for a degree of commonality between the methods for patient diagnosis and evaluation by the teams undertaking this experimental treatment. Daily fluctuations of symptoms make scientific evaluation even more difficult and data had to be compared between centers to achieve sufficient numbers of patients to provide more definitive results in the open trials. An ad hoc international committee formulated a series of recommendations for a common and minimum set of diagnostic and methodological pre- and post-surgery core evaluations, called Core Assessment Program for Intracerebral Transplantations in PD (CAPIT-PD) (Langston *et al.* 1992), which were later refined to allow comparison with new treatments in PD patients, in particular functional neurosurgery such as pallidotomy and deep brain stimulation (Core Assessment Program for Surgical Interventional Therapies, CAPSIT-PD) (Defer *et al.* 1999). The protocol comprises criteria for inclusion of patients, working definitions and aspects of qualitative and quantitative motor tests and no less important, for a fixed time frame of evaluations to obtain a reliable baseline estimate of the pregrafting clinical status and the postgrafting effects for a period long enough to cover the time for the grafted neurons to mature and become functional (after grafting of immature neurons it takes many months, up to one year, before the cells become functionally integrated) (Isacson *et al.* 1995). CAPIT-PD has never been completely embraced by the PD grafting field, partly because the program was considered too laborious (and costly) to carry out in large-scale trials and because grafting was a treatment worth trying rather than as an experimental therapy. However, if all centers that performed neurotransplantation in PD patients over the past decade had used this CAP(S)IT-PD, a wealth of comparative information could have been obtained instead of the present set of incomparable and seemingly conflicting results.

Patient placebo effects and investigator bias are largely eliminated by incorporating in the CAP a series of well-defined objectives, i.e. quantitative measures that are, attained blindly. Such a set of tests performed at (fixed) time points before and after surgery allows, as in human pharmacological studies, comparison of outcomes between different approaches, including standard treatments. So, from a strict methodological point of view, randomized double-blind placebo-controlled studies may be indicated, yet the efficacy of cellular implants in the brain of PD patients can be assessed with a CAP-mediated study design that does not involve sham-operated patients but rather a parallel random-assigned standard-treated reference group of patients.

Next to the ``test bed´´ neurotransplantation clinical trials in PD, trials with neural cell therapy using are also reported patients with HD, AD, MS, ALS, stroke, and epilepsy (Merkel *et al.* 2007). Most of these studies were designed as open trials, but in the case of cellular treatment for HD, a CAP for transplantation studies was established (CAPIT-HD) (Quinn *et al.* 1996). The establishment of disease-specific CAPs dealing with pre- and post-operative evaluations in the above-mentioned brain diseases should be advocated to provide comparisons of treatment approaches. For instance, other experimental surgical interventions in PD, such as placement of electrodes for deep brain stimulation (Benabid 2003), strategic lesions in the outflow pathways of the basal nuclei (Tasker *et al.* 1983), and gene therapeutic interventions as endogene symptomatic treatment or as treatment to stop the degeneration of the dopaminergic nigra cells (Kaplitt *et al.* 2007), could also use this CAP-mediated study design. It may be regarded as unethical not to design such CAPs as they are of value to obviate, or at least diminish, the need for sham control surgery. An additional benefit is that comparison between different experimental methods using the same evaluation protocol can reduce on the number of study subjects.

Informed consent

Animal ``models´´ of neurodegenerative diseases or neurotrauma are only of relative value because they do not mimic the disease in light of a long-term chronic neurodegeneration occuring in humans, nor do they completely match the symptomatology and prognoses in the human situation. Final efficacy of any neurotransplantation approach will thus need clinical trials, that will always impart some risk of negative effects.

It goes without saying that participation in any restorative surgery project must be voluntary and that there is a right to withdraw consent at any time (United Nations 1948; Boer 1994; BMA 1988). In general, one may say that a new experimental approach should be presented in written form to a scientific committee of experts in the field, and should evaluate the proper rationale to justify human experimentation as well as the study design. Neurological patients are, however, vulnerable persons, and often not fully able to give consent. PD patients are usually still able to understand their situation, but late stage HD or AD patients cannot. The assessment of competence/decision-making capacity is therefore a primary responsibility of the investigator. As a general rule, a candidate subject can be considered competent when the nature of the information, the consequences and risks of being a research participant, and the possibility of refusal, are understood. Considering the fact that irreversible experimental surgery is involved, a second opinion on the assessment of competence/decision-making should be sought from a physician who is not involved in the research project. Some patients may have difficulty in expressing choice, and others may be unduly susceptible to the harm and stress of being a research subject. Researchers could minimize this vulnerability by including family members or patient representatives in the decision-making process, as is proposed for neurografting trials in HD patients (Quinn *et al.* 1996). Valid consent is a response to oral and written information. Moreover, informed consent alone can never be an argument to initiate clinical experimentation. Putative efficacy, biosafety, and experimental design are equally important.

CONCLUDING REMARKS

Clinical neuroscience is fast entering an era of experimental cellular and molecular neurosurgery. In particular, stem cell and gene technology are rapidly progressing fields that are likely to permit restorative interventions and will therefore be embraced for the development of new therapeutic strategies in human brain dysfunction. Newspapers and broadcasting media frequently report on these developments, and the use of human ESCs for organ repair is presently a topic of worldwide debate ethical concern and political agendas. The CNS, is structurally heterogeneous which, unlike other organs (i) acts within a different set of physical and mental functions and (ii) is directly or indirectly connected to other substructures in neuronal networks and systems. Neurons connections to other neurons and non-neuronal cells are the basic elements for these functions, which ultimately evokes the human mind. So, surgical implantation of nerve cells for restoration of defects in neural function should be considered with caution and precision so as to preserve physiological functions and cognitive, emotional, and motivational aspects of personhood. The goal therefore is to perform cellular/molecular surgery in such a way that only the neural target is modified for beneficial i.e. therapeutic, effects.

Neurotransplantation is a technique to insert minute amounts of specific neuronal or non-neuronal cells, that either replace lost or dysfunctional brain cells or ameliorate affected neural functions. These interventions have not been shown to adversely interfere with or modulate much of psychologic function. Neural cells of non-human origin structurally integrate within the human brain and functionally integrate similarly, as has been experimentally established in animal-to-animal xenoneurografting (Isacson *et al.* 1995; Isacson & Deacon 1997). However, this is not to say that specific characteristics of personality cannot be altered by cellular implants, whether of human or animal origin. Neuronal networks altered by neural disease, and subsequently structurally or functionally changed by the implantation of minute volume of neural or non-neural cells, will never fully restore CNS morphology in the way that one can completely rebuild an old house.

Definitive breakthroughs in restorative neurosurgery have not been reached in patient studies, although solid claims of beneficial effects are reported for the grafting of immature fetal neurons in the brain of PD (Lindvall *et al.* 1992; Widner *et al.* 1992) and HD patients (Bachoud-Lévi *et al.* 2006). However, both the variability of therapeutic outcome and the logistic, technical, and ethical problems of obtaining enough donor material cannot rubber-stamp this intervention as a therapy. If human stem cells – in particular patients′ autologous stem cells (preventing immunological rejection) – can be cultivated to develop into any kind of neural cell in specified ready-to-integrate states, better surviving, better integrating, and thus therapeutically improved transplants may be achieved. If ESCs do finally prove to be the only optimal source cells to grow such implants, the ethical objections of pro-life community still cannot be circumvented. Nevertheless one might expect that, whenever a solid cell therapy evolves for common serious diseases like PD or AD, large parts of society will embrace this treatment as very beneficial to maintain quality of life.

REFERENCES

Albin, R. L. 2002. Sham surgery controls: intracerebral grafting of fetal tissue for Parkinson′s disease and proposed criteria for use of sham surgery controls. *Journal of Medical Ethics* **28**: 322–5.

Asano, T., Sasaki, K., Kitano Y., Terao, K. & Hanazono, Y. 2006. In vivo tumor formation from primate embryonic stem cells. *Methods in Molecular Biology* **329**: 459–67.

Bach, F. H., Fishman, J. A., Daniels, N. *et al.* 1998. Uncertainty in xenotransplantation: individual benefit versus collective risk. *Nature Medicine* **4**: 141–4.

Bachoud-Lévi, A. C., Gaura, V., Brugières, P. *et al.* 2006. Effect of foetal neural transplants in patients with Huntington's disease 6 years after surgery: a long-term follow-up study. *Lancet Neurology* **5**: 303–9.

Bachoud-Lévi, A. C., Déglon, N. & Nguyen, J. P. 2000. Neuroprotective gene therapy for Huntington's disease using a polymer encapsulated BHK cell line engineered to secrete human CNTF. *Human Gene Therapy* **11**: 1723–9.

Backlund, E. -O., Granber, P. -O. & Hamberger, B. 1985. Transplantation of adrenal medullary tissue to striatum in parkinsonism: first clinical trials. *Journal of Neurosurgery* **62**: 169–73.

Barker, R. A., Kendall, A. L. & Widner, H. 2000. Neural tissue xenotransplantation: what is needed prior to clinical trials in Parkinson's disease? *Neural Tissue Xenografting Project, Cell Transplantation* **9**: 235–46.

Benabid, A. L. 2003. Deep brain stimulation for Parkinson's disease. *Current Opinion in Neurobiology* **13**: 696–706.

Bloch, J., Bachoud-Levi, A. C., Deglon, N. *et al.* 2004. Neuroprotective gene therapy for Huntington's disease, using polymer-encapsulated cells engineered to secrete human ciliary neurotrophic factor: results of a phase I study. *Human Gene Therapy* **15**: 968–75.

BMA (British Medical Association). 1988. BMA Guidelines on the use of fetal tissue. *Lancet* **1**: 1119.

Boer, G. J. 1994. Ethical guidelines for the use of human embryonic or fetal tissue for experimental and clinical neurotransplantation and research. *Journal of Neurology* **242**: 1–13.

Boer, G. J. 1996. The self-restraining ethical guidelines of NECTAR for the clinical neurotransplantation investigations. In Hubig, C. & Poser, C. (eds.) *Cognitio humana – Dynamik des Wissens und der Werte*. Leipzig: XVII Deutscher Kongress für Philosophie, pp. 1420–7.

Boer, G. J. 1999. Ethical issues in neurografting of human embryonic cells. *Theoretical Medicine and Bioethics* **20**: 461–75.

Boer, G. J. 2006. Restorative therapies for Parkinson's disease: ethical issues. In Brudin, P. & Olanow, C. W. (eds.) *Restorative Therapies for Parkinson's Disease*. New York: Springer, pp. 12–49.

Boer, G. J. & Widner, H. 2002. Clinical neurotransplantation: core assessment protocol rather than sham surgery as control. *Brain Research Bulletin* **58**: 547–53.

Borlongan, C. V., Saporta, S., Poulos, S. G., Othberg, A. & Sanberg, P. R. 1998. Viability and survival of hNT neurons determine degree of functional recovery in grafted ischemic rats. *NeuroReport* **9**: 2837–42.

Brundin, P., Nilsson, O. G., Strecker, R. E. *et al.* 1986. Behavioural effects of human fetal dopamine neurons grafted in a rat model of Parkinson's disease. *Experimental Brain Research* **65**: 235–40.

Brundin, P., Karlsson, J., Emgård, M. *et al.* 2000. Improving the survival of grafted dopaminergic neurons: a review over current approaches. *Cell Transplantation* **9**: 179–95.

Cibelli, J. B., Kiessling, A. A., Cunniff, K. *et al.* 2001. Somatic cell nucleus transfer in humans: pronuclear and early embryonic development. *Journal of Regenerative Medicine* **2**: 25–31.

Clark, P. A. 2002. Placebo surgery for Parkinson's disease: do the benefits outweigh the risks? *Journal of Law and Medical Ethics* **30**: 58–68.

CNESVS (National Consultative Ethics Committee For Life Sciences, and Health). 1992. Statement on intracerebral graft of mesencephalic tissue of human embryo origin in patients with parkinsonism for therapeutic experimentation. Paris: Le Comité.

Council of Europe. 1997. Convention for the protection of human rights and dignity of the human being with regard to the application of biology and medicine. *European Treaty Series* **164**.

CPMP Working Party on Efficacy of Medicinal Products. 1990. EEC Note for Guidance: good clinical practice for trials on medicinal products in the European Community. *Pharmacology and Toxicology* **67**: 361–72.

Daar, A. S. 1997. Ethics of xenotransplantation: animal issues, consent, and the likely transformation of transplant ethics. *World Journal of Surgery* **21**: 975–82.

De Wert, G. 2002. The use of human embryonic stem cells for research: an ethical evaluation. *Progress in Brain Research* **138**: 405–70.

De Wert, G., Berghmans, R. L., Boer, G. J. *et al.* 2002. Ethical guidance on human embryonic and fetal tissue transplantation: a European overview. *Medicine, Health Care and Philosophy* **5**: 79–90.

Defer, G. L., Widner, H., Marie, R. M., Remy, P. & Levivier, M. and conference participants. 1999. Core assessment program for surgical interventional therapies in Parkinson's disease (CAPSIT-PD). *Movement Disorder* **14**: 572–84.

Dekkers, W. J. M. & Boer, G. J. 2001. Sham surgery in patients with Parkinson's disease: is it morally acceptable? *Journal of Medical Ethics* **27**: 151–6.

Diederich, N. J. & Goetz, C. G. 2000. Neuropsychological and behavioral aspects of transplants in Parkinson's disease and Huntington's disease. *Brain and Cognition* **42**: 294–306.

Dunnett, S. B., Bjorklund, A. & Lindvall, O. 2001. Cell therapy in Parkinson's disease – stop or go? *Nature Review Neuroscience* **2**: 365–9.

Dunning, J. J., White, D. J. & Wallwork, J. 1994. The rationale for xenotransplantation as a solution to the donor organ shortage. *Pathology and Biology* **42**: 231–5.

EC Directive of the European Parliament, and Council. 2004. Setting standards of quality and safety for the donation, procurement, testing, processing, storage and distribution of human tissues and cells. Brussels, Belgium: 2004/32/EC.

Falkner, F. & Tanner, J. M. ed. 1978. *Human Growth, Vol. 1. Principles and Prenatal Growth.* London: Baillière Tindall.

FIGO. 2003. Research on pre-embryos. In *Recommendations on Ethical Issues in Obstetrics and Gynecology by the FIGO Committee for the Ethical Aspects of Human Reproduction and Women's Health*, pp. 22–3.

Fink, J. S., Schumacher, J. M. & Ellias, S. L. 2000. Porcine xenografts in Parkinson's disease and Huntington's disease patients: preliminary results. *Cell Transplantation* **9**: 273–8.

Flax, J. D., Aurora, S., Yang, C. *et al.* 1998. Engraftable human neural stem cells respond to developmental cues, replace neurons and express foreign genes. *Nature Biotechnology* **16**: 1033–9.

Frank, S., Kieburtz, K., Holloway, R. & Kim, S. 2005. What is the risk of sham surgery in Parkinson disease clinical trials? A review of published reports. *Neurology* **65**: 1101–3.

Freed, C. R., Greene, P. E., Breeze, R. E. *et al.* 2001. Transplantation of embryonic dopamine neurons for severe Parkinson's disease. *New England Journal of Medicine* **344**: 710–9.

Freeman, T. B., Vawter, D., Goetz, C. G. *et al.* 1997. Towards the use of surgical placebo-controlled trials. *Transplant Proceedings* **29**: 1925.

Freeman, Th. B., Vawter, D. E., Leaverton, P. E. *et al.* 1999. Use of placebo surgery in controlled trials of a cellular-based therapy for Parkinson's disease. *New England Journal of Medicine* **341**: 988–91.

Galpern, W. R., Burns, L. H., Deacon, T. W., Dinsmore, J. & Isacson, O. 1996. Xenotransplantation of porcine fetal ventral meencephalon in a rat model of Parkinson's disease: functional recovery and graft morphology. *Experimental Neurology* **140**: 1-3.

Hagell, P., Piccini, P., Bjorklund, A. *et al.* 2002. Dyskinesias following neural transplantation in Parkinson's disease. *Nature Neuroscience* **5**: 627-8.

HMSO (Her Majesty's Stationery Office). (1989). *Review of the Guidance on the Research and Use of Fetuses and Fetal Material (Polkinghorne report)*. Cm 762. London: HMSO.

Isacson, O. & Breakefield, X. O. 1997. Benefits of hosting animal cells in the human brain. *Nature Medicine* **3**: 964-9.

Isacson, O. & Deacon, T. 1997. Neural transplantation studies reveal the brain's capacity for continuous reconstruction. *Trends in Neurological Sciences* **20**: 477-82.

Isacson, O., Deacon, T. W., Pakzaban, P. *et al.* 1995. Transplanted xenogeneic neural cells in neurodegenerative disease models exhibit remarkable axonal target specificity and distinct growth patterns of glial and axonal fibres. *Nature Medicine* **11**: 1189-94.

Kaplitt., M. G., Feigin, A., Tang, C. *et al.* 2007. Safety and tolerability of gene therapy with an adeno-associated virus (AAV) borne GAD gene for Parkinson's disease: an open label, phase I trial. *Lancet* **369**: 2097-105.

Kenny, D. A. 1979. *Correlation and Causality*. New York: Wiley.

Kim, S. Y. H., Holloway, R. G., Frank, S. *et al.* 2006. Volunteering for early phase gene transfer research in Parkinson disease. *Neurology* **66**: 1010-15.

Korecka, J. A., Verhaagen, J. & Hol, E. M. 2007. Cell-replacement and gene-therapy strategies for Parkinson's and Alzheimer's disease. *Regenerative Medicine* **2**: 425-46.

Kraemer, H. C. 2004. Statistics and clinical trial design in psychopharmacology. In Machin, D., Day, S., Green, S., Everitt, B. & George, S. (eds.) *Textbook of Clinical Trials*. New York: Wiley & Sons, pp. 173-83.

Langston, J. W., Widner, H., Goetz, C. G. *et al.* 1992. Core assessment program for intracerebral transplantation (CAPIT). *Movement Disorders* **7**: 2-13.

Larsson, L. C. & Widner, H. 2000. Neural tissue xenografting. *Scandinavian Journal of Immunology* **52**: 249-56.

Lewitzky, M. & Yamanaka, S. 2007. Reprogramming somatic cells towards pluripotency by defined factors. *Current Opinion in Biotechnology* **18**: 467-73.

Lindvall, O. 1999. Cerebral implantation in movement disorders: state of the art. *Movement Disorders* **14**: 201-5.

Lindvall, O., Widner, H., Rehncrona, S. *et al.* 1992. Transplantation of fetal dopamine neurons in Parkinson's disease: one-year clinical and neurophysiological observations in two patients with putaminal implants. *Annals of Neurology* **31**: 155-65.

Linke, D. B. 1993. *Hirnverpflanzung*. Reinbek bei Hamburg: Rowoldt.

London, A. J. & Kadane, J. B. 2002. Placebos that harm: sham surgery controls in clinical trials. *Statistical Methods in Medical Research* **11**: 413-27.

Macklin, R. 1999. The ethical problems with sham surgery in clinical research. *New England Journal of Medicine* **341**: 992-6.

Madrazo, I., Drucker-Colin, R., Diaz, V. *et al.* 1987. Open microsurgical autograft of adrenal medulla to the right caudate nucleus in two patients with intractable Parkinson's disease. *New England Journal of Medicine* **316**: 831-4.

Maitra, A., Arking, D. E., Shivapurkar, N. *et al.* 2005. Genomic alterations in cultured human embryonic stem cells. *Nature Genetics* **37**: 1099-103.

Matthiesen, L. 2002. *Survey on Opinions from National Committees or Similar Bodies, Public Debate and National Legislation in Relation to Human Embryonic Stem Cell Research and Use.* Vols. 1 and 2. Brussels: EC Research Directorate-General.

McLaren, A. 1996. Research on embryos in vitro, the various types of research. Third Symposium on Bioethics, *Medically Assisted Procreation and the Protection of the Human Embryo.* CDBI/SPK 22. Strasbourg: Council of Europe.

McLaren, A. 2001. Ethical and social considerations of stem cell research. *Nature* **414**: 129–31.

McRae, C., Cherin, E., Diem, G. *et al.* 2003. Does personality change as a result of fetal tissue transplantation in the brain? *Journal of Neurology,* **250**: 282–6.

Merkel., R., Boer., G., Fegert, J. *et al.* 2007. *Intervening in the Brain: Changing Psyche and Society. Ethics of Science and Technology Assessment,* vol. 29. Berlin, Heidelberg, New York: Springer, pp. 59–115.

Nuffield Council on Bioethics. 1996. *Animal-to-human Transplants.* London: Nuffield.

Olanow, C. W., Goetz, C. G., Kordower, J. H. *et al.* 2003. A double-blind controlled trial of bilateral fetal nigral transplantation in Parkinson´s disease. *Annals of Neurology* **54**: 403–14.

O´Rahilly, R. & Müller, F. 1987. *Developmental Stages in Human Embryos.* Washington, D.C.: Carnegie Institution of Washington.

Outka, G. 2002. The ethics of human stem cell research. *Kennedy Institute Ethics Journal* **12**: 175–213.

DHSS (Department Of Health, and Social Security). 1972. Peel Report. *The Use of Fetuses and Fetal Material for Research, Report of the Advisory Group.* Her Majesty´s Stationary Office, London.

Quinn, N., Brown, R., Craufurd, D. *et al.* (CAPIT-HD committee) 1996. Core assessment programme for intracerebral transplantation in Huntington´s disease (CAPIT-HD). *Movement Disorders* **11**: 143–50.

Rao, M. 2008. Scalable human ES culture for therapeutic use: propagation, differentiation, genetic modification and regulatory issues. *Gene Therapy* **15**: 82–8.

Rosser, A. E., Zietlow, R. & Dunnett, S. B. 2007. Stem cell transplantation for neurodegenerative diseases. *Current Opinion in Neurology* **20**: 688–92.

Sass, K. J., Buchanan, C. P., Westerveld, M. *et al.* 1995. General cognitive ability following unilateral and bilateral fetal ventral mesencephalic tissue transplantation for treatment of Parkinson´s disease. *Archives in Neurology* **52**: 680–6.

Singer, P. 1990. *Embryo Experimentation. Ethical, Legal and Social Issues.* Cambridge: Cambridge University Press.

Sladek, J. R. & Shoulson, I. 1988. Neural transplantation: a call for patience rather than patients. *Science* **240**: 1386–8.

Tasker, R. R., Siqueira, J., Hawrrylyshyn, P. & Organ, L. W. 1983. What happened to VIM thalamotomy for Parkinson´s disease. *Applied Neurophysiology* **46**: 68–83.

Thomson, J. A., Itskovitz-Eldor, J., Shapiro, S. S. *et al.* 1998. Embryonic stem cell lines derived from human blastocysts. *Science* **282**: 1145–7.

Tuszynski, M. H., Thal, L., Pay, M. *et al.* 2005. A phase 1 clinical trial of nerve growth factor gene therapy for Alzheimer disease. *Nature Medicine* **11**: 551–5.

United Nations. 1948. *Universal Declaration of Human Rights. Yearbook of the United Nations 1948–49.* New York: Department of Public Information, United Nations.

Widner, H., Tetrud, J., Rehncrona, S. *et al.* 1992. Bilateral fetal mesencephalic grafting in two patients with parkinsonism induced by 1-methyl-4-phenyl-1,2,3,6-tetrahydropyridine (MPTP). *New England Journal of Medicine* **327**: 1556–63.

Wolf, E., Zakhartchenko, V. & Brem, G. 1998. Nuclear transfer in mammals: recent developments and future perspectives. *Journal of Biotechnology* **65**: 99–110.

World Medical Association Declaration of Helsinki. 2000. Ethical: ethical principles for medical research involving human subjects. *Journal of the American Medical Association* **284**: 3043–5.

10

Neurogenetics and ethics
How scientific frameworks can better inform ethics

K. FITZGERALD & R. WURZMAN

INTRODUCTION

The extraordinary increase in scientific knowledge achieved in the past century has generated numerous challenges for ethics. As a result, the field of bioethics has expanded, with an increased emphasis on a need for scientific advances to be accompanied by an examination of the humanistic implications of biomedical research.

In this regard, the intersection of ethics and neurogenetics is exceptionally significant because it connects the tensions found in discussions regarding brain–mind distinctions with the difficulties encountered in delineating mental health. At this intersection, epistemological issues arise as researchers and health care professionals attempt to relate human experiences – such as pain, suffering, illness, conscience, or even the awareness of self-existence – to physical correlates – such as genetic sequence variations and protein deposits – and vice versa. Hence, this intersection of ethics and neurogenetics involves a combination of issues that cannot be adequately interpreted, understood, or addressed from any single vantage point.

To explicate the dynamics of this intersection of ethics and neurogenetics, this chapter will focus on certain specific areas of neurogenetics – behavioral genetics, pharmacogenomics, and genetic testing – in order to reveal how scientific understanding and its accompanying assumptions can better facilitate the ethical decision-making process. Particular attention will be given to the problematic

Scientific and Philosophical Perspectives in Neuroethics, ed. J. J. Giordano & B. Gordijn. Published by Cambridge University Press. © Cambridge University Press 2010.

effects and consequences a reductionistic scientific framework can have at this intersection of neurogenetics and ethics, and to how a more integrative approach, such as an emergentistic framework, can be used to address these issues more completely.

Behavioral genetics and pharmacogenomics often produce tensions within the relationship between science and ethics as a result of a mismatch between the epistemological approach of some neuro-genetic research methodologies and the clinical conclusions that are derived from these methodologies. This mismatch arises from over-simplification, (genetically) deterministic conclusions, and faulty reasoning about biological causality, that all affect ethical reasoning and decision-making.

Science, as a human endeavor, proceeds within an epistemo-logical framework that involves an inevitable reciprocity between the specific goals of the research and the broader effects that research outcomes can have on the understanding, and relative meaning, of human flourishing and well-being (Allchin 1998). Scientific reduction-ism – the narrowing or limiting of relevant information to scientific data only – can be particularly problematic in neurogenetics because the use of only scientific concepts in interpreting research data directly affects the larger constructs of what it means ``to be human´´, both biologically and behaviorally. Hence, both the human research subject, and subsequent patients, can be reduced to their neurogenetic features alone resulting in the loss of attention to many other aspects of their self-awareness that inform their sense of healthiness, as well as their sense of identity and sense of self-worth.

For example, pain conclusions based on purely reductionist models can affect clinical attitudes and opinions (e.g. the genetic ``ingraining´´ and refractoriness of chronic pain), clinical decision-making, the clinical relationship, and even how individual and societal responsibility and culpability are regarded in the treatment and interpretation of pain. One research strategy of both behavioral gen-etics and pain genetics is to emphasize heritability data. This approach is primarily a quantitative description of the variability in trait distri-butions in a sample of individuals that can be associated with genetics or the environment, which then can be used to describe the origin of the trait in individuals as genetic or environmental, or both (Lerner

2004; Collins *et al.* 2000). This emphasis on heritability data can negatively affect clinical practice.

Treatment decisions about whether to employ social, psychological, and/or behavioral interventions versus pharmacological or biological interventions (or both) depend in part upon whether the patho-etiology is regarded as biological (including genetic), psychological or environmental, or some combination of these elements. Inappropriate clinical decision-making may result from reductive genetic methodologies because they frequently are interpreted in a way that blurs or ignores the distinction between description and explanation. This confusion is caused by using a description of the variability (genetic or environmental) to *explain* the variability itself (Lerner 2004).

An example of this confusion is that heritability methodologies have repeatedly identified the gene for the serotonin transporter (hSERT) and polymorphisms in its promoter region (5HTTLPR) as linked to bipolar disorder, major depression, anxiety-related dimensions, and violent suicidal behavior (Plomin & McGuffin 2003). Similar research approaches have described low serotonin turnover (reflected in amounts of 5-HIAA (a marker of serotonin levels) in cerebrospinal fluid (CSF)), to be associated with ``... the mediation of negative emotions, impulsive aggressive behavior, increased use of alcohol and nicotine, increased food consumption, increased sympathetic and parasympathetic nervous system outflow, and altered neuroendocrine function ...´´ (Williams *et al.* 2003). These results have led to conclusions that the ``... altered CNS serotonergic function is a driver of the clustering of negative moods, risky health behaviors, and altered biological functions that increase disease risks in certain individuals and groups – for example, lower socioeconomic status (SES)´´ (Williams 1994, 1998). These reductionistic heritability studies have led some to portray the serotonin-influenced behaviors solely and even uniformly as determined by one´s serotonergic genotype.

Genetic studies of chronic pain have similarly shown phenomena related to pain perception to be varyingly associated with different racial, ethnic, and cultural groups, as well as familial clustering(s) of pain perception and illness (for a review of studies, see A. J. MacGregor, 2004). While interpretations of these findings have weighted the influences of family environment over shared genetic factors, some methodologies can bias conclusions so as to reinforce the importance of genetic influences. For instance, animal studies that have examined genotypes contributing to pain thresholds and other phenotypic pain traits with genotype and pharmacogenetic research purporting a relationship between genotype and analgesia effects – both of which are necessarily assessed behaviorally – seem to emphasize genetic sources over environmental ones for such differences in pain reactivity (Mogil 2004). Even though room is left to consider modification by environmental factors, these studies still lead to a strong genetic determinism because most environmental factors are only nominally under an individual's control (e.g. the social environment of the family-of-origin). Therefore, applying these research conclusions to patient treatment can detrimentally diminish the perception that individuals suffering from chronic pain can actively further their own healing. The patient's (pain) behavior is seen as significantly, if not entirely, predetermined with little actual control over it by the self and/or rational mind.

Alternatively, such research could – and, we offer, should – be interpreted to implicate a biological variable (e.g. serotonin) in these psychological and behavioral traits across a diverse population, but only as one of many possible factors that affect the observed variability of the traits (Horowitz 2000; Lerner 2004; Collins *et al.* 2000). Hence, the problem with using a reductionistic hereditarian methodology is that it only evaluates the relative influence of genes or environment, and consequently such results do not sufficiently establish that the specific genes investigated are the primary determinants of a behavioral, psychological, or pain disorder (Parens 2004). Supporting an alternative notion of synergy among effectual variables, the effects of polymorphisms in 5HTTLPR on serotonin availability, as well as the association of genotype and phenotype with the abnormal behaviors studied, seems to be affected by independent interactions between serotonin alleles and other factors such as biogeographical ancestry, ethnicity, gender, and social factors (Lerner 2004; Williams *et al.* 2003). It is likely that similar independent interactions would be found between such factors and the genetic polymorphisms associated with chronic pain (e.g. the gene coding for catechol-*o*-methyltransferase (*COMT*)).

If one attempts to articulate a single, general interpretation of clinical status incorporating both genetic information and independent relationships with social variables, one could posit that genotype may contribute to sensitivity to different features in the environment (Parens 2004; Lerner 2004; Horowitz 2000). This means that gene–environment quantifications must be considered in specific contexts, and not as isolated measurements for a given trait. If genes are understood primarily as determinants of environmental sensitivity, instead of the trait itself, then non-linear and dynamic relationships among biological factors and social factors are inferred. This more integrative understanding of the causes of behavior render underlying biological, psychological and social factors neither entirely self-controlled nor predetermined. Hence, black-and-white interpretations of behavior are avoided (Horowitz 2000).

Because over-simplification can be especially harmful in pharma-cogenomic and behavioral genetics studies – particularly those evalu-ating social or group factors with respect to the genetic contribution to developing abnormal phenotypes – caution must be taken when inter-preting research results to protect against the danger of over- or under-estimating the relevance and effect(s) of psychosocial and behavioral factors (Parens 2004; Lerner 2004). Without an approach that considers integrated biopsychosocial variables, conclusions may err in the direc-tion of genetic determinism, or blaming particular psychosocial envir-onments (which are themselves dynamically interrelated to biological and systemic social factors). In guarding against these types of conclu-sions (e.g. those that would disproportionately blame genetics for health disparities, such as disability resulting from chronic disease in some groups) it is important to acknowledge that a broader definition of health versus illness and disease remains a social construction (Parens 2004).

The ethical implications of reductionism and causal interpret-ations of neurogenetic data may be most far-reaching upon the prac-tice of pain medicine (and similarly the psychiatric aspects of pain and pain care), given the current state of the science that informs ethical decision-making in broad medical, legal, and societal contexts. The reductive nature of much of pain medicine (and biological psychiatry) is also vulnerable to erroneous conclusions of causal relationships between genes and behavior. For example, when clinical benefits are observed during pharmacotherapy, the cause of the condition is often hypothesized to involve the mechanism of the drug as it is understood (Brown 2003; Klernam 1984).

The primary problem of this type of logic is that it involves an error called *ex juvantibus* reasoning, which directly connects the cause of an illness to the effectiveness of a treatment (Kraepelin 1921). In actuality, there is no way to validly reach an explanation about the physical cause of pheomenological illness merely from the effects of a drug. This claim by no means denies the involvement of neurobiology in the mechanism of pain or psychopathology, nor does it deny any functionality related to the drug's targets and the system in which they are embedded. The claim is simply that the fact of clinical improvement cannot directly provide information about a causal mechanism for the illness, nor can clinical improvement be directly attributed to the activity of the drug.

The classic example of this situation is the efficacy of diuretics in treating congestive heart failure. Although diuretics act directly on the kidneys and not the heart, congestive heart failure is not caused by renal dysfunction. Rather, the kidneys are normal, and diuretics exert their therapeutic effects in the renal system only as an indirect means to decrease the burden on the heart by eliminating excess water and electrolytes (Brown 2003; Valenstein 1998). Yet inasmuch as genes are related to neurotransmitter system functions, causal conclusions derived from the action of psychotropic medications may be easily extended to causal conclusions about the genes that control the activity of those neurotransmitters that are pharmacological targets. A case in point is the emphasis upon the genes related to opioid function as a potential focus of understanding the causes of pathological pain.

Thus pharmacogenomic data, especially as it complements neurogenetic data, is often interpreted as validating the focus upon neurotransmitter dysfunction as the organic root of many pain disorders, despite growing evidence that the situation is far more complex. For example, pharmacogenomic animal studies are seen to implicate genotype as a causal factor in pain disorders. This conclusion is based on differences in nociceptive responses between different populations of genetically near-identical rats. As such, these studies often fail to address how such results translate to humans, who are genetically more diverse – much less how nocisponsivity in rats relates to the qualitative pain experience of rats or humans. While these experiments validly implicate genetics in phenotypic differences of certain neurotransmitter receptors known to mediate the effects of analgesic drugs, the assertion that these genes are integral to functional phenotypes of pain ignores the explanatory gap between physical mechanism and phenomenal experience. Moreover, as such animal studies solely address nociceptive processing (i.e. physical processing and response to the presence of noxious physical stimuli) and analgesia; they do not address the complex and multidimensional experience of pain.

Furthermore, reductionistic interpretations of pharmacogenomic studies tend to employ an implicit assumption that the mechanism for analgesia effects a direct reversal of (or interference in) the processes that generate physical pain. On the contrary, evidence suggests that analgesia – while reducing responsiveness to pain – utilizes

pathways, receptors, and mechanisms different from those of nociceptive processes. Whereas nociception can be mostly thought of as a
``bottom-up´´ process (e.g. processing and integration of peripheral
stimuli), analgesics may function in a more ``top-down´´ fashion by
engaging diverse networks (such as those mediating emotional and
cognitive responses to pain) that alter or override nociceptive afference
to decrease sensitivity, perceptivity, or reactivity to noxious stimuli. A
more integrated and dynamic conception of the neurophysiologic etiology of pain and analgesia would serve as a better foundation to address
the complexity of pain phenotypes, and accordingly would better
inform the ethical practice of pain medicine (Giordano 2006, 2007,
2008).

INFLUENCE OF EPISTEMOLOGY ON CLINICAL PRACTICE: ETHICAL CONSEQUENCES

Pharmacogenomic data, influenced by *ex juvantibus* reasoning, can
inappropriately provide a conceptual link to causally and directly
attribute pain disorders to genetics. This situation reflects a broader
biological reductionism regarding pain experience that ultimately can
affect how patients with pain are viewed, assessed, treated, and valued.
Treatment approaches are heavily influenced by the dictum that biological etiologies require biological interventions (i.e. usually drugs,
e.g. antibiotics for infections) (Brown 2003). In addition, the emphasis
upon the organic basis of neuropsychiatric disorders extends to pain
medicine so as to favor a comparable ``disease´´ model for pain, as
opposed to conceptions that would portray pain as an illness, thus
elevating the experience of the functional effects of pain to a relatively
greater significance (Giordano 2006). In contrast, research in pain
medicine implicitly aims to understand the phenomenological, as well
as the physical, causes of pain. However, to effectively do so, investigators must be vigilant against what is known as ``type physicalism´´
that attempts to relate a phenomenal experience to an equivalent and
uniform psychological event.

   Neurogenetic data are considered to significantly support ``dis-
ease´´ models within a reductionist epistemology because of the way in
which reductionism relates biological mechanisms to causality. When
pharmacogenomic studies identify a gene that is related to another
gene identified by using behavioral genetic techniques, and if a
therapeutic agent is known to interact with the gene product or gene
itself, it becomes very tempting to conclude that abnormalities in

systems in which the gene product is embedded are the ``cause´´ of the clinical syndrome. In this way, reductionism tends to implicate genetics as a direct and efficient cause in any demonstrably biological system. Following from the assumption that a pain disorder can be understood in predominantly physical terms, pain research has somewhat disproportionately focused upon the mechanisms of nociception in the hope that new and better treatments may be developed as the further elucidation of neural substrates provides viable therapeutic targets. However, this approach has led to pain disorders becoming increasingly compartmentalized as a medical problem to be treated primarily with pharmacological strategies, thereby risking the diminishment of the importance or relevance of the psychological and/or behavioral components of pain. An example of this tendency is the current favoring of analgesic drugs over behavioral and cognitive interventions.

The principal problem with this situation is that pharmacological interventions alone may not represent the optimal care of the pain patient, and this regard should elicit consideration of both the ethical rightness and the goodness of treatment. Optimal patient care requires critically evaluating the neurogenetic evidence and the context of the paradigm from which it was derived (i.e. reductionism). It may also be necessary to consider alternatives to the reductionistic strategy, such as emergentism. The epistemological approach of emergence is grounded in the possibility that the conceptions of fundamental causes of phenomena at a less complex level cannot account for phenomena at progressively higher levels of complexity (e.g. the chemistry of nucleic acids explaining the properties of DNA in genetics). The emergence of new properties and causality at higher complexities, and their relationship to the properties and causality of less complex levels of scientific inquiry, is explained by incorporating non-linear causality (Horowitz 2000). This non-linear causality locates the fundamental cause of mechanism within the appropriate complexity level of the system´s processes (Crutchfield 2008; Bruntrup 1998). Accordingly, although genes are still an important element in any biological process, their role cannot be taken in isolation from other elements at both higher and lower levels of system complexity. Hence, in emergentist frameworks neurogenetic links to psychological or behavioral disorders do not have sufficient causal significance to explain fully the condition, and thus the reductionistic disease model is not supported.

How biological causality is regarded illustrates one way in which an epistemological framework can affect ethics. Conclusions drawn from and within a particular epistemological approach may also impact medical treatment, the way the legal system handles illness, and how society at large determines responsibility for wellness. Ethical problems arising from reductionism can also extend to clinical applications of neurogenetics, perhaps most prominently neurogenetic testing. Reducing behavior to genetics implies that it would be appropriate to diagnose or predict the course of a neuropsychiatric disorder based solely upon molecular variables (Brown 2003). The fact that enormous resources are currently devoted to elucidating genes involved in neuropsychiatric disorders is evidence of the popularity of this belief. It becomes worthwhile to question whether employing such resources is desirable if these findings may not actually enhance treatment or produce wellness. Knowing ``a gene for´´ an illness cannot necessarily predict or address the phenomenologically individualistic nature of the disorder – for instance, the specific manifestation of maldynia as the illness amalgam of organic pathophysiology, cognitive coping patterns, learned behavioral responses, and the subjective mental experience that these entail. If the procedure for translating genetics to an individual´s phenomenal manifestation of illness is not forthcoming, then testing for genetic risk factors may not deliver upon the hopes vested in such procedures. Again, the medical challenge of addressing and controlling pain, especially chronic pain, may provide an example that facilitates the delineation of the factors that can mitigate the direct applicability of neurogenetic testing to diagnosis and treatment.

First, the complex etiology of pain and the individuality of pain experience make it unlikely that knowledge of genotype alone would affect treatment decisions for patients. Even being able to predict analgesic sensitivity to various drugs based on genotype would not predict (at least not with as much sensitivity as anticipated or desired) how effective the analgesic would be when social, cognitive, and behavioral contributions to pain experience are also significant factors. Genetic markers of analgesic sensitivity are at best incomplete indicators of how effective a drug will be in a given individual.

Second, genetic testing for a particular pain disorder is redundant to the clinical presentation of pain. Hence, the benefit would need to be information that might be useful for guiding treatment strategies if research endeavors are able to relate genotypic differences to diagnosis and differential efficacies of specific treatments. At this time, it is questionable whether such genetic information alone would be sufficient to categorize pain (and pain patients) in this way.

Third, issues concerning the ethics of pre-symptomatic testing for genetic disorders must be considered. Even when the presence of the gene clearly and reliably predicts a certain disease, the use(s), applications, and limitations of this information can evoke profound ethical consequences. For example, consensus holds that individuals at risk for adult-onset disorders should not be tested during childhood (in the absence of symptoms) because this raises the possibility of stigmatization within the family and in other social settings, and may have serious educational and career implications (Bloch & Hayden 1990; Harper & Clarke 1990). Chronic pain is estimated to incur billions of dollars annually in health care and disability compensation costs (Bennett 1999). Because of this situation, potential pain patients might be singled out by insurance companies, employers, and other third parties as higher-risk individuals who might incur financial or productivity losses. Ethical considerations regarding confidentiality, stigmatization, and the legal protection of genetic information would thus be acutely relevant to pain disorders, especially because they tend to be both chronic and generally non-life-threatening. In addition, the knowledge that an individual has a ``pain disorder gene´´ might lead to an over-reaction to or minimization of pain experience in detrimental ways, both for the individual and for family and friends.

Finally, the presence of a ``positive´´ test result for genes related to chronic pain disorders might alter the probability of a patient´s developing the disorder by influencing the patient´s behaviors as well as the attitudes and predictions of pain physicians, thus affecting not only treatment decisions, but also the manner in which understanding of severe or intractable pain is communicated to the patient. This probability might be especially large if communication and treatment begins in the early stages of pain. In this situation the variables that are affected by diagnosis, prognosis, and treatment choice could be affected in ways that directly influence therapeutic outcomes by instigating potential nocebo effects.

INTEGRATING BRAIN–MIND PHENOMENA IN AN ETHIC OF NEUROGENETICS

Explaining mental phenomena by using biology, primarily or solely, carries implications for people´s conceptions of what it means to be healthy and human, the experience of which is phenomenally distinguished more than biologically distinguished. If explanations of the phenomenal aspects of human disease are necessary for health care to ethically utilize scientific understanding of disease entities, a reductive approach to neurogenetics is ultimately too limited. This limitation is clear epistemologically because there is simply no guarantee that a sufficient explanation will be forthcoming when all the biological functional details are amassed. Without an appropriately sufficient explanation of the phenomenal features of patient experience, neurology and psychiatry become relatively disempowered to address these phenomena, including human suffering, in those illnesses for which a biological approach is singularly employed. At the level of the individual, mental phenomena are ultimately what characterize patients´ experience of illness and shape the way that they identify with it, and relate themselves to their experience of illness. A given understanding of illness as tied into one´s individual human identity can affect the way a person copes with suffering as well as participates in healing activities.

Methodological reductionism, as applied to neuroscience, postulates that the mind can be reduced to physical brain processes. As a philosophy, reductionism is dependent upon a value system concerning the relationship between the brain and the mind. In tracing the historical evolution of that belief, one finds that it arose out of a shift in philosophical values concerning the transition from the scientific notion of body and soul to brain and mind, and ultimately to the modern neuroscientific notion of brain–mind wherein the two may become ontologically identical. Yet in the context of mental and behavioral health, brain and mind should not be ontologically identical, since, for example, the experience of refractory maldynic pain is by definition ontologically distinct from the organic brain, as mentioned above.

In a reductive medicine, where mental phenomena are reduced to neuroscience and the mind is identified as the brain, conflating the notions of illness and disease becomes almost inevitable. Illness refers more to the phenomenal aspects of suffering, whereas disease refers more to the biophysical pathology. Although the two can exist independently, a reductive approach to neurogenetics tends to conflate them – as evident in the use of the phrase ``the biochemical basis for mental illness´´. If the phenomenal is to be reducible, it cannot be explained outside of the context of biochemistry. Thus, applying reductionism to mental illness phenomena has consequences for our subsequent interpretations of brain and mind; attempts to explain mental aspects of illness phenomena become restricted to neurophysiological mechanisms.

Problems arise because the meaning of mental health cannot be inferred or deduced from neurophysiological activity. Instead, this meaning includes the phenomenal features of mind, such as emotion, feelings, and thoughts, and especially illness-related suffering (Edel 1961). The *telos* of medicine depends on an understanding of this meaning. Judgments in ethics do and should rely on scientific results, but problems arise when the sole point of reference is scientific information. Any kind of relevant information that contextualizes the lives and actions of human beings by illuminating human nature, social relations, experiences, and potential – in other words, mean-ingful information – is relevant for an ethics of neurogenetics and mental health. If psychological, social, and environmental variables are of more dynamic importance than granted by reductionism, reduc-tionism may lead to the disempowering of patients that might other-wise be able to control significant variables leading to their state of illness. In order to reflect the complexity of the human condition, and protect against such disempowerment, more integrated and emergent theories are warranted.

Perhaps not surprisingly, one can argue that integrating ethics with neurogenetics is akin to integrating mind and brain. A flawed understanding about the relationship of neurogenetics and illness would be mirrored in a flawed appreciation for the complexity and non-linear causality of the mind/brain interaction. If this complexity is not appreciated on the level of understanding how illness occurs, then it certainly will not be appreciated in judging how to appropriately care for those who experience such illness.

CONCLUSION

Medicine is an inter-subjective endeavor, as is applied ethics, and both deal with scientific information as it regards some of the most personal and powerful aspects of the patient's self-understanding and self-worth. Pragmatically, applying theories of normative ethics along with ethically grounded daily clinical practice to the cutting-edge advances of neuroscience and biomedicine requires the incorporation of this rapidly expanding scientific knowledge into basic health care decision-making (Edel 1961). A flawed understanding regarding the relationship of neurogenetic research to mental or behavioral illness could well result in the choice of a less effective, or even harmful, treatment approach, and also lead to an inappropriate communication of genetic determinism to patients and the public. To ensure that assessments of risks and ethical consequences of actions in neuromedicine are accurate, the epistemological framework for understanding pain should reflect a scientific model that accounts for the functional integration of neurogenetic, perceptive, social, and experiential variables that contribute to pain disorders.

REFERENCES

Allchin, D. 1998. Values in science and in science education. In Fraser, B. J. & Tobin, K. G. (eds.), *International Handbook of Science Education*, vol. 2. Dordrecht: Kluwer Academic Publishers, pp. 1803–92.

Bennett, R. M. 1999. Emerging concepts in the neurobiology of chronic pain: evidence of abnormal sensory processing in fibromyalgia. *Mayo Clinic Proceedings* **74**: 385–98.

Bloch, M. & Hayden, M. R. 1990. Opinion: predictive testing for Huntington disease in childhood: challenges and implications. *American Journal of Human Genetics* **46**: 1–4.

Brown, T. 2003. Reductionism and the circle of the sciences. In Brown, T. & Smith, L. (eds.) *Reduction and the Development of Knowledge*. Mahwah, NJ: Lawrence Erlbaum Associates. (Available from: Questia. Accessed November 1, 2007.)

Bruntrup, G. 1998. Is psycho-physical emergentism committed to dualism? The causal efficacy of emergent mental properties. *Erkenntins* **48**(2–3): 131–51.

Collins, W. A., Maccoby, E. E., Steinberg, L., Hetherington, E. M. & Bornstein, M. H. 2000. Contemporary research on parenting: the case of nature and nurture. *American Psychologist* **55**: 218–32.

Crutchfield, J. P. 2008. Is anything ever new? Considering emergence. In Bedau, M. A. & Humphreys, P. (eds.) *Emergence*. Cambridge, MA: The MIT Press, pp. 269–86.

Edel, A. 1961. *Science and the Structure of Ethics*. Chicago, IL: University of Chicago Press. (Available from: Questia. Accessed November 1, 2007.)

Giordano, J. 2006. Understanding pain as disease and illness: part one. *Practical Pain Management* **6**(6): 70–3.

Giordano, J. 2007. A big picture: neurogenesis, pain and the reality and ethics of medicine. *Practical Pain Management* **7**(2): 37–52.

Giordano J. 2008. Complementarity, brain~mind, and pain. *Forschende. Komplementärmedizin* **15**: 71–3.

Harper, P. S. & Clarke, A. 1990. Should we test children for ``adult'' genetic diseases? *Lancet* **335**: 1205–6.

Horowitz, F. D. 2000. Child development and the PITS: simple questions, complex answers, and developmental theory. *Child Development* **71**: 1–10.

Klernam, G. L. 1984. History and development of modern concepts of affective illness. In Post, R. M. & Ballenger, J. C. (eds.) *Neurobiology of Mood Disorders*. Baltimore, MD: Williams & Wilkins, pp. 1–19.

Kraepelin, E. 1921. *Manic Depressive Insanity and Paranoia*. Edinburgh: E & S Livingstone.

Lerner, R. M. 2004. Genes and the promotion of positive human development: hereditarian versus developmental systems perspectives. In Coll, C. G., Bearer, E. L. & Lerner, R. M. (eds.) *Nature and Nurture: The Complex Interplay of Genetic and Environmental Influences on Human Behavior and Development*. Mahwah, NJ: Lawrence Erlbaum Associates. (Available from: Questia. Accessed November 1, 2007.)

MacGregor, A. J. 2004. The heritability of pain in humans. In Mogil J. S. (ed.) *The Genetics of Pain: Progress in Pain Research and Management*, vol. 28. Seattle: IASP Press, pp. 151–69.

Mogil, J. S. 2004. Complex trait genetics of pain in the laboratory mouse. In Mogil, J. S. (ed.) *The Genetics of Pain: Progress in Pain Research and Management*, vol. 28. Seattle: IASP Press, pp. 123–49.

Parens, E. 2004. Genetic differences and human identities: on why talking about behavioral genetics is important and difficult. *Hastings Center Report Special Supplement* **34**(1): S1–S36.

Plomin, R. & McGuffin, P. 2003. Psychopathology in the postgenomic era. *Annual Review of Psychology* **54**: 205–28.

Valenstein, E. S. 1998. *Blaming the Brain*. New York: The Free Press.

Williams, R. B. 1994. Neurobiology, cellular and molecular biology, and psychosomatic medicine. *Psychosomatic Medicine* **56**: 308–15.

Williams, R. B. 1998. Lower socioeconomic status and increased mortality: early childhood roots and the potential for successful interventions. *Journal of American Medical Association* **279**: 1745–6.

Williams, R. B., Marchuk, D. A., Gadde, K. M. *et al.* 2003. Serotonin-related gene polymorphisms and central nervous system serotonin function. *Neuropsychopharmacology* **28**: 533–41.

11

Neuroimaging
Thinking in pictures

J. VANMETER

INTRODUCTION

Functional neuroimaging techniques, such as functional MRI (fMRI), positron emission tomography, and others have proven to be powerful methods for examining brain function that have led to major advances in our understanding of the brain and various neurological conditions. fMRI has provided researchers with a non-invasive tool to delineate basic neurophysiological processes and found use in clinical applications such as pre-surgical mapping of important functional areas that can guide neurosurgical cases. More thought-provoking examples include identifying a distinct response to romantic love, different from sexual arousal (Aron *et al.* 2005) and the development of an fMRI-based neural feedback system to improve management of pain (deCharms *et al.* 2005).

Since 1992 there has been an exponential increase in the number of papers published on fMRI (Bandettini 2007). This is in part due to the fact that fMRI as a technique only began to be used in the early 1990s but also due to the ready availability of MRI scanners capable of conducting these studies. Correspondingly, there has been an explosion of media coverage of this branch of neuroscience, driven in part by the compelling portrayal of these results with the pictures and movies to which these techniques readily lend themselves (Racine *et al.* 2005). Neuroscientific explanations combined with richly detailed and beautiful pictures depicting the results from fMRI experiments have been shown to increase the perceived validity of a finding even when the underlying science is questionable (McCabe & Castel 2008; Weisberg

Scientific and Philosophical Perspectives in Neuroethics, ed. J. J. Giordano & B. Gordijn. Published by Cambridge University Press. © Cambridge University Press 2010.

et al. 2008). Indeed, the power of the picture to persuade is exemplified by the following quote from a recent PBS documentary on brain fitness: "... we know this to be true because we can see pictures of the brain" (Brown 2008).

Putting the scientific findings from fMRI studies into a proper context and conveying the nuances of the researchers' interpretation of their own data requires a level of exposition and discussion that is typically not possible in the format of most forms of popular media. As with any scientific measurement technique there are inherent limitations that have important implications regarding what the data convey and the inferences that can be made. Furthermore, the experimental design and the methods used to process the data introduce additional constraints and limitations on the interpretation of the results. Finally, there is a tendency, both in the media's coverage but also to a certain extent in the scientific literature, to extrapolate from the results of a single study based on a relatively small number of subjects to overly broad statements and unsupported claims about the implications of those results.

The remainder of this chapter focusses on functional MRI, as this technique more than any other has created an explosion in neuroimaging, especially as it has been reported in the media. An overview of what is measured by using fMRI and the methods for processing the data are given as a background for a discussion of the limitations of fMRI. This is followed by specific examples of how the results from studies using fMRI have been presented in the mass media.

WHAT IS CAPTURED BY FMRI?

fMRI requires an MRI scanner with the ability to acquire several images corresponding to slices through the brain at a rate of 10–50 milliseconds per slice. Each collection of 2D slices is treated as a unit, referred to as a volume. During the fMRI scan, a series of volumes are collected while the subject or patient is instructed to perform some cognitive or motoric task. Since fMRI is a non-quantitative technique, a comparison of two or more conditions is required. By matching each condition the subject was performing to the corresponding volume, it is possible to identify regions of the brain that have changes in MRI signal intensity, taken to correspond to the neuronal activity induced by the task. However, it is not possible to determine by visual examination of the raw images where these changes occurred. This is because changes in neuronal activity produce a very small change in the MRI signal intensity, typically of the order of 0.1%–0.5%. Thus, to extract the task-related signal change, each condition is repeated as many as 20–100 times.

What causes the changes in MRI signal during neuronal activity? The most commonly used fMRI method is based on changes in oxygenation of hemoglobin (red blood cells) that in turn induce changes in the MRI signal. This method, called the BOLD (Blood Oxygenation Level Dependent) contrast method, relies on the differential effect that hemoglobin has on the MRI signal, depending on whether it is carrying an oxygen molecule (Ogawa *et al.* 1990). In particular, deoxygenated hemoglobin (a red blood cell with its oxygen molecule extracted) produces a weak disturbance in the surrounding magnetic field whereas oxygenated hemoglobin has little or no effect on the MRI signal. When neurons become active their metabolism is fueled by glucose and oxygen. The neurovasculature responds to an increase in neuronal activity by increasing the flow of blood to that area of the brain. Both increased neuronal activity and blood flow contribute to changes in the local concentration of deoxygenated hemoglobin.

An increase in neuronal activity produces a complicated cascade of events that affect the oxygenated state of hemoglobin, the nature of which is not completely understood. The initiation of neuronal activity requires the use of the locally available oxygen, resulting in an immediate increase in deoxygenated hemoglobin. This is followed by an increase in blood flowing into the area, peaking about 6 seconds after the initial activity. The increase in blood flow results in the delivery of more oxygen than is actually required by the active neurons, leading to an overall increase in oxygenated hemoglobin and a decrease in deoxygenated hemoglobin. While it may seem counterintuitive, the net effect of the increase in blood flow that occurs with neuronal activity is an overabundance of oxygenated hemoglobin and a decrease in deoxygenated hemoglobin, producing an increase in the MRI signal (Kwong *et al.* 1992). However, other factors can lead to changes in the BOLD signal, including changes in the rate at which oxygen is extracted from the blood as well as relative changes in blood volume.

Several issues are important to the interpretation of fMRI data, including the temporal and spatial resolution of the raw data. The temporal resolution of fMRI is typically of the order of seconds (assuming several slices are acquired); in the context of neuronal activity, this is relatively poor. Spatial resolution is typically a couple of cubic millimeters and thus the neuronal activity captured by using fMRI represents the aggregate activity of millions of individual neurons. It is possible to achieve either higher temporal resolution, by collecting only a handful of slices, or higher spatial resolution at the expense of temporal resolution and/or a loss of overall signal.

FMRI: FROM RAW DATA TO MAPS OF ACTIVATION

Extracting the fMRI signal changes from the raw fMRI volumes requires a number of complicated steps. The fundamental method of processing fMRI data proceeds on a voxel-by-voxel basis whereby the changes in the MRI signal across time are correlated with the changes in the stimulation paradigm at each individual voxel. In many instances the data from several subjects are combined together also on a voxel-by-voxel basis. This data processing technique is generally referred to as Statistical Parametric Mapping (Friston *et al.* 2007). Below, the preprocessing and statistical analysis steps that are used in a typical analysis are described, along with the changes that the data undergo and the implications each has on the interpretation of the final results.

Data preprocessing

To process the data on a voxel-by-voxel basis, any head motion that occurred over the course of the scanning session must be removed. If there is motion of the brain across time, then examination of a given cardinal coordinate will correspond to different locations in the brain between volumes, thus negating the possibility of using a voxel-by-voxel analysis. This step in the preprocessing chain is referred to as Realignment or Motion Correction and uses one of several image registration algorithms to align the brain in each volume with the position of the brain in the first volume or some other representative volume (Woods *et al.* 1998). These algorithms examine the intensities in the pair of images to determine the set of spatial transformations required for alignment. Typically, a "rigid-body" transformation is used with parameters consisting of rotations about each of the three axes and translations in each axis. Once the transformation parameters have been determined, they are applied by using an interpolation algorithm to create a reformatted volume. The brain in the resulting realigned volume is then in the same position as the first volume within the accuracy of the registration algorithm.

Issues that can arise from motion correction include the very real possibility that not all of the motion has been removed from the time series. This residual motion will naturally lead to a reduction in statistical power, especially around the edges of an area of activation, decreasing our ability to detect smaller areas of activation. In addition, spatial resolution is further reduced when the interpolation algorithm is applied, as these algorithms use some form of a weighted average of the neighboring voxels to reformat the realigned volume. Thus, this part of the data preprocessing chain has two unwanted side effects: (1) decreased detectability of signal changes; and (2) decreased spatial resolution. In general, the benefits of motion correction outweigh these problems.

A common method for combining data across subjects and localizing the changes in the neuronal activity to specific anatomic regions is to transform each person's individual brain into a reference space such as the Talairach atlas (Talairach & Tournoux 1988). These methods, referred to as Spatial Normalization, deform the images from each subject by using a combination of linear and non-linear transformations, which again requires interpolation and results in another decrement in spatial resolution (Ashburner *et al.* 1997).

The final step in the preprocessing of the fMRI data is to apply a smoothing kernel, such as a Gaussian weighting function, to each of the volumes. This removes local spatial noise and helps to compensate for less than perfect spatial normalization by spreading areas of activation, increasing the potential overlap between subjects. Naturally, this step reduces spatial resolution and can produce a reduction in the magnitude of activation by decreasing the difference in signal between two conditions.

Statistical analysis

Typically, a parametric statistical test is applied at each voxel in the brain, including *t*-tests, correlations, and general linear models, to identify those voxels in which the MRI signal changes relate to alterations in the conditions of the task. In many studies, changes common across subjects and differences between groups of subjects are examined by using another level of statistical tests. Inferences about the areas active in a given population are typically performed with a mixed-effects analysis, whereby summary statistics such as the mean difference between two conditions from each subject corresponding to a fixed-effects analysis are combined in second-stage random-effects analysis. Use of this two-stage approach allows for inferences to be applied to the group from which the subjects are drawn. It is worth noting that the overwhelming majority of results reported are based on some form of group analysis; this inherently glosses over and ignores individual differences in the patterns of activation, which can be considerable.

The last stage of the analysis is to generate the tables and pictures depicting the areas of activation found in the statistical analysis. This procedure overlays areas determined to be significant onto either a mean high-resolution structural scan from the subjects included in the study or, more commonly, a prototypical high-resolution scan from a normal volunteer. Key to generating these tables and pictures is deciding the appropriate statistical cut-off to use. As in many disciplines the only uniformly accepted standard is that the statistical cut-off should result in no more than a 5% chance of erroneously attributing activation to an area where none really exists. The fact that a statistical test is being performed at each and every voxel, which can number as high as several hundred thousand, leads to a severe problem, referred to in statistics as the problem of multiple comparisons. In essence, each additional statistical test greatly increases the likelihood that spurious and artifactual changes in the MRI signal will be identified as significantly activated. The multiple comparisons problem is dealt with by using a variety of corrections, many of which take into account the fact that the underlying and induced smoothness of the data increases the spatial dependency of the signal from voxel to voxel (Logan & Rowe 2004). Other correction methods use permutation testing (Nichols & Holmes 2002) or techniques such as false discovery rate borrowed from other disciplines that deal with large amounts of data, such as genetics (Genovese *et al.* 2002). Although these techniques are widely available it is unfortunately not uncommon to see published data that have not been corrected for multiple comparisons, primarily because these corrections would lead to a null result. This is especially true in situations where the number of subjects used in the experiment is relatively small, the experimental design is contrasting two very closely related conditions, or the difference between two populations of subjects is small.

Interpretation of the results

Since the BOLD signal is non-quantitative, no meaningful interpretation can be assigned to the signal observed during a single cognitive process performed by a subject. Rather, any fMRI experiment requires the comparison of signals arising from two or more tasks. This technique, referred to as the *subtraction method*, is used to identify areas of activity. Ideally, the process of interest differs from the control task, which is used as the reference or baseline, by a single cognitive process. For example, to examine whole word reading a possible control task might be false font strings, which consist of letter-like components formed from lines and arcs. In this case, the false font strings control for the visual processing that is common to both tasks leaving only reading processes following the subtraction of the two tasks. Fundamental to these experimental designs is the *assumption of pure insertion* whereby it is assumed that the insertion of a single cognitive process into a control task does not change other processes. Unfortunately, this assumption does not always hold. Jennings and colleagues found an interaction between how a subject was asked to respond and activation for a semantic task compared with a letter judgment task (Jennings *et al.* 1997). As the experimental design determines what can be inferred from the results of the study, careful consideration is required.

Several other factors can influence the results of a study. Variations in the BOLD signal have been found to be correlated with the number of hours of sleep a subject had the night before (Habeck *et al.* 2004), decrease with caffeine use (Perthen *et al.* 2008), increase with higher arterial carbon dioxide concentration (Wise *et al.* 2004), and decrease with nicotine use (Hahn *et al.* 2007). Task difficulty and differences in level of attention required to complete a task can have a major impact on results, leading to the activation of executive and attentional networks that may not be involved in the cognitive process of interest (Culham 2006; O'Craven *et al.* 1997). Differences in the difficulty of the task are of special concern when comparing different populations of subjects (Matthews *et al.* 2006). For instance, if a task is difficult for Alzheimer subjects but relatively easy for elderly controls then it is likely that areas such as the anterior cingulate cortex (attention) and the dorsal lateral prefrontal cortex (executive function) will be activated in the patient group, regardless of the cognitive task, and possibly not in the controls.

STUDIES EXEMPLIFYING ETHICAL AND SCIENTIFIC CONCERNS

Two examples where the use of the results from fMRI have raised ethical and scientific concerns include the commercialization of fMRI in the form of a lie detector and the supposed predictive value of fMRI in determining preferences or reactions to television advertising and perceptions of presidential candidates.

fMRI as a new lie detector

One of the more controversial and potentially far-reaching applications of fMRI is in the area of deception detection. It has been the goal of many institutions, especially in relation to national security concerns but also in the judicial arena, to come up with a better lie detector. The possibility that fMRI, by showing what is occurring in a person's brain, could be used to determine whether an individual was telling the truth is naturally very compelling, especially given the impact that the pictures from fMRI can have. To date two corporations have been formed around this idea: No Lie MRI, Inc. and Cephos Corporation. The mass media has taken great interest in the work of these companies, resulting in several almost uniformly positive stories. ABC News aired a report on No Lie MRI and how they were able to "prove" that a man did not commit arson (Stone 2007). In several of these stories, the reporters themselves were scanned and the detection of their lying in the controlled experimental setting was demonstrated, leading to amazed reactions by those same reporters (Ritter 2006).

A number of peer-reviewed studies on the use of fMRI for deception detection have been published (Bhatt *et al.* 2009; Kozel *et al.* 2004; Langleben *et al.* 2005). The general consensus is that several areas of the brain are reliably identified in these studies: the anterior cingulate cortex (ACC), prefrontal cortex, and parietal cortex. Although these studies provide evidence of the potential application of fMRI to detect deception, there are a number of technical and ethical issues that should be carefully considered. Technical issues include uniqueness of the neural signature, individual variability, and applicability of the laboratory experiments to real-world scenarios. Individual differences can arise from personality and psychological factors such as psychopathy (Bhatt *et al.* 2009).

The uniqueness of the neural signature attributed to deception is questionable since the same areas of the brain that show greater activation during deception are involved in a wide range of other cognitive processes. Of particular note is the ACC, given its role as a regulator of top-down executive focus and how it can be influenced by emotional salience (Bush *et al.* 2000). Further, the ACC plays a significant role when it comes to monitoring errors, task difficulty, and motivation. In a real-world application of this technique in situations

where the risks associated with failing the test carry serious consequences, motivation will undoubtedly be a major factor. As of yet there
is no way to distinguish activation in the ACC due to deception from
activation caused by a high degree of motivation to pass the test.

An additional issue is the limited testing of this technique on
individual subjects. All but two of the published studies have been
based on the results from group-level analyses, which necessarily
ignore subject-to-subject variability. It is important to understand that
in any given fMRI study there is considerable variability across subjects
and not all subjects reliably produce statistically measurable differences in the BOLD signal (McGonigle *et al.* 2000). One study to examine
the accuracy of this fMRI-based deception detection found an accuracy
of 88% on an individualized basis in 22 subjects (Davatzikos *et al.* 2005).
However, nearly all of the data from all the subjects studied were used
to train the SVM (support-vector machine) classifier. In another study,
90% accuracy was found in a test of 61 subjects, half of whom were
used to construct the classifier (Kozel *et al.* 2005). Together these studies
suggest that it is possible, at least in these controlled experimental
settings, to determine deception on an individual basis by using fMRI,
though certainly not with 100% accuracy. For fMRI to become an
accepted deception detection procedure, several more studies would
need to be conducted to reproduce and extend these findings.

Real-world applicability is another important issue, as the
translatability of the results from the laboratory setting is questionable. Necessarily, the experimental designs used to date involve scenarios in which both the subject and experimenter know that the
subject will make a false response at some point during the experiment. However, a false response is not necessarily equivalent to lying.
Further, these studies have involved scenarios in which the stakes do
not compare with those that could be expected in a death penalty case
or credibility assessment for national security. In those situations, it is
reasonable to assume that an innocent suspect would exhibit a high
degree of brain activity, unrelated to deception, that could overlap with
the putative areas of the brain involved in deception, especially in
areas of attention and executive function. In comparison, the low-
stakes experimental designs used in the published fMRI experiments
do not provide the emotional context or the potential consequences
that exist in these more serious situations (Sip *et al.* 2008).

Beyond the technical challenges there are a number of legal and
ethical concerns with the use of fMRI for the purpose of deception
detection. Legal issues include threats to privacy and the self-

incrimination clause of the Fifth Amendment (Stoller & Wolpe 2007). Of note is whether an fMRI lie-detection scan would be considered by the judiciary to be equivalent to physical evidence such as a blood or handwriting sample, which is not protected by the Fifth Amendment, or consistent with the protection of testimonial evidence, which is protected (Stoller & Wolpe 2007). Privacy concerns are clear and raise questions as to whether there is a right to privacy regarding one's cognitive processes and internal thoughts (Wolpe *et al.* 2005).

"Instant science" versus peer-review

Given the impact that the pictures generated from fMRI studies can have, they are often included in print or online articles and television reports. In some cases these reports overstate the results and make claims that are beyond the scope of what can be reasonably inferred from the data. Although it is understandable that reporters seek angles that will have the greatest impact, it is incumbent upon the scientists to work with the reporters to put the results in the proper context. An unfortunate trend that has emerged in recent years is when scientists circumvent the peer-review process and report their findings directly to the media. These reports have included examining the response in individual subjects to various Super Bowl commercials and, more recently, attempts to ascribe the feelings individual voters have towards different presidential candidates based on the results from fMRI scans (Iacoboni 2006; Iacoboni *et al.* 2007).

In 2006, Marco Iacoboni from the University of California, Los Angeles, scanned subjects using fMRI as they viewed different commercials from Super Bowl XL, which they had not seen previously. The reported aim of the study was to test whether there is "a disconnect between what people say about what they like – and the real, underlying deeper motives". The specifics of the experiment provided by the researchers have been limited to the number of subjects (5) and the number of advertisements used (24). Other critical details such as how many times each advertisement was shown, what control task was used, whether the results are from a group or single-subject analysis, the statistical cut-off used, to name a few, were not reported. Rather than providing these standard details of the experimental design, the researchers instead tout this as the "very first attempt at doing 'instant-science'". As one might expect, the results of this study were widely reported in the media, including most national morning news programs (Iacoboni 2006).

The results that were reported from this study include a ranking of the commercials based on some statistical analysis of the fMRI data and beautifully rendered pictures of the results. Using these results, the researchers claimed that the Disney advertisement featuring the winning quarterback was declared the ``winner'' whereas the Burger King and FedEx advertisements were deemed ``losers'' (Iacoboni 2006). Exactly how these rankings were determined has not been disclosed and is not self-evident. Nonetheless, the researchers claim that the high level of activity in the anterior cingulate cortex, dorsolateral prefrontal cortex, orbito-frontal cortex, and ventral striatum were ``positive markers of brain responses to the ad'' (Iacoboni 2006). The exact location, the spatial extent, and statistical level of each area of activation were not provided. However, the authors did provide some very broad interpretations, including the following: ``female subjects may give verbally very low `grades' to ads using actresses in sexy roles, but their mirror neuron areas seem to fire up quite a bit, suggesting some form of identification and empathy'' (Iacoboni 2006). Interestingly, the basis for these claims and even how many of the five subjects were female was lacking.

Although this kind of research into the effect of advertising on the motivation of individual consumers and how they influence buying decisions certainly can have scientific merit, it is nonetheless disappointing that this study has never been published in a peer-reviewed journal. It is probable that the fact that this study was done in partnership with FKF Applied Research, Inc., a company that is attempting to commercialize this technique as a tool for marketing research, referred to as neuromarketing, was a major factor in the decision about how to disseminate this research.

Similarly, this type of instant publication of results has been extended into the area of political preferences and the emotional bases thereof. Published as an Op-Ed piece in the *New York Times* on November 11, 2007, Iacoboni and his collaborators presented the results of an experiment that examined 20 potential voters' responses to politically based stimuli such as the names of the major political parties and photographs or videos of major presidential candidates (Iacoboni *et al.* 2007). Based on the areas activated in some or all of the subjects, the authors made very broad interpretations of the results, drawing inferences such as differences between males' and females' reactions to photographs and videos of Hillary Clinton. To wit, the authors' conclusions regarding voters' reaction to Mrs. Clinton: ``When viewing images of her, these voters exhibited significant activity in the anterior cingulate cortex, an emotional center of the brain that is aroused when a person feels compelled to act in two different ways but must choose one˝. Although this interpretation of the activation in the anterior cingulate cortex is plausible, there are a number of alternate explanations that could be equally valid: even something as simple as increased attention on the part of the subjects during these video clips. Since the format of an Op-Ed piece does lend itself to longer expositions, the details of the experimental design that would aid a reader in evaluating the conclusions that the authors make are lacking. In response, several leading neuroscientists wrote a letter to the editor strongly rebuking the authors for their mostly unsubstantiated inferences regarding mental states and the lack of details about the experiments (Aron *et al.* 2007). As with the Super Bowl commercial experiment, this study was conducted in collaboration with the principles of the neuromarketing firm FKF Applied Research, Inc. Likewise, this experiment has not been published in a scientific journal.

CONCLUSION

Functional MRI has the ability to examine neuronal processing and thus provide amazing insights into how the brain works, leading to both valuable neuroscience advancements and clinical benefits. The beautiful and eye-catching pictures that can be generated from these experiments are powerfully persuasive and handily help to convince readers of the results being presented in papers. This tendency is greatly amplified when data are presented in various media where images and movies of the brain can grab the attention of consumers, which is naturally to the advantage of the journalist and media outlet. This, combined with the limited science background of most journalists and in some instances with overselling by researchers, can lead to serious misperceptions of the certainty and generalizability of the results.

It is necessary to be mindful of what is measured by each neuroimaging technique and its limitations. In the case of fMRI, the underlying signal is derived from changes in the state of the oxygenation of the blood, which is generally well correlated with blood flow changes and in turn neuronal activity. However, several factors other than neuronal activity can create changes in the BOLD signal. Further, this dependence on hemodynamic changes necessarily limits the temporal and spatial resolution that can be achieved by using fMRI. The different stages of processing that the data go through leads to further limitations as to what can be inferred from the experimental results. These limitations need to be carefully considered in areas such as deception detection and neuromarketing, where the ethical use of this and related neuroimaging techniques is only beginning to be examined.

REFERENCES

Aron, A., Badre, D., Brett, M. *et al.* 2007. *Politics and the Brain.* New York: *New York Times.*

Aron, A., Fisher, H., Mashek, D. J. *et al.* 2005. Reward, motivation, and emotion systems associated with early-stage intense romantic love. *Journal of Neurophysiology* **94**: 327–37.

Ashburner, J., Neelin, P., Collins, D. L., Evans, A. & Friston, K. 1997. Incorporating prior knowledge into image registration. *Neuroimage* **6**: 344–52.

Bandettini, P. 2007. Functional MRI today. *International Journal of Psychophysiology* **63**: 138–45.

Bhatt, S., Mbwana, J., Adeyemo, A. *et al.* 2009. Lying about facial recognition: an fMRI study. *Brain and Cognition* **69**: 382–90.

Brown, E. 2008. *The Brain Fitness Program.* (Running time 100 min.)

Bush, G., Luu, P. & Posner, M. I. 2000. Cognitive and emotional influences in anterior cingulate cortex. *Trends in Cognitive Sciences* **4**: 215–22.

Culham, J. C. 2006. Functional neuroimaging: experimental design and analysis. In Cabeza, R. & Kingstone, A. (eds.) *Handbook of Functional Neuroimaging of Cognition.* Cambridge, MA: The MIT Press, pp. 53–82.

Davatzikos, C., Ruparel, K., Fan, Y. *et al.* 2005. Classifying spatial patterns of brain activity with machine learning methods: application to lie detection. *Neuroimage* **28**: 663–8.

deCharms, R. C., Maeda, F., Glover, G. H. *et al.* 2005. Control over brain activation and pain learned by using real-time functional MRI. *Proceedings of the National Academy of Sciences, USA* **102**: 18626–31.

Friston, K. J., Ashburner, J. T., Kiebel, S. J., Nichols, T. E. & Penny, W. D. 2007. *Statistical Parametric Mapping: The Analysis of Functional Brain Images.* New York: Academic Press.

Genovese, C. R., Lazar, N. A. & Nichols, T. 2002. Thresholding of statistical maps in functional neuroimaging using the false discovery rate. *Neuroimage* **15**: 870–8.

Habeck, C., Rakitin, B. C., Moeller, J. *et al.* 2004. An event-related fMRI study of the neurobehavioral impact of sleep deprivation on performance of a delayed-match-to-sample task. *Brain Research Cognitive Brain Research* **18**: 306–21.

Hahn, B., Ross, T. J., Yang, Y. *et al.* 2007. Nicotine enhances visuospatial attention by deactivating areas of the resting brain default network. *Journal of Neuroscience* **27**: 3477–89.

Iacoboni, M. 2006. *Who Really Won the Super Bowl? The Story of an Instant-Science Experiment.* www.edge.org/3rd_culture/iacoboni06/iacoboni06-index.html

Iacoboni, M., Freedman, J., Kaplan, J. *et al.* 2007. *This is your Brain on Politics.* New York: *New York Times.*

Jennings, J. M., McIntosh, A. R., Kapur, S., Tulving, E. & Houle, S., 1997. Cognitive subtractions may not add up: the interaction between semantic processing and response mode. *Neuroimage* **5**: 229–39.

Kozel, F. A., Johnson, K. A., Mu, Q. *et al.* 2005. Detecting deception using functional magnetic resonance imaging. *Biological Psychiatry* **58**: 605–13.

Kozel, F. A., Revell, L. J., Lorberbaum, J. P. *et al.* 2004. A pilot study of functional magnetic resonance imaging brain correlates of deception in healthy young men. *Journal of Neuropsychiatry and Clinical Neuroscience* **16**: 295–305.

Kwong, K. K., Belliveau, J. W., Chesler, D. A. *et al.* 1992. Dynamic magnetic resonance imaging of human brain activity during primary sensory stimulation. *Proceedings of the National Academy of Sciences, USA* **89**: 5675–9.

Langleben, D. D., Loughead, J. W., Bilker, W. B. *et al.* 2005. Telling truth from lie in individual subjects with fast event-related fMRI. *Human Brain Mapping* **26**: 262–2.

Logan, B. R. & Rowe, D. B. 2004. An evaluation of thresholding techniques in fMRI analysis. *Neuroimage* **22**: 95–108.

Matthews, P. M., Honey, G. D. & Bullmore, E. T. 2006. Applications of fMRI in translational medicine and clinical practice. *Nature Reviews Neuroscience* **7**: 732–44.

McCabe, D. P. & Castel, A. D. 2008. Seeing is believing: the effect of brain images on judgments of scientific reasoning. *Cognition* **107**: 343–52.

McGonigle, D. J., Howseman, A. M., Athwal, B. S. *et al.* 2000. Variability in fMRI: an examination of intersession differences. *Neuroimage* **11**: 708–34.

Nichols, T. E. & Holmes, A. P. 2002. Nonparametric permutation tests for functional neuroimaging: a primer with examples. *Human Brain Mapping* **15**: 1–25.

O'Craven, K. M., Rosen, B. R., Kwong, K. K., Treisman, A. & Savoy, R. L. 1997. Voluntary attention modulates fMRI activity in human MT-MST. *Neuron* **18**: 591–8.

Ogawa, S., Lee, T. M., Nayak, A. S. & Glynn, P. 1990. Oxygenation-sensitive contrast in magnetic resonance image of rodent brain at high magnetic fields. *Magnetic Resonance Medicine* **14**: 68–78.

Perthen, J. E., Lansing, A. E., Liau, J., Liu, T. T. & Buxton, R. B. 2008. Caffeine-induced uncoupling of cerebral blood flow and oxygen metabolism: a calibrated BOLD fMRI study. *Neuroimage* **40**: 237–47.

Racine, E., Bar-Ilan, O. & Illes, J. 2005. fMRI in the public eye. *Nature Reviews Neuroscience* **6**: 159–64.

Ritter, M. 2006. *Brain-Scan Lie Detectors Coming in Near Future.* www.foxnews.com/story/0,2933,183294,00.html

Sip, K. E., Roepstorff, A., McGregor, W. & Frith, C. D. 2008. Detecting deception: the scope and limits. *Trends in Cognitive Sciences* **12**: 48–53.

Stoller, S. E. & Wolpe, P. R. 2007. Emerging neurotechnologies for lie detection and the fifth amendment. *American Journal of Law and Medicine* **33**: 359–75.

Stone, G. 2007. *See a Lie Inside the Brain.* ABC News.

Talairach, J. & Tournoux, P. 1988. *Co-Planar Stereotaxic Atlas of the Human Brain.* New York: Thieme Medical Publishers.

Weisberg, D. S., Keil, F. C., Goodstein, J., Rawson, E. & Gray, J. R. 2008. The seductive allure of neuroscience explanations. *Journal of Cognitive Neuroscience* **20**: 470–7.

Wise, R. G., Ide, K., Poulin, M. J. & Tracey, I. 2004. Resting fluctuations in arterial carbon dioxide induce significant low frequency variations in BOLD signal. *Neuroimage* **21**: 1652–64.

Wolpe, P. R., Foster, K. R. & Langleben, D. D. 2005. Emerging neurotechnologies for lie-detection: promises and perils. *American Journal of Bioethics* **5**: 39–49.

Woods, R. P., Grafton, S. T., Holmes, C. J., Cherry, S. R. & Mazziotta, J. C. 1998. Automated image registration: I. General methods and intrasubject, intramodality validation. *Journal of Computer Assisted Tomography* **22**: 139–52.

12

Can we read minds?
Ethical challenges and responsibilities in the use of neuroimaging research

E. RACINE, E. BELL & J. ILLES

Can we read minds? Can neuroimaging serve as a new form of lie-detector or reveal the essence of who we are? Should we be fearful that in the near future our personal thoughts will become publicly available through neuroimaging? Popular science and the media in particular have emphasized the mind-reading powers of neuroimaging. Questionable practices relying on such beliefs have begun to surface. Although appealing, these beliefs expose functional neuroimaging to potential abuse, and the equation between neuroimaging and mind-reading betrays the sophisticated nature of tools such as functional magnetic resonance imaging (fMRI) and positron emission tomography (PET). At stake is a potential misunderstanding of the true capabilities of functional neuroimaging – a misunderstanding that can be perpetuated if the mind-reading paradigm is not thoroughly examined.

The goal of this chapter is not to consider the numerous ethical challenges in neuroimaging research in detail, since many general overviews have been published (Downie & Marshall 2007; Illes *et al.* 2007; Marshall *et al.* 2007; Racine & Illes 2007a). Instead, it specifically reviews ethical and social challenges related to the interpretation of functional neuroimaging research, in and outside of clinical care, in order to critically examine the mind-reading potential of functional neuroimaging. This popular portrayal of neuroimaging must be addressed in the context of a balanced discussion of risks and ethical issues related to neuroimaging and neuroscience.

Scientific and Philosophical Perspectives in Neuroethics, ed. J. J. Giordano & B. Gordijn. Published by Cambridge University Press. © Cambridge University Press 2010.

We first briefly review some key aspects of fMRI and then present an overview of emerging uses of functional neuroimaging, in particular focussing on its applications in neurosurgery, chronic disorders of consciousness, and lie detection to provide context for our discussion. We then review why and how interpretation is a key epistemological and ethical challenge, intertwined in modern functional neuroimaging research with the historical investigation of brain function. The final discussion section addresses ethical and scientific responsibilities in matters of scientific integrity, public involvement, and self-reflection.

A PATHWAY TO BRAIN FUNCTION: AN OVERVIEW OF
FUNCTIONAL MAGNETIC RESONANCE IMAGING (FMRI)

As reviewed elsewhere (Illes & Racine 2005; Illes *et al.* 2006), powerful functional neuroimaging tools have been introduced throughout the twentieth century. The most prominent tools to date, electroencephalography (EEG), magnetoencephalography (MEG), PET, single photon emission computed tomography (SPECT), and fMRI, have provided a continuous stream of information about human behavior since the late 1920s, when the possibilities of actually measuring and mapping brain activity alongside behavior were first realized. The different techniques for measuring brain function each have relative advantages and disadvantages. fMRI is likely to have the greatest enduring effect on our society outside the realm of academia and medicine, given trade-offs between the various forms of functional neuroimaging, temporal and spatial resolution, and its non-invasive nature.

The discovery of fMRI in the 1990s enabled the mapping of neural function by measuring correlated hemodynamic changes in the brain. Revealing active brain regions, the blood-oxygenation-level-dependent (BOLD) contrast, relies on a dynamic set of events occurring in the brain coupled with neural activity, including changes in blood flow, blood volume, and blood oxygenation, which are measurable by fMRI scan (Nair 2005). Almost all functional neuroimaging studies involve comparison or subtraction methods between two controlled conditions, heavy statistical processing, and computer-intensive data reconstructions to produce the colorful activation maps with which we have become familiar. fMRI is no different; the activation maps produced by fMRI reflect indirect effects of neural activity on local blood flow under constrained experimental conditions. A typical fMRI experiment requires that participants engage in an experimental task (mental process of interest) and a control (baseline or comparison) task.

When engaging in these tasks during scanning, brain areas involved in their execution become active and a cascade of hemodynamic events, detectable by fMRI, results in a measurable increase in the MRI signal in activated regions. An assessment of brain activity during the mental process of interest then resides in statistical comparisons across the entire brain (separated into cubic elements or voxels), of the signal level between the control task and the experimental task. Those brain regions, or voxels, which meet statistical significance at a set threshold level, differentiate areas where the signal is statistically greater in the active versus control task. These regions are labeled in a color-coded map to represent active brain areas, and are generally overlaid onto a structural image.

EMERGING RESEARCH AND APPLICATIONS OF FUNCTIONAL NEUROIMAGING IN CLINICAL MEDICINE AND COGNITIVE SCIENCE

A century of imaging work has yielded information about brain function; fMRI has emerged as a powerful tool in these investigations over the past fifteen years. fMRI has frequently been used to explore the neural basis of sensory function or motor behaviors or in cognitive neuroscience to investigate memory, attention, language, and problem-solving. In a comprehensive literature review, one of us (JI) demonstrated a steady expansion of fMRI studies, alone or in combination with other imaging modalities, with evident social and policy implications, including studies of lying and deception, human cooperation and competition, brain differences in violent people, genetic influences, and variability in patterns of brain development (Illes *et al.* 2003a).

A similar evolution of fMRI has occurred in the clinical setting. The use of fMRI to map basic sensory or motor cortex prior to surgical intervention has been extended to map critical regions involved in language (Tharin & Golby 2007). Additionally, fMRI has been used to test the integrity of auditory processing pathways in people who are candidates for cochlear implants (Bartsch *et al.* 2006). Other active efforts to use the technology in clinical settings have focussed on the potential for diagnosis or treatment management in Alzheimer's disease (AD) and psychiatric illness (Paquette *et al.* 2003; Bondi *et al.* 2005; Fleisher *et al.* 2005; Chen *et al.* 2007; Fu *et al.* 2007). Promises that fMRI will lead to new drug discovery in a number of neurological disorders have also been made (Paulus & Stein 2007). Moreover, in the past few years, the potential of fMRI to determine levels of consciousness in minimally conscious or vegetative state patients has been examined in several studies; measures of brain function may, in the future, allow monitoring of rehabilitation interventions in these patients (Giacino *et al.* 2002; Schiff *et al.* 2005; Owen *et al.* 2006; Di *et al.* 2007).

It is evident that fMRI research has advanced rapidly across clinical and non-clinical domains with the potential to advance the understanding of both disordered and healthy brain processes. Emerging uses of fMRI continue to expand the landscape of use for this tool. In order to launch our discussion of the importance of interpretation in fMRI applications, we describe in more detail three emerging areas of fMRI investigation: presurgical mapping, detection of consciousness in severe brain injury, and lie detection. We will frame our discussion of scientific, social, and cultural interpretation challenges in fMRI around these three examples.

Brain mapping in presurgical assessment

Presurgical mapping of brain function is perhaps one of the most obvious clinical extensions of fMRI; it stems directly from the ability of fMRI to yield maps of brain function. The presurgical assessment of patients by using fMRI is a relevant issue, with the creation of two new clinical billing codes established by the American Medical Association in January 2007, designed for neuropsychologists and physicians who carry out fMRI mapping in patients. Other previously developed presurgical methods to map the areas of the cortex controlling sensory, motor, or language behaviour, such as intracranial stimulation (the gold standard method) (Tharin & Golby 2007) and/or Wada testing for language lateralization, are still employed. However, there are limitations in the presurgical mapping process to each of these techniques. Wada testing is invasive and carries a risk of stroke (1%), and the anesthesia of one hemisphere to observe function in the other can cause distress in patients (Tharin & Golby 2007). Intracranial stimulation is also an invasive technique, and generally requires that patients undergo a craniotomy wider than is needed for the surgical resection itself (Tharin & Golby 2007). Additionally, intracranial stimulation is disadvantaged by the fact that preoperative decisions about specific areas to resect cannot be made until the patient has already undergone craniotomy, and therefore does not allow preoperative planning (Tharin & Golby 2007).

fMRI has been tested across many studies for its potential in noninvasive presurgical mapping, with mixed success compared with previously established methods for the same purpose. fMRI has been shown to successfully map the motor cortex, in comparison to intra-cranial stimulation (Tharin & Golby 2007). Majos and colleagues (2005) report that the correlation between fMRI and intracranial stimulation mapping of motor cortex is 84%, based on their study of 33 patients. Others have also shown agreement (12 of 19 patients) between fMRI and PET to localize motor cortex for presurgical mapping (Krings *et al.* 2002). A recent review by Sunaert (2006) reports a success rate of approximately 80%–85% for presurgical fMRI in motor mapping. How-ever, the sensitivity of fMRI in the detection of critical cortical regions in higher-order cognitive tasks is less well established (Hirsch *et al.* 2000; Rutten *et al.* 2002). Some researchers have shown that fMRI maps are not always well correlated with intracranial electrical stimulation maps of language in patients (Roux *et al.* 2003); other studies have supported a good correspondence of language lateralization determination in fMRI compared with the Wada test (Binder *et al.* 1996; Desmond & Chen 2002; Kloppel & Buchel 2005). There is also a lack of evidence to support fMRI as a tool to map memory lateralization in presurgical mapping (Book-heimer 2007). Overall, however, preoperative fMRI mapping has been shown to have an impact on earlier established treatment plans by allowing a more aggressive therapeutic approach, shortening surgical time, increasing the size of resected brain regions, and decreasing craniotomy size (Petrella *et al.* 2006).

Detection of consciousness in brain injury

Over the past few years, fMRI studies investigating brain response in severely brain-injured patients have emerged. These studies have common objectives: to use fMRI to test for responsiveness, awareness, or remaining cognitive function in these patients. The management of patients with severe brain injury, in particular, is challenging, and the misdiagnosis of vegetative patients is surprisingly frequent (Childs *et al.* 1993; Andrews *et al.* 1996). Neuroimaging studies, which suggest that brain maps distinguish between the vegetative and minimally con-scious states, may be able to detect the presence of residual con-sciousness in patients with severe brain injury. The investigation by Di and others (2007) of brain activity in response to a person's own spoken name, revealed distinguishing patterns of activation between the vegetative state (wakeful, unaware) and the minimally conscious state (awake, some awareness, and responsive behaviors). Patients in a minimally conscious state exhibited greater widespread activation of higher-order processing areas. Two patients in the vegetative state who showed more extensive activation relative to their counterparts were diagnosed as minimally conscious 3 months post-scan. Further support of enduring brain activity in the persistent vegetative state to the patient's own name has been demonstrated in a case study (Staffen *et al.* 2006) and the preservation of some functional awareness in the vegetative state has also been supported in the fMRI study of one patient by Owen *et al.* (2006). In the latter study, the subject's brain activation patterns were tested on two motor imagery tasks and compared to activation maps obtained in healthy controls completing the same tasks. The authors report that the neural patterns observed in the patient were "indistinguishable from those observed in healthy volunteers" (Owen *et al.* 2006). Pending further proof that fMRI is able to evaluate the presence of conscious awareness, some researchers have suggested that fMRI may translate into a useful addition to rehabilitation monitoring in patients with disorders of consciousness (Giacino *et al.* 2006; Laureys *et al.* 2006).

Lie detection

In applications of fMRI that bridge cognitive science and law, some advancement in studying social attitudes, affect, reasoning, and emotional control have the potential to change approaches to truth verification and lie detection. Langleben *et al.* (2002), for example, used fMRI to study neural patterns associated with deception. In their landmark experiment, volunteers were instructed to either truthfully or falsely confirm or deny having a playing card in their possession. When subjects gave truthful answers, fMRI showed increased activity in visual and motor cortex. When they were deliberately deceptive, additional activations were measured in areas including the anterior cingulate cortex to which monitoring of response conflict and inhibition of response have been attributed (Langleben *et al.* 2002). In the future, therefore, we may not only be able to discern whether an individual is being deceptive, but also whether the deception was premeditated or not. More recently, Langleben *et al.* (2005) have demonstrated the detection of lie from truth in *individual* subjects during their previously employed card-holding paradigm, with an accuracy of 78%. This is a potentially important advancement in lie detection by fMRI. Although distinguishing brain patterns between lie and truth in a group advances our understanding of brain function, this does not easily translate to the testing of one person. Instead, in order to apply fMRI as a lie detection tool, it would have to allow for the testing and determination of lie vs. truth in a single individual, as Langleben *et al.* (2005) have reported.

The first sections of this chapter introduced fMRI and explored some of the contributions of fMRI to the clinical and non-clinical investigation of brain processes. Given this dynamic evolution, the attribution of both scientific and social meaning to functional neuroimaging research deserves attention, particularly as fMRI begins to have an impact on clinical decision-making, and imparts new knowledge about psychosocial aspects of behavior. In a previous paper, we (ER and JI) argued that ethical, legal and social challenges in neuroimaging research were intertwined with such epistemological issues. Examining what we should do (ethics) is fundamentally tied to what we interpret neuroscience data to mean (epistemology) (Illes & Racine 2005). Fundamentally, the challenge related to the interpretation and use of functional neuroimaging is twofold and includes both scientific and sociocultural considerations. Challenges of interpretation lead to ethical responsibilities that we explore in the final section of this chapter.

Scientific interpretation

The challenge of interpretation largely relates to the simplicity of the visual format of neuroimages (Beaulieu 2002), a simplicity that can mask the complex scientific and technological processes underlying the constructions of such images (Beaulieu 2001). Brain activation maps depicting brain function in task performance are much more complicated than the commonly used metaphor of a ``window into the brain´´ suggests. Numerous constraints exist preventing any such general simplification: the way in which the fMRI signal is derived, the ambiguous relationship between structure and function, the variability in study design, and the complexity of statistical analysis. These are all factors that shape a scientifically sound interpretation of fMRI images (Illes *et al.* 2006).

Challenge in deriving meaning from signals

Techniques like fMRI rely on metabolic correlates of neural activity, not the activity itself. Images are constructed based on BOLD contrast, which is an indirect measure of a series of processes. A human subject performs a behavioral task, for example imagining playing tennis or a repetitive finger-tapping task. Neuronal networks across the brain are activated to initiate, coordinate, and sustain this activity. Neurons require large amounts of energy in the form of ATP (adenosine triphosphate) to sustain their metabolic activity and since the brain does not store its own energy, it must make ATP from the oxidation of glucose. Increased blood flow is required to deliver the necessary glucose and oxygen (bound to hemoglobin) to maintain this metabolic demand. Since the magnetic properties of oxyhemoglobin and deoxyhemoglobin are different, they show different signal intensities on an MRI scan. When a brain region is more metabolically active, more oxygenated hemoglobin is recruited to that area; this results in a local increase in MR signal or BOLD contrast (Illes *et al.* 2006).

The challenge of deriving meaning from physiological signals is well illustrated in research on the detection of consciousness in severely brain-injured patients. For example, in addition to structural brain injuries, it is possible that patients in a vegetative or minimally conscious state exhibit key neurophysiologic changes, which could impact the acquisition of a meaningful signal (Laureys *et al.* 2006). The presence, or extent, of hemodynamic coupling dysfunction in these patients is still not yet well established. In fact, PET studies have demonstrated reduced cortical metabolism in vegetative patients, which is up to 60% reduced from healthy subjects. This metabolic deficit worsens as patients remain in the vegetative state, and by the time patients are in a persistent vegetative state they only maintain 30%–40% of normal cortical metabolic function (Laureys *et al.* 2004). In fact, there is some evidence to support the idea that minimally conscious patients maintain normal metabolic coupling, whereas vegetative patients do not (Laureys *et al.* 2006). Moreover, if oxygen utilization is altered in traumatic brain injury this would significantly impact key features of the BOLD signal. While more ATP is formed by the conversion of glucose in the presence of oxygen, this process can also occur in an anaerobic fashion, and it is unclear whereas more anaerobic processes occur in brain-injured patients, compared with healthy individuals (Laureys *et al.* 2004).

Deriving meaning from the fMRI signal is also a challenge when evaluating fMRI data taken from a single subject, as might be the case when fMRI is used eventually as a lie detector. Variability in blood flow is especially relevant here because, as with many other physiological processes in the human body, blood flow is influenced by many factors including the properties of the red blood cells, the integrity of the blood vessels, and the strength of the heart muscle, in addition to the age, health, and fitness level of the individual. Fluctuations in any of these variables are known to affect the signal measured and result in misinterpretation of a signal change.

Equating structure and function

As functional neuroimaging relies on task-dependent activations under highly constrained conditions (Desmond & Chen 2002; Kosik 2003), equating structure and function is somewhat analogous to equating genes and function. This is fraught with challenges, especially where many internal and external factors can affect the BOLD signal (Kosik 2003) and introduce both intra and inter-subject variability in the measured signal across subjects (Illes *et al.* 2006). For example, eye-blink paradigms have been shown to activate the hippocampal formation and the cingulate gyrus; however, lesions of the hippocampal formation do not eradicate eye-blink conditioning (Desmond & Chen 2002). There are two alternative interpretations for this result. Either the hippocampus is involved in some aspect of eye-blink conditioning, but not necessary to elicit the behavioral result, or the hippocampal activations are false positives. A false positive activation may lead to erroneous conclusions that brain areas are associated with a function when in fact they are not. Therefore, fMRI results do not definitively demonstrate that a brain region is involved in a task but rather that it is activated during the task (Rosen *et al.* 2002; Illes *et al.* 2006).

The challenge of equating structure with function is well exemplified by the use of fMRI in presurgical mapping of function. There are significant differences in the ways in which intracranial stimulation and fMRI relate structure and function in the brain. During preoperative language mapping, intracranial stimulation of the cortex disrupts the function of the stimulated brain region, and therefore offers information about the necessity of the brain region in performing language tasks (Tharin & Golby 2007). Electrical stimulation of a brain region necessary for language will disrupt some behavioral capacity of language in the patient, and therefore should be avoided in resection. Rather, fMRI testing preoperatively depicts areas of the brain *involved* in the function being tested (Sunaert 2006). Detecting areas of the brain activated by a language task using fMRI does not reveal any information about which areas are particularly necessary or sufficient for language (Tharin & Golby 2007). The difference between these two techniques is an essential consideration because localizing areas of the brain involved but not necessary to function, using fMRI, may lead a surgeon to avoid resecting tissue. This avoidance may be an unnecessary precaution and lead to poorer outcomes for a patient left with a partially resected tumor.

Designing an fMRI experiment

Part of the science and art of fMRI is designing an experimental task that is simple and specific so that behavioral responses can be attributed to an isolated mental process and not confounded by other functions, a concept known as functional decomposition. The design of the psychophysical task itself is crucial for research reliability and validity. Given the subtraction paradigm underlying fMRI experiments, care must be taken when comparing results from different fMRI studies and when extending results outside the scope of the research environment. Just because two studies both used tasks probing the regions of the brain responsive to fear does not mean that the activation maps can necessarily be directly compared. Along the same lines, an image generated from a single subject (example: lie detection for an individual) cannot be readily compared to an image representing the average of a group of normal subjects who performed a similar behavioral task (Illes *et al.* 2006).

What task best demonstrates the presence of consciousness? This question highlights a crucial challenge in our ability to detect consciousness using fMRI in vegetative or minimally conscious patients. In order to identify which patients maintain conscious awareness, an fMRI task which will capture consciousness is required. There have been a variety of tasks explored to detect consciousness in brain-injured patients, including testing their response to their own name (Staffen *et al.* 2006; Di *et al.* 2007), to language and speech comprehension (Coleman *et al.* 2007), and to mental imagery tasks (Owen *et al.* 2006). Unfortunately, it is difficult to determine even if brain activity patterns are similar in healthy controls whether brain activation patterns are willfully produced or rather automatic responses of the brain (Owen & Coleman 2007). It seems that a mental imagery task like the one administered by Owen and colleagues (2006) may have the most potential to delineate conscious experience in patients. Reliable and distinct brain activity patterns have been shown to occur during such tasks where healthy subjects ``imagine playing tennis´´ or ``imagine visiting the rooms in your home,´´ and vegetative patients may maintain these activation patterns (Owen *et al.* 2006; Boly *et al.* 2007). Using this task, it has been suggested, would allow patients to be tested for their ability to understand instructions and carry out purposefully different mental actions, without needing to make outward behavioral responses, of which they may be incapable (Owen & Coleman 2007).

Task selection for fMRI used in presurgical mapping is also a complex issue. The literature presents many variations of language tasks used in the presurgical mapping of function using fMRI. In fact, some research has suggested that correlations with intracranial stimulation and detection of language areas improves when using functional imaging of *two* language tasks (Roux *et al.* 2003). Task selection in presurgical mapping is of utmost importance and patients risk serious consequences if tasks are either too non-specific or too restrictive. Identifying areas of brain activation based on non-specific language tasks could result in a preoperative plan that leaves too much cortex deemed ``off-limits´´ to the surgeon, whereas a restrictive task could fail to identify areas of the cortex involved in higher-order language processes. Moreover, it is well established that performance during an fMRI task will impact resulting brain activation maps. Therefore, tasks should be designed to take into account a patient´s performance level and it has even been suggested that patients should meet an established criteria for performance before scanning (Sunaert 2006).

Statistical analysis of fMRI data

As described by Illes *et al.* (2006), among the most challenging issues in neuroimaging is the selection of the statistical treatment of neuroimaging data. There are several stages of processing that are performed on fMRI data. First, preprocessing prepares the data for statistical analysis. This often includes correcting for motion artifacts, normalizing or transforming the images of each subject´s brain into a common stereotactic coordinate system, and smoothing with a Gaussian filter. Second, a general linear model (GLM) regression determines for each subject the degree to which changes in signal intensity for each voxel (cubic volume of the brain image) can be predicted by a reference waveform that represents the timing of the behavioral task. The final stage is population inference. This step involves using the GLM results for each subject in a random effects model for making inferences to the population, or inferences regarding differences in the population. With this method, activation differences between experimental conditions or groups can be assessed over all brain regions and results can be reported in a standardized coordinate system. Commercial and freely available software packages for data analysis are widely used, but differences exist in the specific implementation of the statistics.

When the results from the GLM and the random effects model are combined, the result is a statistical parameter map of brain activity. This activation map is typically color-coded according to the probability value for each voxel. An important challenge in fMRI analysis occurs because of multiple comparisons. Across the brain, many tens of thousands of statistical comparisons are computed in the GLM, which limits current practices of correcting for multiple comparisons to decrease the number of false positives. Lowering the threshold will create more regions that are statistically significant, whereas raising the threshold will reduce the number of significant regions. The choice of the threshold is largely determined by convention among researchers, rather than absolute standards. This thresholding procedure can have significant implications for the interpretation of the brain activation maps, and if it is too strict will result in increased false negative results.

The impact of statistical analysis on the application of functional neuroimaging is significant. A high potential for false negatives or false positives in the interpretation of fMRI data presents an additional challenge for mapping brain function prior to surgical intervention. Sunaert (2006) has highlighted how important these errors are in preoperative decision-making. The presence of false positives (detecting areas of activity that are not truly activated by the task), may result in a surgeon's decreasing the size of resection to avoid this area, even though in truth the area need not be avoided and the patient may be left with unresected tumor. On the contrary, false negatives (not detecting areas of activity that are involved in the task), can result in the surgeon being misinformed about sparing a specific region, leaving the patient with a functional deficit.

It is a particular challenge to estimate neural activity using fMRI in the individual, rather than across a group. In response to basic sensory or motor tasks, BOLD signal change may reach a magnitude of up to approximately 6% (Huettel et al. 2004). In higher level cognitive procedures, BOLD signal change may be of much lesser magnitude (Huettel et al. 2004). The detection of brain activity in discrete brain processes relies largely on the ability to increase power while decreasing the amount of variability and error that might be present in the data. In most fMRI studies, statistical power is increased by averaging multiple subjects' brain maps. However, there has recently been some suggestion that fMRI may be used to detect deception in the *individual* subject (Langleben *et al.* 2005). Statistical testing at the individual level needs to take into account the fact that the signal may be weak and contaminated by within-subject variability.

Social and cultural interpretation

We have highlighted the existence of several fundamental scientific challenges in the interpretation and use of functional neuroimaging data. We now explain how, at the social and cultural level, the interpretation of functional neuroimaging data poses a second set of challenges, illustrated by the triad concepts of neuro-essentialism, neuro-realism, and neuro-policy (Racine *et al.* 2005). These challenges interact with scientific issues in complex ways, and sound scientific interpretation could still be subject to socio-cultural over-interpretations. As Dorothy Nelkin wrote regarding press coverage of the recombinant DNA controversy in the mid 1970s, "[t]he way people perceive research and interpret costs and benefits may be influenced less by the details of scientific evidence than by media messages" (Nelkin 2001). Consequently, current risks of over-interpretation of neuroimages in the form of interrelated neuro-essentialist and neuro-realist messages may lead to misuses of brain scans that lure patients, consumers, or juries into premature uses of neurotechnology (Racine *et al.* 2005).

Neuro-essentialism

The concept of neuro-essentialism signifies interpretations of the brain as the self-defining essence of a person, a secular equivalent to the soul (Table 12.1). The brain thus becomes a shorthand for concepts (e.g. the person, the self) that may serve to express other features of the individual not ordinarily found in the concept of the brain. In the public domain, neuro-essentialism is a combination of biological reductionism and enthusiasm for neuroscience research. The reductionist component takes various forms such as the equation of brain and personhood, the localization of personality traits or illness, or the subtle replacement of the grammatical subjects by the brain (Racine *et al.* 2005).

Closely associated with the various forms of neuro-essentialism, we find enthusiasm for neuroscience research and the "secrets" that neuroscience can reveal about ourselves. For example, according to print media, neuroimaging technologies allow for the exploration of

Table 12.1 *Examples of neuro-essentialism, neuro-realism, and neuro-policy in media reporting of neuroimaging research*

Neuro-essentialism

``With more powerful imaging devices and new genetic information, scientists are exploring the secrets of the organ that makes humans unique'' (Colburn 1999).

``One of the most striking findings came in 1997, when a team of researchers from the University of California at San Diego found what they called the ``God module'' in the brain'' (Cook 2001).

Neuro-realism

``Brain scan can catch a lie'' (Anonymous 2004).

``It's hard to fight an enemy (mental illness) you can't see ( . . . ). This will make it as easy to see sickness in the mind as it is to see a broken bone in the body'' (Anonymous 1999). ``The fMRI gives us a window into the human brain''

(Fackelmann 2001). ``The brain can't lie: Brain scans can reveal how you think and feel, and even how you might behave. No wonder the CIA and big business are interested'' (Sample & Adam 2003).

Neuro-policy

``The breakthroughs are so rich in insights for parents and so pregnant with possibilities for health care and public policy that the nation has become absorbed with the scientific intricacies of what happens inside a baby's head. News magazines spew articles replete with heart-melting images of babies and mind-boggling diagrams of their brains. TV specials draw us into the arcane world of synapse formation. Parents contemplate reading Shakespeare to their infants'' (Cummins 1997).

``Overall, a woman's brain, like her body, is 10 percent to 15 percent smaller than a man's, yet the regions dedicated to higher cognitive functions such as language are more densely packed with neurons. (. . .) recognizing some of these differences can make a difference in our daily lives'' (Hales 1998).

``As new research raises possibility that police recruits could be screened for bias, some experts argue US study's conclusions are misplaced: Inside the mind of a racist: scans may reveal brain's hidden centres of prejudice'' (Adam 2003).

Updated from: Racine *et al.* (2005)

``the secret, uncharted areas of the brain'', and the identification of ``the individual sources of all our thoughts, actions and behaviour'' (Dobson 1997). The brain is also portrayed as ``the mystery we still can't penetrate'' (Hall 2001), an ``enigma'' (Connor 1995) and the ``terra incognita that lies between our ears'' where one can find ``the keys to the kingdoms of memory, of thought, of desire, of fear, of the habits and skills that add up to who we each are´´ (Hall 1999). Neuroscience will therefore reveal ``life´s ultimate mystery: our conscious inner selves´´ (Connor 1995) and is presented as science ``gone in search of the soul´´ (Hellmore 1998). Not surprisingly, emerging evidence based on experiments involving the comparison of lay understandings of neuroimaging evidence in comparison to other scientific illustrations suggest that neuroimages are particularly convincing (McCabe & Castel 2007; Weisberg *et al.* 2007).

In contrast to sweeping neuro-essentialism, we note that inter-pretations of what we are and what is our ``essence´´ relies not only on scientific frameworks, but also on cultural and anthropological ones. Consider concepts such as ethical decision-making, cooperation, altru-ism, normal social behavior, and mythical experience. Investigations carried out by fMRI to delineate the neural processes involved in these tasks are based on specific understandings of these concepts. The cul-tural influence in the interpretation challenge is clear, seeing that these concepts can be understood in diverse manners (Morris 1994).

Neuro-realism

The concept of neuro-realism identifies lay interpretations implying that neuroimaging research yields direct data on brain function (Table 12.1). Observed brain activation patterns can become accordingly the ultimate proof that a phenomenon is real, objective, and effective (e.g. in the case of health interventions such as hypnosis and acupuncture), despite the complexities of data acquisition and image processing involved (Racine *et al.* 2005).

Neuro-realist interpretations of functional imaging results occur in various forms of claim: attributing mind-reading powers to neuro-imaging; suggesting that neuroimaging can provide a ``visual proof´ or give insight into the true nature of a phenomenon; and describing neu-roimaging as a ``window into the brain´´ or a tool that produces pictures and movies of the brain ``at work´´. In addition to these print media examples, one can see that, in some popular science work, neuroscience tools are depicted as a direct route to our inner selves, making them candidates that could eventually replace introspective methods bound to become cultural relics of another age according to this interpretation.

> For a hundred years, much of Western society has assumed that the most powerful route to self-knowledge took the form of lying on a couch, talking about our childhoods. The possibility entertained in this book is

that you can follow another path, with equally insightful results: going under the fMRI [functional Magnetic Resonance Imaging] scanner, or hooking up to a neurofeedback machine, or just reading a book about brain science

Johnson 2004.

Current neuro-realism has interesting historical counterparts. The media heralding of ``diagnoscopy´´ in the early twentieth century, a pre-EEG electrophysiological technique developed by Zachar Bissky and that was to be used for electric personality profiling (e.g. for vocational guidance) represents one such fine example. Diagnoscopy determined personality profiles based on the stimulation of reaction zones on the surface of the head. When touched with a detecting electrode, an electric circuit emitted a graded (more-or-less loud) tone (Borck 2001). A diagnoscopic examination of a set of 50 reaction zones could be outputted as a graph showing the development of various personality traits. Historian of neuroscience Cornelius Borck provides further evidence of historical neuro-realism: ``the press typically glorified diagnoscopy as a new visualizing tool and characterized it as an x-ray machine of the soul´´ (Borck 2001). Here is a journalistic account published by the writer Emil Ludwig in the *Berliner Illustrierte Zeitung* in 1926 and quoted by Borck. Note the parallel with Jonhson´s contemporary claim of a new grammar based on neuroscience cited earlier as well as its neuro-realist connotations:

> After completion of the investigation in less than half an hour, I took the sheet with an excitement beyond curiosity, and looked at the winding line, similar to a temperature or weather curve, which resulted by connecting the individual values in the scale from 1 to 4 at each point. I juxtaposed to this charade a legend in form of an explication of each point in psychical terms … I read how fantasy and logic, how constructive thinking, color sense and orientation, mathematics and techniques are represented in myself in degrees of normal, less, or more than normal. I read whether volition and determination, mysticism or neurasthenia, idleness, stinginess, parsimony, selfishness, sexuality, violent temper, diligence, accuracy, eagerness, velocity of thinking and acting were weak or strong in me
>
> Borck 2001.

The enthusiastic early neuro-realist reception of the electroencephalography of Hans Berger in print media and the subsequent enthusiasm of journalists undergoing mind-reading EEG examinations for the first time constitutes another example of historical neuro-realism. In 1930, one could have read in an article written by Walter Finkler on the ``electrical scriptures of the brain´´ and published in the

July 4, 1930 issue of *The Neues Wiener Journal* that, ``The scientists working with this apparatus are mind readers, they literally read the thoughts of the human guinea-pig with the silver electrodes in his head´´ (Borck 2001). Such statements are strikingly similar to current neuro-realist media messages (Table 12.1).

Neuro-policy

Rapid transfer of neuroscience research may also be made especially appealing when results seem to reflect the essence and the true nature of various phenomena (Table 12.1). Currently, there are numerous target domains for this phenomenon, called neuro-policy (Racine *et al.* 2005). These include education and childhood development programs, courtrooms, and direct sales of neuroimaging services (Illes & Kirschen 2003; Illes *et al.* 2004). The print media also include claims that neuroimaging results inform policies and social practices. Other claims bear on the use of neuroimaging to provide insight on the conduct of one´s life and new wisdom based on neuroscience´s revelations.

Neuro-policy connects with the historical roots of phrenology. The early phrenologist Gall possessed exquisite skills in neuroanatomy and, with Spurzheim, he made remarkable contributions to the integrative understanding of the central nervous system based on comparative anatomy and pre-Darwinian evolutionary principles (Clarke & Jacyna 1987). However, his writings were largely popularized and disseminated in the United States by the Fowler brothers, who had keener business flair than Gall and Spurzheim. Orson and Lorenzo Fowler promoted phrenology as a self-improvement practice that would allow individuals to overcome mental shortcomings. The article ``Phrenology made easy´´, published in the literary *Knickerbocker Magazine* (June 2, 1838), defended phrenology as a practical approach to understanding and reforming negative character traits and argued for its wide application to child-rearing, education, and marriage choices. In *Familiar Lessons on Physiology Designed for the Use of Children and Youth in Schools and Families*, Dr. Lydia Folger Fowler (Mrs. Lorenzo Fowler) argued that ``a correct knowledge of the laws and principles of Physiology and Phrenology is undoubtedly the most effectual medium for children to know themselves, mentally and physically´´ (Fowler 1855). Phrenologists also used popular magazines such as *Ladies Magazine* and *The New Yorker* to laud and disseminate the merits of their approach.

Another historical example of neuro-policy is the promotion by neuroscientists Oskar and Cécile Vogt of cerebral characterology to identify abilities, characteristics, and talents (``characterological profiling´´) based on an individual´s brain features. The Vogts were influenced by Paul Fleshig´s and August Forel´s view of neuroscience that made it ``the highest science of the human in man´´. They also accepted the fundamental role those mentors attributed to neuroscience in social management, and eventually eugenics. In particular, the Vogts used work in the field of cytoarchitechtonics, the systematic mapping of neuronal cell types, to provide a physical grounding for character trait profiling. In the scientific environment of the period, cultural progress was projected into the human cortex. Accordingly, the Vogts believed that, ``man will increasingly become a brain animal´´, and therefore the dangers of illness had to yield to the development of a ``brain hygiene´´, cited in Hagner (2001). In the context of this brain hygiene project, the Vogts collected ``elite´´ and ``criminal´´ brains. They did not hesitate to use print media to raise awareness of the newly founded Kaiser Wilhelm Institute or to showcase some of their provocative research, such as a study of Lenin´s brain.

Contemporary examples of neuro-policy are subtler than those of phrenology and characterology but tap into similar popular interpretations about brain function, the power of neurotechnology to read minds, and the *prima facie* authority of science. For example, the use of neuroimages in the context of childhood policies or education has given rise to unrealistic expectations conveyed in the media (Bruer 1998; Thompson & Nelson 2001). In the US some centers are offering SPECT scans to help diagnose ADHD or Alzheimer´s disease in spite of limited scientific support (Illes *et al.* 2003b). Whole-body and brain scans are offered on the Internet even though their clinical value is questionable (Illes *et al.* 2003b; Racine *et al.* 2007b). Other products (e.g. toys) or educational intervention strategies, in particular for under-achieving children, are marketed as being supported by brain-based neuroimaging research (e.g. showing seductive before-and-after scans). One can read the following statement in a patient brochure that sells neuroimaging on the Internet without physician referral.

> A SPECT scan allows patients to see a physical representation of their problems that is accurate and reliable and helps to increase compliance. It can influence a patient´s willingness and ability to accept and adhere to the treatment program. They can better understand that not treating anxiety, depression, rage, ADD, etc. is similar to not wearing the correct prescription glasses.
>
> Amen 2006.

This review of some current and historical scientific and sociocultural challenges in functional neuroimaging research shows the importance of connecting epistemology and ethics. It also illustrates the extent and magnitude with which neuroscience research and its mind-reading interpretation are penetrating society at large, and generating a need to renew a number of relevant scientific and ethical responsibilities.

NEUROETHICAL RESPONSIBILITIES

The methodological complexity of neuroimaging justifies substantial qualifications about the conditions under which knowledge is produced and interpreted. The public portrayal of mind-reading with neuroimaging does not fully convey this complexity. As we have described here and elsewhere (Racine & Illes 2006), the simple appearance of neuroimages may veil unsuspected complexity – from the specialized medical equipment needed to acquire a scan, to the array of parameters used to elicit activations and the statistical thresholds set to draw out meaningful patterns, to the expertise required for the objective interpretation of the maps themselves. Hence, public involvement and outlook on consequences of the technology are identified in ethical discussion of genomics (Racine 2002) and are also becoming part of the ethical landscape of functional neuroimaging research (Table 12.2).

Responsiveness

The need for responsiveness can be illustrated by the aggressive, direct-to-consumer marketing of neuroimaging services that has surfaced particularly in North America in the past 5 years. There is a growing dissemination of neuroimaging devices and services in the non-clinical for-profit sector (Racine & Illes 2008). Without physician referral, across the United States and Canada today, consumers may purchase for themselves or their loved ones CT head scans, if they fear they have had a stroke, or functional scans with SPECT, to obtain assessments of attention and memory. Recent years have also seen the appearance of lie detection fMRI scans, marketed direct to businesses and legal professionals over the internet (e.g. NoLie MRI: http://www.noliemri.com/). What obligations do neuroimagers have regarding legitimate or nefarious goals to which neuroimaging might contribute? In the absence of clear deontological obligations to consumers, how would

Table 12.2 *Emerging neuroethical responsibilities in neuroimaging research*

Responsibilities	Actions	Sample responses
Responsibility-responsiveness	Consider the interests of human subjects in an increasingly complex research environment	Respond to and inform about claims presented in direct-to-consumer advertising of neuroimaging services.
Civic and democratic responsibility	Adopt a broad outlook on the social consequences and implications of neuroscience	Provide a balanced presentation of the merits and limits of functional neuroimaging when interacting with media.
Prospective responsibility	Consider the future and off-label use of neuroscience and its applications	Promote ethical reflection on the possibilities of emerging uses of neuroimaging.
Self-reflection	Reflect on precedent	Analyze the history of neuroscience to better understand the current challenges related to understanding brain function and possible solutions.

Adapted from Racine and Illes (2006).

market forces and profit imperatives challenge traditional researcher roles? What are the principles that entrepreneurial neuroimagers must adhere to in order to properly inform consumers? Respecting autonomy in the context of the open market may be insufficient. New levels of responsiveness are vital to inform patients and public about the clinical benefits of functional neuroimaging in a consumerist environment.

Civic and democratic responsibility

We have highlighted the numerous challenges in public understanding and transfer of knowledge related to neuroimaging research. We have observed that neuroscientists, like physicists and geneticists, are increasingly aware of their social and civic responsibilities in fostering public education and dialogue on brain research. This is in part, we believe, one of the contributions that neuroethics has already made (Illes *et al.* 2005; Leshner 2005; Racine *et al.* 2005). However, making the public more aware of both the excitement surrounding neuroimaging research and its limits, at the same time, is challenging even for the most committed and articulate researchers. Analysis of the media shows that, in the case of fMRI, proper interpretation of data, validity, and limitations of research are prime concerns and outweigh (in sheer numbers) ethical issues (Racine *et al.* 2005). Instances of frank neuro-essentialism, neuro-realism, and neuro-policy are not rare (Racine *et al.*, 2005). In this context, what can be we expect in terms of epistemo-logical awareness? With the existence of many views about mind and brain, neuroethics will have to foster discussions among neuroscien-tists whose methods may vary and when interpretations of results differ. These discussions must build on meaningful dialogue with scholars in the humanities about concepts like deception, conscious-ness, and moral decision-making – which will benefit from interdis-ciplinary input. Open dialogue with the public is no less necessary given that different cultural and religious perspectives subject findings to different interpretations and ethical boundaries. Responsible dis-semination of information through the media and public education are also essential to close the gap between scientists and concerned citi-zens, especially as the complexity and abstractness of results increase and studies tackle topics such as decision-making and consciousness. Great competence and skills are needed to perform neuroimaging research (Rosen *et al.* 2002), but comparable skills are also needed in scientific communication to transfer the subtleties and the uncer-tainties of neuroimaging results calling upon a wide array of scientific and neuroethical responsibilities (Racine & Illes 2006).

Prospective responsibility

With an increasing number of studies that provide insights into con-sciousness, altruism, moral decision-making, and economics, the dimension of prospective responsibility defines how we can tackle future uses of neuroimaging. The challenge in engaging in discussion about potential and even future uses of biomedical science is the sheer difficulty of predicting which areas will translate into real-world clin-ical or non-clinical uses. One can only consider here how concerted clinical trials in stroke (Savitz & Fisher 2007) and Parkinson's disease (Ravina *et al.* 2003), despite efforts to predict efficient therapies, have been overpowered by this feat. But to remain silent in front of advances in neuroscience would probably be worse, as scenarios would not be proactively prepared or discussed. For example, who will have access to the applications of neuroimaging based on cutting-edge research? How will physicians and patients incorporate these new types of data into their clinical and moral reasoning about diagnosis, prognosis, and decision-making? Access to advanced technologies by the privileged only, whether for diagnosis, for medical intervention, or for a competitive neurocognitive edge, will only further upset an already delicate and hardly acceptable *status quo*. While in the past technology and ethics have in some cases leapfrogged each other, bioethicists and neuroscientists will be well served by working gracefully together to understand the power of a visual image and the impact it can have on people and collectively on society.

Self-reflection

Remembering the past can help us prepare for the future (Racine & Illes 2006). Historical precedent illustrates how some researchers in neuroscience have been involved in infamous acts (Shevell 1999). Contrary to this cruelty is the illustrious history of neuroscience. Great neuroscientists have positively changed humanity by bringing a deepened understanding of the nervous system and the development of therapies and compassionate attitudes to neurological and psychiatric illness (Fins 2008). There are challenges to personal reflection in all fields of research. However, certain events such as the introduction of the humanities into the medical curriculum (medical humanities) may broaden the education of researchers and physicians and foster the development of skills in critical and constructive self-reflection.

CONCLUSION

This chapter reviewed scientific and sociocultural challenges in the interpretation of neuroimaging that inform its sound and ethical use. Far from being a simple mind-reading device, fMRI is a sophisticated research tool. The examples of frontier research we discussed illustrate the promises of neuroimaging and the work still needed to understand brain function. As research advances, researchers become aware of the limits of available tools and the need for ongoing technological refinement to achieve their goals. In parallel, ethics must not itself over-interpret the mind-reading capabilities of neuroimaging to nurture its own agenda. Doing so may spark unfounded fears and controversies that jeopardize the challenging scientific quest for knowledge. In tandem, ethics-informed science and science-informed ethics can contribute to a balanced appreciation of the potentials of neuroscience for health and humanity.

REFERENCES

Adam, D. 2003. Inside the mind of a racist: scans may reveal brain's hidden centres of prejudice. *The Guardian*, Nov. 17, London, http://www.guardian.co.uk.
Amen, D. G. 2006. "Why SPECT?" http://amenclinics.com. Retrieved May 4, 2006.
Andrews, K., Murphy, L., Munday, R. & Littlewood, C. 1996. Misdiagnosis of the vegetative state: retrospective study in a rehabilitation unit. *British Medical Journal* **313**: 13–16.
Anonymous. 1999. Laser device offers peek at brain breakthrough, may help in diagnosis of Alzheimer's patients. *Omaha World Herald*, Nov. 30.
Anonymous. 2004. Brain scan can catch a lie. *The Houston Chronicle*, Houston, Nov. 30, p. 10.
Bartsch, A. J., Homola, G., Biller, A., Solymosi, L. & Bendszus, M. 2006. Diagnostic functional MRI: illustrated clinical applications and decision-making. *Journal of Magnetic Resonance Imaging* **23**: 921–32.
Beaulieu, A. 2001. Voxels in the brain. *Social Studies of Science* **31**: 1–45.
Beaulieu, A. 2002. Images are not the (only) truth: brain mapping, visual knowledge and iconoclasm. *Science, Technology and Human Values* **27**: 53–87.
Binder, J. R., Swanson, S. J., Hammeke, T. A. *et al.* 1996. Determination of language dominance using functional MRI: a comparison with the Wada test. *Neurology* **46**: 978–84.
Boly, M., Coleman, M. R., Davis, M. H. *et al.* 2007. When thoughts become action: an fMRI paradigm to study volitional brain activity in non-communicative brain injured patients. *Neuroimage* **36**: 979–92.
Bondi, M. W., Houston, W. S., Eyler, L. T. & Brown, G. G. 2005. fMRI evidence of compensatory mechanisms in older adults at genetic risk for Alzheimer disease. *Neurology* **64**: 501–8.
Bookheimer, S. 2007. Pre-surgical language mapping with functional magnetic resonance imaging. *Neuropsychology Review* **17**: 145–55.
Borck, C. 2001. Electricity as a medium of psychic life: electrotechnological adventures into psychodiagnosis in Weimar Germany. *Science in Context* **14**: 565–90.
Bruer, J. T. 1998. The brain and child development: time for some critical thinking. *Public Health Reports* **113**: 388–98.
Chen, C. H., Ridler, K., Suckling, J. *et al.* 2007. Brain imaging correlates of depressive symptom severity and predictors of symptom improvement after antidepressant treatment. *Biological Psychiatry* **62**: 407–14.
Childs, N. L., Mercer, W. N. & Childs, H. W. 1993. Accuracy of diagnosis of persistent vegetative state. *Neurology* **43**: 1465–7.
Clarke, E. & Jacyna, L. S. 1987. *Nineteenth-Century Origins of Neuroscience Concepts*. Berkeley, CA: University of California Press.
Colburn, D. 1999. The infinite brain; people used to think the brain was static and inevitably declined with age. Actually, the brain never stops changing – and we never stop learning. *The Washington Post*, Sept. 28, Washington, p. Z12.

Coleman, M. R., Rodd, J. M., Davis, M. H. *et al.* 2007. Do vegetative patients retain aspects of language comprehension? Evidence from fMRI. *Brain* **130**: 2494–507.

Connor, S. 1995. Science; The last great frontier. The brain is the ultimate enigma. Now, after centuries of study by philosophers and scientists, some of its deepest secrets are being unveiled. *The Independent,* May 21, London, p. 52.

Cook, G. 2001. Plumbing the mystery of prayer with the instruments of science. *The Boston Globe*, May 3, Boston, p. A2.

Cummins, H. J. 1997. What's on baby's mind? Researchers studying how an infant's brain develops are intrigued by what's going on in the heads of their tiny subjects. *Star Tribune*, Aug. 27, Minneapolis, p. 6A.

Desmond, J. E. & Chen, S. H. A. 2002. Ethical issues in the clinical application of fMRI: factors affecting the validity and interpretation of activations. *Brain and Cognition* **50**: 482–97.

Di, H. B., Yu, S. M., Weng, X. C. *et al.* 2007. Cerebral response to patient's own name in the vegetative and minimally conscious states. *Neurology* **68**: 895–9.

Dobson, R. 1997. Navigating the maps of the mind; the latest advancements in mind mapping will bring us closer to solving the age-old mysteries of the brain. *The Independent*, Mar. 9, London, p. 40.

Downie, J. & Marshall, J. 2007. Pediatric neuroimaging ethics. *Cambridge Quarterly of Healthcare Ethics* **16**: 147–60.

Fackelmann, K. 2001. $3 million brain scanner is new weapon in drug fight. *USA Today*, Feb. 1, McLean, p. 9D.

Fins, J. J. 2008. A leg to stand on: Sir William Osler and Wilder Penfield's "Neuroethics." *American Journal of Bioethics* **8**: 37–46.

Fleisher, A. S., Houston, W. S., Eyler, L. T. *et al.* 2005. Identification of Alzheimer disease risk by functional magnetic resonance imaging. *Archives of Neurology* **62**: 1881–8.

Fowler, L. F. 1855. *Familiar Lessons on Physiology: Designed for the Use of Children and Youth in Schools and Families.* New York: Fowler & Wells.

Fu, C. H., Mourao-Miranda, J., Costafreda, S. G. *et al.* 2007. Pattern classification of sad facial processing: toward the development of neurobiological markers in depression. *Biological Psychiatry* **63**: 656–62.

Giacino, J. T., Ashwal, S., Childs, N. *et al.* 2002. The minimally conscious state: definition and diagnostic criteria. *Neurology* **58**: 349–53.

Giacino, J. T., Hirsch, J., Schiff, N. & Laureys, S. 2006. Functional neuroimaging applications for assessment and rehabilitation planning in patients with disorders of consciousness. *Archives of Physical Medicine and Rehabilitation* **87**: S67–76.

Hagner, M. 2001. Cultivating the cortex in German neuroanatomy. *Science in Context* **14**: 541–63.

Hales, D. 1998. Gray matters. *Columbus Dispatch*, July 29, Columbus, p. 1G.

Hall, C. T. 2001. Fib detector; study shows brain scan detects patterns of neural activity when someone lies. *The San Francisco Chronicle*, Nov. 26, San Francisco, p. A10.

Hall, S. S. 1999. Journey to the center of my mind. *The New York Times*, June 6, New York, p. 122.

Hellmore, E. 1998. She thinks she believes in God. In fact, it's just chemical reactions taking place in the neurons of her temporal lobes; science has gone in search of the soul. *The Observer*, May 3, London, p. 20.

Hirsch, J., Ruge, M. I., Kim, K. H. *et al.* 2000. An integrated functional magnetic resonance imaging procedure for preoperative mapping of cortical areas associated with tactile, motor, language, and visual functions. *Neurosurgery* **47**: 711–21; discussion 721–2.

Huettel, S. A., Song, A. W. & McCarthy, G. 2004. *Functional Magnetic Resonance Imaging.* Sunderland, MA: Sinauer Associates.

Illes, J., Blakemore, C., Hansson, M. G. *et al.* 2005. International perspectives on engaging the public in neuroscience. *Nature Reviews Neuroscience* **6**: 977–82.

Illes, J., Fan, E., Koenig, B. *et al.* 2003b. Self-referred whole-body CT imaging: current implications for health care consumers. *Radiology* **228**: 346–51.

Illes, J., Kann, D., Karetsky, K. *et al.* 2004. Advertising, patient decision making, and self-referral for computed tomographic and magnetic resonance imaging. *Archives of Internal Medicine* **164**: 2415–19.

Illes, J., Kirschen, M. P. & Gabrieli, J. D. 2003a. From neuroimaging to neuroethics. *Nature Neuroscience* **6**: 205.

Illes, J. & Kirschen, M. (2003). New prospects and ethical challenges for neuroimaging within and outside the health care system. *American Journal of Neuroradiology* **24**: 1932–4.

Illes, J. & Racine, E. 2005. Imaging or imagining? A neuroethics challenge informed by genetics. *American Journal of Bioethics* **5**: 5–18.

Illes, J., Racine, E. & Kirschen, M. 2006. A picture is worth a thousand words, but which one thousand? In Illes, J. (ed.) *Neuroethics: Defining the Issues in Research, Practice and Policy.* Oxford: Oxford University Press, pp. 149–68.

Illes, J., Rosen, A., Greicius, M. & Racine, E. 2007. Prospects for prediction: ethics analysis of neuroimaging in Alzheimer´s disease. *Annals of the New York Academy of Sciences* **1097**: 278–95.

Johnson, S. 2004. *Mind Wide Open: Your Brain and the Neuroscience of Everyday Life.* New York, NY: Scribner.

Kloppel, S. & Buchel, C. 2005. Alternatives to the Wada test: a critical view of functional magnetic resonance imaging in preoperative use. *Current Opinion in Neurology* **18**: 418–23.

Kosik, K. S. 2003 Beyond phrenology, at last. *Nature Neuroscience* **4**: 234–39.

Krings, T., Schreckenberger, M., Rohde, V. *et al.* 2002. Functional MRI and 18F FDG-Positron Emission Tomography for presurgical planning: comparison with electrical cortical stimulation. *Acta Neurochirurgica* **144**: 889–99.

Langleben, D. D., Schroeder, L., Maldjian, J. A. *et al.* 2002. Brain activity during simulated deception: an event-related functional magnetic resonance study. *NeuroImage* **15**: 727–32.

Langleben, D. D., Loughead, J. W., Bilker, W. B. *et al.* 2005. Telling truth from lie in individual subjects with fast event-related fMRI. *Human Brain Mapping* **26**: 262–72.

Laureys, S., Giacino, J. T., Schiff, N. D., Schabus, M. & Owen, A. M. 2006. How should functional imaging of patients with disorders of consciousness contribute to their clinical rehabilitation needs? *Current Opinion in Neurology* **19**: 520–7.

Laureys, S., Owen, A. M. & Schiff, N. D. 2004. Brain function in coma, vegetative state, and related disorders. *Lancet Neurology* **3**: 537–46.

Leshner, A. I. 2005. It´s time to go public with neuroethics. *American Journal of Bioethics* **5**: 1–2.

Majos, A., Tybor, K., Stefanczyk, L. & Goraj, B. 2005. Cortical mapping by functional magnetic resonance imaging in patients with brain tumors. *European Radiology* **15**: 1148–58.

Marshall, J., Martin, T., Downie, J. & Malisza, K. 2007. A comprehensive analysis of MRI research risks: in support of full disclosure. *Canadian Journal of Neurological Sciences* **34**: 11–17.

McCabe, D. P. & Castel, A. D. 2008. Seeing is believing: the effect of brain images on judgments of scientific reasoning. *Cognition,* **107**: 343–52.

Morris, B. 1994. *Anthropology of the Self. The Individual in Cultural Perspective.* Colorado: Pluto Press.

Nair, D. G. 2005. About being BOLD. *Brain Research: Brain Research Reviews* **50**: 229–43.

Nelkin, D. 2001. Beyond risk: reporting about genetics in the post-Asilomar press. *Perspectives in Biology and Medicine* **44**: 199–207.

Owen, A. M. & Coleman, M. R. 2007. Functional MRI in disorders of consciousness: advantages and limitations. *Current Opinion in Neurology* **20**: 632–7.

Owen, A. M., Coleman, M. R., Boly, M. *et al.* 2006. Detecting awareness in the vegetative state. *Science* **313**: 1402.

Paquette, V., Levesque, J., Mensour, B. *et al.* 2003. ``Change the mind and you change the brain´´: effects of cognitive-behavioral therapy on the neural correlates of spider phobia. *Neuroimage* **18**: 401–9.

Paulus, M. P. & Stein, M. B. 2007. Role of functional magnetic resonance imaging in drug discovery. *Neuropsychology Reviews* **17**: 179–88.

Petrella, J. R., Shah, L. M., Harris, K. M. *et al.* 2006. Preoperative functional MR imaging localization of language and motor areas: effect on therapeutic decision making in patients with potentially resectable brain tumors. *Radiology* **240**: 793–802.

Racine, E. 2002. Éthique de la discussion et génomique des populations. *Éthique Publique* **4**: 77–90.

Racine, E., Bar-Ilan, O. & Illes, J. 2005. fMRI in the public eye. *Nature Reviews Neuroscience* **6**: 159–64.

Racine, E. & Illes, J. 2006. Neuroethical responsibilities. *Canadian Journal of Neurological Sciences* **33**: 269–77.

Racine, E. & Illes, J. 2007a. Emerging ethical challenges in advanced neuroimaging research: review, recommendations and research agenda. *Journal of Empirical Research on Human Research Ethics* **2**: 1–10.

Racine, E. & Illes, J. 2008. Neuroethics. In Singer, P. & Viens, A. (eds.) *Cambridge Textbook of Bioethics.* Cambridge: Cambridge University Press, pp. 495–503.

Racine, E., Van der Loos, H. Z. A. & Illes, J. 2007b. Internet marketing of neuroproducts: new practices and healthcare policy challenges. *Cambridge Quarterly of Healthcare Ethics* **16**: 181–94.

Ravina, B. M., Fagan, S. C., Hart, R. G. *et al.* 2003. Neuroprotective agents for clinical trials in Parkinson´s disease: a systematic assessment. *Neurology* **60**: 1234–40.

Rosen, A. C. & Gur, R. C. 2002. Ethical considerations for neuropsychologists as functional magnetic imagers. *Brain and Cognition* **50**: 469–81.

Roux, F. E., Boulanouar, K., Lotterie, J. A. *et al.* 2003. Language functional magnetic resonance imaging in preoperative assessment of language areas: correlation with direct cortical stimulation. *Neurosurgery* **52**: 1335–45; discussion 1345–7.

Rutten, G. J., Ramsey, N. F., van Rijen, P. C., Noordmans, H. J. & van Veelen, C. W. 2002. Development of a functional magnetic resonance imaging protocol for intraoperative localization of critical temporoparietal language areas. *Annals of Neurology* **51**: 350–60.

Sample, I. & Adam, D. 2003. The brain can´t lie. *The Guardian,* Nov. 20, London, p. 4.

Savitz, S. I. & Fisher, M. 2007. Future of neuroprotection for acute stroke: in the aftermath of the SAINT trials. *Annals of Neurology* **61**: 396–402.

Schiff, N. D., Rodriguez-Moreno, D., Kamal, A. *et al.* 2005. fMRI reveals large-scale network activation in minimally conscious patients. *Neurology* **64**: 514–23.

Shevell, M. I. 1999. Neurosciences in the Third Reich: from ivory tower to death camps. *Canadian Journal of Neurological Sciences* **26**: 132–38.

Staffen, W., Kronbichler, M., Aichhorn, M., Mair, A. & Ladurner, G. 2006. Selective brain activity in response to one's own name in the persistent vegetative state. *Journal of Neurology, Neurosurgery and Psychiatry* **77**: 1383–4.

Sunaert, S. 2006. Presurgical planning for tumor resectioning. *Journal of Magnetic Resonance Imaging* **23**: 887–905.

Tharin, S. & Golby, A. 2007. Functional brain mapping and its applications to neurosurgery. *Neurosurgery* **60**: 185–201; discussion 201–2.

Thompson, R. A. & Nelson, C. A. 2001. Developmental science and the media. *American Psychologist* **56**: 5–15.

Weisberg, D. S., Keil, F. C., Goodstein, J., Rawson, E. & Gray, J. R. 2008. The seductive allure of neuroscience explanations. *Journal of Cognitive Neuroscience* **20**: 470–7.

13

Possibilities, limits, and implications of brain–computer interfacing technologies

T. HINTERBERGER

INTRODUCTION

A major characteristic of the information era is the continuous increase in interconnectedness created by a worldwide electronic network: the Internet. Thus, through such electronic linkage, our minds move closely together even if spatially separated by thousands of miles. In this scenario the computer usually creates an interface between us and the digital world. An ultimate connectedness between our minds and the information pool of the Internet can be fantasized within a science fiction scenario as represented in the movie *The Matrix*. Brain–mind operation could be connected to a computer, which might afford an opportunity to enter a direct interaction with a virtual world. Such brain – machine interfaces would have to fulfill a two-directional task: one is to give the human user the opportunity to communicate with the system by sending signals to the computer (which can be achieved either by voluntary control of a computer, or by a computer's ability to engage and interpret our thoughts); the other is brain stimulation by a device in order to let us experience the virtual world. Whereas the first task attempts to replace the keyboard and mouse of a computer, the second tries to substitute the computer screen and audio system. Current multimedia consumer technology already offers great possibilities available in the modern home cinema. In terms of the information transfer rate of such visual and auditory stimulating systems, one should note that they require a far higher information flow compared with the control devices

Scientific and Philosophical Perspectives in Neuroethics, ed. J. J. Giordano & B. Gordijn. Published by Cambridge University Press. © Cambridge University Press 2010.

(e.g. mouse and keyboard) of a computer. This means that offering an experiential virtual world requires us to satisfy the visual and auditory senses. Currently, direct brain stimulation does not offer a perception of content-related images or sound, and research in this field remains in its infancy. However, neuroprosthetic approaches can replace parts of ocular function; for example, the function of the retina was successfully imitated by a retina implant (Chow *et al.* 2004; Winter *et al.* 2007) and cochlear implants can replace some tasks of the auditory system (Seligman & Shepherd 2004; Shepherd 2004).

However, rather than linking us to a cyber world, such implants are currently solely utilized in medical applications to assist patients with disabilities to regain abilities by partly replacing the lost functionality of the visual or auditory system. For such patients, it is important that this technology be applied carefully in order to prevent psychological distress by overstimulation caused by malfunction of a stimulating implant (a simple example is the problem of acoustic feedback in some hearing aids).

A BRIEF HISTORY OF BCI RESEARCH

In 1942 Curt Siodmak published a novel entitled *Donovan's Brain* about a millionaire whose brain was kept alive after ``a fatal'' plane crash. As the brain, per se, could not express itself, the scientist in this story formulated the problem: ``... If I could find ... a code which translates the relation between the reading of the encephalograph and the mental image ... the brain could communicate with me''. This idea of direct brain–computer communication is a central goal in BCI research. However, what was first required was the possibility of real-time processing and feedback, which could extract a meaningful signal from the data stream in order to control a communication interface. Even if analog biofeedback devices, as were offered for the so-called Alpha-training that was popular in the 1970s, were used, any ``intelligent'' feedback systems needed to engage a computer, and this would not be available for another decade.

With the possibility of digital EEG, investigating evoked responses became a focus in brain research. The raw EEG signal does not reveal a typical response pattern upon a single presentation of a specific event; hence computer-aided averaging of several similar events had to be used for the detection of any event-related potential (ERP). One of the first useful brain–computer communication systems actually used the principle of detecting ERPs, via a P300-driven spelling device published by Farwell & Donchin (Farwell and Donchin 1988). The P300 is a positive wave that occurs about 300 ms after presentation-onset of a meaningful or novel visual or auditory stimulus in humans.

The BCIs of the 1990s were dominated by a different approach. Event-related desynchronization of the sensory/motor and mu-rhythms, and its role in an operant conditioning feedback paradigm, were first employed in 1977 (Pfurtscheller & Aranibar 1977; Sterman 1977). The sensory/motor rhythm (SMR) is a resting state of 12–15 Hz, whereas the mu-rhythm has a slightly lower frequency range of 8–12 Hz (and is also referred to as the motor alpha rhythm). With each movement of a limb, this rhythm becomes desynchronized, as evidenced by a decrease in EEG amplitude over the corresponding brain area. One should note that even imagination of movement (without performing actual movement) desynchronizes those rhythms significantly. Therefore, Pfurtscheller constructed BCIs in which individuals can learn to control a computer solely by imagining hand or foot movements (i.e. by voluntarily altering the synchronization and desynchronization of those rhythms that the computer can detect from single-trial EEG during the task) (Pfurtscheller et al. 1996; Kalcher et al. 1996; Flotzinger et al. 1994). Similar methods were used in BCI research by Wolpaw and his group (Wolpaw & McFarland 1994).

A third approach was undertaken by Birbaumer et al. in Tübingen in the late 1990s using slow cortical potentials (SCPs) as a control signal. Operant conditioning of SCP self-regulation using a computerized feedback system was a major focus of that group. The learned ability to self-regulate SCP-shifts toward a negative or positive potential was first successfully used in epilepsy patients for seizure control (Kotchoubey et al. 1996). This type of two-directional control ability can also be used to respond and transmit information to a computer across a menu of choices. This was the basic principle underlying the development of the so-called Thought-Translation-Device (TTD) developed by the author and colleagues (Birbaumer et al. 1999; Kübler et al. 2001; Hinterberger et al. 2001, 2003b, 2004, 2007). The TTD was designed for verbal communication (Perelmouter et al. 1999) by isolating letters from a selection tree using binary brain responses. It was applied in completely paralyzed patients who suffered from amyotrophic lateral sclerosis (ALS), which in its final state can lead to a locked-in syndrome in which the patient can be fully conscious without having any means of communication (as there is no voluntary muscle control). The TTD was the first BCI that offered late-stage ALS patients the ability to write messages (Birbaumer et al. 1999; Kübler et al. 2001). Thus, we can see that the 1990s were dedicated to evaluating those SCP- and mu-rhythm-based BCIs that might be useful as orthotic devices in paralyzed patients.

From 2000, the number of BCI research centers increased dramatically, and algorithms and communication paradigms became increasingly more sophisticated. Detection algorithms were refined, new classification algorithms were developed and tested, and the number of selection classes could be increased from 2 to at least 3–5. In addition, BCIs were developed for various signal types besides the EEG, and invasive technologies offered new methods for brain interfacing.

CURRENT STATE OF THE ART

Non-invasive technologies

BCIs based on EEG currently offer the widest range of applications, because of (1) the validity of EEG as a well studied method (2) the relative affordability of equipment, and (3) the portability and ease of use of EEG systems.

SCP-driven BCIs (such as the TTD) have been shown to facilitate function(s) in paralyzed patients. However, BCI communication speed is slow, and as not more than two or three states can be successfully discriminated, most patients do not achieve high (>90%) control accuracy, and not all patients can learn to self-regulate SCPs. While more advanced classification algorithms for SCPs (Hinterberger et al. 2003a, 2004) seemed to solve such problems, some patients successfully learned to regulate neuronal activity and engage feedback and feedforward BCI. This was also shown with fMRI/SCP self regulation tasks (Hinterberger et al. 2003a, 2005). But what can the SCP tell us about someone´s brain state? Basically, SCPs appear to depict readiness (i.e. the *Bereitschaftspotential*); voluntary regulation of the SCPs can require extensive training that may take weeks to acquire. Interestingly, those patients who are successful SCP regulators report individually different mental strategies to achieve these goals.

Considerable effort is devoted to the further development of SMR and mu-rhythm-driven BCIs, as well as more general BCIs controlled by oscillatory brain signals. Similarly, a three-choice task was tested by Hinterberger and Studer to control a robot using a Support Vector Machine (SVM) classifier that could direct movement based upon imagined/planned movement of the tongue, or hand. Wolpaw et al. have successfully shown that the mu-rhythm allows for graded cursor control and thus not only binary, but also 4- or 5-goal orientation using one-dimensional cursor manipulation for communication. Using oscillatory activity from two different frequencies, Wolpaw and McFarland (1994) achieved two-dimensional graded cursor control, and recently presented a BCI engaging a computer mouse (McFarland *et al.* 2008). A comparison study of several different discrimination tasks showed that there might be a limit of four classes, and that different mental strategies can be used to engage EEG-based direction to separate them. Moreover, Anderson *et al.* (2007) reported reliable classification of five different mental tasks (mental writing, counting, calculating, rotating, and resting) in an asynchronous BCI (i.e. a continuous classification of the brain states without pacing), and this type of rapid advancement seems to be *de rigueur* for the field.

The P300 approach of Donchin for direct brain communication has undergone something of a revival during recent years (Wang *et al.* 2005). Using stepwise linear discriminant analysis (SWLDA) the P300 spelling system allowed for up to 90% or greater accuracy for letter selection out of a 6×6 matrix without extensive training (Sellers *et al.* 2006). It was also shown that P300-driven BCIs can be used in paralyzed patients to a certain extent (Sellers & Donchin 2006; Nijboer *et al.* 2008). The application of current BCI technology to other non-invasive recording methods has been demonstrated for the magnetoencephalography (MEG) (Lal *et al.* 2005b) and also for near infrared spectroscopy (NIRS) (Sitaram *et al.* 2006).

Invasive technologies

A major problem of EEG and MEG measurements is that each electrode senses the summated activity of millions of neurons that may have widely dissimilar functions. This dramatically obfuscates information content, and the signal acquisition through the cranium only further attenuates signal clarity. Thus, invasive techniques attempt closer positioning of electrodes to the actual neuronal sources in order to increase available information content and clarity. The electrocorticogram (ECoG) is a signal measured from electrodes that are placed subdurally on the surface of the cortex, and which provides higher frequencies compared with EEG. BCIs for EEG operation can be used with ECoG and do not require alteration of algorithms, owing to the similarity of the signals (Leuthardt *et al.* 2004, 2006). More invasive techniques are mostly studied in non-human primates. Implanted grids of needle electrodes can be used to directly measure the local field potentials (LFPs) surrounding neurons. Nicolelis showed that it is possible to reconstruct the trajectory of a three-dimensional arm movement of a monkey from the LFPs of only a few hundred neurons or fewer (Nicolelis 2001, 2003).

Imaging technologies

Modern imaging techniques, such as functional magnetic resonance imaging (fMRI), provide information about activation or deactivation of specific brain areas within a resolution of a few millimeters. With increasing computational power, the blood oxygen level-dependent (BOLD) response of a particular brain area can be used in real-time feedback systems with a delay of about one second. Weiskopf *et al.* (2004) presented a real-time fMRI-based BCI that engaged feedback-mediated self-regulation of the supplementary motor area (SMA) and parahippocampal place area (PPA). Posse *et al.* (2003) reported self-induced amygdalar activation using real-time fMRI. However, despite these somewhat promising results, immediate feedback of an fMRI-detected neuronal process cannot be achieved because the hemodynamic BOLD response is delayed by about 3–8 seconds. Therefore, the advantage of an fMRI-based BCI lies not in temporal resolution, but in the specificity of the signal.

RANGE OF APPLICATIONS

Most BCIs follow the idea of translating an intention into an action; this can be a word, a movement, a switch, etc. However, the method or strategy a BCI user employs for expressing his/her idea to the computer does not (and need not) match the action. As matter of fact, in most cases it does not. For example, one can write words by imagining left and right hand movements. Actually, we do the same when typing on a keyboard, as our finger movements towards the letters have nothing to do with the content of our written words. Thus, we can say that basically, BCIs attempt to supplant the motor system of the brain, and not ``read the thoughts´´ of our minds.

A point of possible exception is related to the use of neuro-prostheses. Here it makes sense to connect an imagination strategy as closely as possible to the actual movement of the prosthesis. Taylor (2007) used intracortical microelectrodes on motor areas of a monkey to show that it was possible to learn how to use cortical signals to control assistive devices, such as a 3D cursor and a robotic arm. Birbaumer and Cohen (2007) trained partly paralyzed stroke patients in an

MEG-driven BCI to regain movement abilities. Another neuromotor prosthesis was designed by Hochberg *et al.* (2006) and used an implanted 96 channel microelectrode array in the primary motor cortex of a tetraplegic patient three years after a spinal cord injury. The decoded signals could be used to move a cursor on a screen for tasks such as opening emails or operating TV switches. In addition, the subject was able to neuronally control a prosthetic hand and robotic arm with this technology. EEG-based neuroprosthesis experiments in wheelchair control were conducted by Leeb *et al.* (2007) and Pfurtscheller *et al.* (2003). There are no current iterations of BCI with 100% accuracy, and in this regard it is worth mentioning that, to date, the best brain–machine interface is our neuromotor system itself. The brain is highly reliable, fast, and able to direct complex movements in ways to which none of the current BCI systems can compare. Still, for paralyzed patients a BCI can be of huge help and support.

POTENTIAL ETHICAL CONSIDERATIONS

The possibility of ``reading the mind directly from the brain'' is certainly contentious, yet remains threatening because of concerns about protection of privacy. Such privacy of thoughts provides an inner security, in part by enabling a personal ``discretionary'' space that allows the latitude to think in a prospective way about possible intentions and actions before actually behaving (although, this may, in fact, be something of an illusion). Implicitly, this is the realm of moral consideration and perhaps of ``character''. The privacy of thinking allows the possibility of pre-considering and reflecting upon actions, leads to insight, and hopefully enables us to act in responsible ways. Such volition, whether actual or apparent, imparts a decisional ``feeling'' of who we ``are'', who we want to be, and how to relate in and to our social environment. However, our thinking, feelings, and emotions create something of a hidden reality. This subjectivity essentially determines the quality of life, and therefore it is of high value, and in this way warrants respect and protection. We must wonder how neurotechnology might affect this privacy, and the value(s) we place upon it.

For several decades it has been possible to view autonomic changes in arousal level by measurement of the EDA (electrodermal activity), a correlate of changes in emotional state that has often been used for lie detection. Measuring EDA thus can be regarded as a kind of ``observation of intent'' – with all the possibilities of misinterpretation that are inherent in systems' and observer dissonance(s). These incongruities are well-known and accepted, and the validity (and value) of EDA is contentious. However, we invest considerable faith (and apprehension) in those technologies that are newest, and most novel, and progress in neuroscience (i.e. our understanding of the brain and mind) has been fueled by neurotechnology, and so in many ways this becomes a self-justifying paradigm.

Given the rapid advances in neurotechnology, and the relative faith that we place in its capabilities, the question now is: to what extent could the translation of brain neurophysiology be modeled into an interpretable method to unlock the boundaries and privacy of thoughts? Up to now, communicating thought via a BCI required the strong engagement of the user in order to allow computer discrimination of different brain states that might be provoked through mental strategies. Synchronous BCIs demand the user's skill in disciplined cooperation with the computers' timing structure. Even a passively controlled BCI, such as the P300 speller, requires the user to focus an item on the screen that has to be chosen voluntarily. To be sure, asynchronous BCIs would offer a higher possibility of ``reading thoughts'' because the computer continuously attempts to classify brain dynamics into predefined ``mind'' – or intentional – states. At present, those predefined states could be a number of different thoughts, and these must be trained to evoke any valid outcomes, through numerous repetitions that require a significant commitment by the patient. But, after having adapted an asynchronous BCI system to an individuals' EEG response, the device *is* actually able to detect a set of specific neural activities – thoughts – which are expressed in a particular way.

The goal of this chapter is not to explicitly address the ethical issues, questions, and problems that surround BCI technology, but rather to briefly illustrate how this technology (and its applications) might give rise to those issues and questions that are so well addressed elsewhere in this book. Concerns about the possibility of uncovering the private space of thoughts, and the potential ways in which this information could be used – to both positive and negative effect and ends – spawns real, potential, and imagined ethical, legal, and social issues. The precedent for these concerns has been set by the Internet (through home pages and community websites), and has made apparent the realities of unintended or non-consensual access to personal data. This reveals on a very public level that the issue of information privacy and thought protection is both viable and contentious and will probably become one of the greatest challenges facing the information society of the twenty-first century. Sooner or later we must reach a consensus about the limitations upon access to, and distribution of private information in order to allow persons to feel ``free'' as well as ``safe'' in such a technological world. Similar to other scientific developments, it is primarily the responsibility of science to study, address, and respond to the ethical, legal, and social challenges. But science in general, and neurotechnology more specifically, are not confined to the ivory tower. To date, BCIs have been primarily used in clinical applications, but one can easily envision the use of such devices by the military, by the automotive and aeronautical industry, and even by the general public. Given both the enhanced power of more advanced BCIs, and the very real possibility of their more broad use, we must keep in mind that basic ethical integrity must be maintained. Irrespective of use, what is needed is some strategy and set of tactics that guarantees that current and future use of BCIs is both prudent and good. However, in light of increasingly pluralized societies and the possible penetrance of neurotechnology into various realms of such societies, it may be that the only way to ensure (at least to some extent) ethical considerations is to develop and adapt an inclusive paradigm of both technological innovation and ethical, legal, and social reflection.

CONCLUSIONS

The current state of the art in BCIs is oriented toward a goal of sensing brain signals in an attempt to give humans an alternative opportunity to express themselves in, and engage, their environment. Current BCIs require the commitment of a user to enable and engage the machine, and while the computer can approximate the occurrence of a predefined imaginary task, the accuracy of such sensing remains variable, to a great extent. Thus, we are still quite far from uncovering the specific content of ``thoughts'' by using BCI technology. Even if some fMRI studies report a high predictability of particular changes in specific brain structures during some well-defined mental task, the inverse challenge of ``revealing'' a mental action or thought from an fMRI image is far more difficult, as the corresponding activation patterns show high inter-individual variability, and require constant conditions for a successful replication. In EEG research it is known that a set of classification parameters often cannot be applied from one session to another. So, although it seems to be relatively easy to detect changes (e.g. activation of the insular cortex during emotional states), it is much harder to intuit and predict what those changes ``mean'' in various contexts. Therefore, we can say that reading contents from a brain is a skill – if not an art – that is still in its infancy and, like any infant, is both developing and somewhat self-referent. The goal, therefore, is to work to ensure that this development is sound, and that this new entity effaces its self-reference, so as to `get along well with others´´, both in science and in society. Clearly, this requires a durable, `two-parent´´ approach that must entail both neuroscience and neuroethics.

REFERENCES

Anderson, C. W., Kirby, M. J., Hundley, D. R. & Knight, J. N. 2007. Classification of time-embedded EEG using short-time principal component analysis. In G. Dornuege et al. (eds.) *Towards Brain-Computer Interfacing*. Cambridge, MA; London: MIT Press, pp. 261–77.

Birbaumer, N. & Cohen, L. G. 2007. Brain-computer interfaces: communication and restoration of movement in paralysis. *Journal of Physiology* **579**: 621–36.

Birbaumer, N., Ghanayim, N., Hinterberger, T. *et al.* 1999. A spelling device for the paralysed. *Nature* **398**: 297–98. doi:10.1038/18581.

Chow, A. Y., Chow, V. Y., Packo, K. H. *et al.* 2004. The artificial silicon retina microchip for the treatment of vision loss from retinitis pigmentosa. *Archives of Ophthalmology* **122** (4): 460–9. doi:10.1001/archopht.122.4.460.

Farwell, L. A. & Donchin, E. 1988. Talking off the top of your head: toward a mental prosthesis utilizing event-related brain potentials. *Electroencephalography and Clinical Neurophysiology* **70**(6): 510–23.

Flotzinger, D., Pfurtscheller, G., Neuper, C., Berger, J. & Mohl, W. 1994. Classification of non-averaged EEG data by learning vector quantisation and the influence of signal preprocessing. *Medical and Biological Engineering and Computing* **32**(5): 571–6.

Hinterberger, T., Kaiser, J., Kübler, A., Neuman, N. & Birbaumer, N. 2001. The thought translation device and its applications to the completely paralyzed. In H. H. Diebner, T. Druckrey & P. Weibel (eds.) *Sciences of the Interfaces*. Tübingen: Genista-Verlag, pp. 232–40.

Hinterberger, T., Kübler, A., Kaiser, J., Neuman, N. & Birbaumer, N. 2003a. A brain-computer-interface (BCI) for the locked-in: comparison of different EEG classifications for the Thought Translation Device. *Clinical Neurophysiology* **114**: 416–25.

Hinterberger, T., Mellinger, J. & Birbaumer, N. 2003b. The Thought Translation Device: structure of a multimodal brain-computer communication system. In *Proceedings of the 1st International IEEE EMBS Conference on Neural Engineering, Capri Island, Italy, March 20–22, 2003*, pp. 603–6.

Hinterberger, T., Nijboer, F., Kübler, A. *et al.* 2007. Brain computer interfaces for communication in paralysis: a clinical-experimental approach. In G. Dornhege *et al.* (eds.) *Towards Brain–Computer Interfacing*. Cambridge, MA: MIT Press.

Hinterberger, T., Schmidt, S., Neuman, N. *et al.* 2004. Brain-computer communication and slow cortical potentials. *Special Issue on Brain-Computer Interfaces of the IEEE Transactions on Biomedical Engineering* **51**: 1003–18.

Hinterberger, T., Veit, R., Strehl, U. *et al.* 2003c. Brain areas activated in fMRI during self-regulation of slow cortical potentials (SCPs). *Experimental Brain Research* **152**: 113–22.

Hinterberger, T., Veit, R., Wilhelm, B. *et al.* 2005. Neuronal mechanisms underlying control of a brain-computer interface. *European Journal of Neuroscience* **21**: 3169–81.

Hinterberger, T., Widmann G., Lal, T. N. *et al.* 2008. Voluntary brain regulation and communication with electrocorticogram signals. *Epilepsy and Behavior* **13**: 300–6.

Hochberg, L. R., Serruya, M. D., Friehs, G. M. *et al.* 2006. Neuronal ensemble control of prosthetic devices by a human with tetraplegia. *Nature* **442**(7099): 164–71. doi:10.1038/nature04970.

Kalcher, J., Flotzinger, D., Neuper, C., Gölly, S. & Pfurtscheller, G. 1996. Graz brain-computer interface II: towards communication between humans and computers based on online classification of three different EEG patterns. *Medical and Biological Engineering and Computing* **34**(5): 382–8. doi:10.1007/BF02520010.

Kotchoubey, B., Schneider, D., Schleichert, H. *et al.* 1996. Self-regulation of slow cortical potentials in epilepsy: a retrial with analysis of influencing factors. *Epilepsy Research* **25**(3): 269–76.

Kübler, A., Neuman, N., Kotchoubey, B., Hinterberger, T. & Birbaumer, N. 2001. Brain-computer communication: self-regulation of slow cortical potentials for verbal communication. *Archives of Physical Medicine and Rehabilitation* **82**: 1533–9.

Lal, T. N., Hinterberger, T., Widmann, G. *et al.* 2005a. Methods towards invasive human brain computer interfaces. In *Advances in Neural Information Processing Systems, Vol. 17*. Cambridge, MA: MIT Press, pp. 737–44.

Lal, T. N., Schröder, M., Hill, J. *et al.* 2005b. A brain computer interface with online feedback based on magnetoencephalography. In *The 22nd International Conference on Machine Learning, Bonn, Germany, 2005*.

Leeb, R., Friedman, D., Müller-Putz, G. R. *et al.* 2007. Self-paced (asynchronous) BCI control of a wheelchair in virtual environments: a case study with a tetraplegic. *Computational Intelligence and Neuroscience*: **79642**. doi:10.1155/2007/79642.

Leuthardt, E. C., Miller, K. J., Schalk, G., Rao, R. P. N. & Ojemann, J. G. 2006. Electrocorticography-based brain computer interface – the Seattle experience. *IEEE Transactions on Neural Systems and Rehabilitation Engineering: A Publication of the IEEE Engineering in Medicine and Biology Society* **14**(2): 194–8. doi:10.1109/TNSRE.2006.875536.

Leuthardt, E. C., Schalk, G., Wolpaw, J. R., Ojemann, J. G. & Moran, D. W. 2004. A brain–computer interface using electrocorticographic signals in humans. *Journal of Neural Engineering* **1**(2): 63–71.

McFarland, D. J., Krusienski, D. J., Sarnacki, W. A. & Wolpaw, J. R. 2008. Emulation of computer mouse control with a noninvasive brain-computer interface. *Journal of Neural Engineering* **5**(2): 101–10. doi:10.1088/1741-2560/5/2/001.

Nicolelis, M. A. 2001. Actions from thoughts. *Nature* **409**(6818): 403–7. doi:10.1038/35053191.

Nicolelis, M. A. L. 2003. Brain-machine interfaces to restore motor function and probe neural circuits. *Nature Reviews Neuroscience* **4**(5): 417–22. doi:10.1038/nrn1105.

Nijboer, F., Sellers, E. W., Mellinger, J. *et al.* 2008. A P300-based brain-computer interface for people with amyotrophic lateral sclerosis. *Clinical Neurophysiology: Official Journal of the International Federation of Clinical Neurophysiology* **119**(8): 1909–16. doi:10.1016/j.clinph.2008.03.034.

Perelmouter, J., Kotchoubey, B. & Kübler, A. 1999. Language support program for thought-translation-devices. *Automedica* **18**: 67–84.

Pfurtscheller, G. & Aranibar, A. 1977. Event-related cortical desynchronization detected by power measurements of scalp EEG. *Electroencephalography and Clinical Neurophysiology* **42**(6): 817–26.

Pfurtscheller, G., Stancák, A. & Neuper, C. 1996. Event-related synchronization (ERS) in the alpha band – an electrophysiological correlate of cortical idling: a review. *International Journal of Psychophysiology: Official Journal of the International Organization of Psychophysiology* **24**(1–2): 39–46.

Pfurtscheller, G., Müller, G. R., Pfurtscheller, J., Gerner, H. J. & Rupp, R. 2003. 'Thought' – control of functional electrical stimulation to restore hand grasp in a patient with tetraplegia. *Neuroscience Letters* **351**(1): 33–6.

Posse, S., Fitzgerald, D., Gao, K. *et al.* 2003. Real-time fMRI of temporolimbic regions detects amygdala activation during single-trial self-induced sadness. *NeuroImage* **18**(3): 760–8.

Seligman, P. M. & Shepherd, R. K. 2004. Cochlear implants. In K. Horch & G. Dhillan (eds.) *Neuroprosthetics*. New Jersey: World Scientific, pp. 878–904.

Sellers, E. W. & Donchin, E. 2006. A P300-based brain-computer interface: initial tests by ALS patients. *Clinical Neurophysiology: Official Journal of the International Federation of Clinical Neurophysiology* **117**(3): 538–48. doi:10.1016/j.clinph.2005.06.027.

Sellers, E. W., Krusienski, D. J., McFarland, D. J., Vaughan, T. M. & Wolpaw, J. R. 2006. A P300 event-related potential brain-computer interface (BCI): the effects of matrix size and inter stimulus interval on performance. *Biological Psychology* **73**(3): 242–52. doi:10.1016/j.biopsycho.2006.04.007.

Shepherd, R. K. 2004. Central auditory prostheses. In K. Horch & G. Dhillon (eds.) *Neuroprosthetics*. New Jersey: World Scientific, pp. 1103–14.

Sitaram, R., Zhang, C., Guan, C. *et al.* 2006. Temporal classification of multi-channel near-infrared spectroscopy signals of motor imagery for developing a brain–computer interface. *NeuroImage* **34**(4): 1416–27.

Sterman, M. B. 1977. Sensorimotor EEG operant conditioning: experimental and clinical effects. *Pavlovian Journal of Biological Science* **12**(2): 63–92.

Taylor, D. M. 2007. The importance of online error correction and feed-forward adjustment in brain-machine interfaces for restoration of movement. In *Towards Brain-Computer Interfacing*. Cambridge, MA: MIT Press, pp. 161–73.

Wang, C., Guan, C. & Zhang, H. 2005. P300 brain-computer interface design for communication and control applications. *Conference Proceedings: Annual International Conference of the IEEE Engineering in Medicine and Biology Society. IEEE Engineering in Medicine and Biology Society. Conference* **5**: 5400–3. doi:10.1109/IEMBS.2005.1615703.

Weiskopf, N., Mathiak, K., Bock, S. W. *et al.* 2004. Principles of a brain-computer interface (BCI) based on real-time functional magnetic resonance imaging (fMRI). *IEEE Transactions on Biomedical Engineering* **51**(6): 966–70.

Winter, J. O., Cogan, S. F. & Rizzo, J. F. 2007. Retinal prostheses: current challenges and future outlook. *Journal of Biomaterials Science. Polymer Edition* **18**(8): 1031–55. doi:10.1163/156856207781494403.

Wolpaw, J. R. & McFarland, D. J. 1994. Multichannel EEG-based brain-computer communication. *Electroencephalography and Clinical Neurophysiology* **90**(6): 444–9.

14

Neural engineering
The ethical challenges ahead

B. GORDIJN & A. M. BUYX

Most current research efforts in neural engineering focus on restoring health and functionality of the nervous system. In addition, there is considerable interest in developing neural engineering technologies for the purpose of enhancement. In the short term, the bulk of the neural engineering applications will likely continue to focus on curing disease and reinstating lost functions. In the medium or long term, however, the focus of neural engineering might slowly but surely shift from therapy towards enhancement. Although neural engineering has a huge potential to relieve suffering, its further development is likely to trigger difficult ethical questions as well. These challenges will have to be adequately dealt with so as to guarantee responsible further development and appropriate use of neural engineering technologies.

INTRODUCTION

Neural engineering is a promising new field of research that employs an engineering approach to the study, reinstatement, and enhancement of a wide range of nervous system functions. The first international neural engineering conference was held in Capri, Italy, in 2003. A year later the field's first academic journal, *The Journal of Neural Engineering*, was established.[1] Though new, neural engineering synthesizes a broad range of older fields, such as experimental neuroscience, clinical neurology,

[1] See the website of the *Journal of Engineering*: http://www.iop.org/EJ/journal/JNE. (Accessed on March 1, 2008.)

Scientific and Philosophical Perspectives in Neuroethics, ed. J. J. Giordano & B. Gordijn. Published by Cambridge University Press. © Cambridge University Press 2010.

computational neuroscience, electroconvulsive therapy, electrical engineering, robotics, computer engineering, and materials science.

Most current research efforts in neural engineering focus on curing disease and reinstating lost functions of the nervous system. Besides, several recent research initiatives demonstrate a significant interest in the development of neural engineering technologies for the purpose of enhancing human traits. This chapter sketches how, after achieving safe technologies and substantial therapeutic successes, future research efforts in neural engineering will probably focus increasingly on enhancing desirable traits. The ethical analysis in this chapter focusses on the ethical challenges that might ensue from this development.

INCREASING THERAPEUTIC OPTIONS

A variety of different neural engineering strategies have been developed to increase the therapeutic options for patients with sensory, motor, cognitive, and mood deficits. As an illustration of the sheer range of neural engineering, a few examples are given of methods explored and topics addressed by current research.

Transcranial magnetic stimulation (TMS) is a non-invasive technology that employs rapidly changing magnetic fields, which induce electric fields in the brain. A variety of clinical applications of TMS are currently being studied, such as its merits in treating migraine headaches, severe depression, auditory hallucinations, drug-resistant epilepsy, and tinnitus. Although research in this area is in its infancy, evidence seems to be mounting that TMS is an effective treatment for depression and auditory hallucinations (see, for example, Avery *et al.* 2006; Poulet *et al.* 2005).

Cranial electrotherapy stimulation (CES) influences the brain's functions by passing micro current levels of electrical stimulation across the head via electrodes clipped to the ear lobes. The Food and Drug Administration (FDA) approved CES for the treatment of anxiety, depression, and insomnia (Gilula & Kirsch 2005).

Deep brain stimulation (DBS) involves craniotomy for implantation of a brain pacemaker that interferes with neural activity at the target site by electrical stimulation. The FDA approved DBS in 1997 as a treatment for Parkinson's disease as well as essential tremor. In 2003 it was permitted as a treatment for dystonia. Additionally, there are indications that DBS may also alleviate symptoms in patients suffering from treatment-resistant clinical depression or obsessive–compulsive disorder (Mayberg *et al.* 2005; Greenberg *et al.* 2008).

Brain prostheses (BPs) are devices replacing damaged brain tissue, thereby restoring brain function. An interesting example is the artificial hippocampus, developed by a team led by Theodore Berger. Damage to the hippocampus can cause inability to form new memories. The artificial hippocampus is a chip that is meant to perform all the functions of a normal hippocampus, thereby enabling new memory formation. It was tested successfully on tissue from rats' brains. However, before trials with human subjects can begin, further tests on living animals will have to be done (Graham-Rowe 2003).

Neural prostheses (NPs) are devices that employ electrical stimulation of the nerves in order to restore functions lost as a result of neural damage. Currently, several NPs are used in clinical practice, such as implantable NPs to restore hearing, bladder control, and respiration (Prochazka *et al.* 2001). The cochlear implant is the most widespread used to date. It is a surgically implanted electronic device that works by directly stimulating any functioning auditory nerves inside the cochlea with electrical impulses. In addition, many other NPs are under study or in development. Important ongoing research, for example, concerns retinal implants. With these sight prostheses scientists hope to enable patients with defective sensory cells to see (Weiland & Humayun 2006).

Brain–computer interfaces (BCIs) intercept neural impulses in the brain and establish a direct communication pathway with a computer. Neural signals can be registered either by electrodes on the scalp (electroencephalography), by the cortical surface (electrocorticography), or by a brain implant. An important objective of BCI research is non-muscular communication and control of devices, which might evidently benefit people who are paralyzed. Both non-invasive BCIs, which aim to derive the user's intent from scalp-recorded EEG activity, and more invasive BCIs are being studied and tested in humans. In 1998, Kennedy and Bakay were first to install a brain implant in a human that enabled a patient with a ``locked-in syndrome´´ to control a computer cursor (Kennedy & Bakay 1998). Recently, another patient, paralyzed from the neck down, became the first person to control an artificial hand using an invasive BCI (Leigh *et al.* 2006). BCIs could also, in principle, work the other way round. They have been investigated with a view to their potential of directly affecting brain activity. In rats, radio-controlled electrodes have been shown to influence and direct behavior by stimulating cortical representation areas of left and right whiskers and a ``reward center´´ of the hypothalamus (Talwar *et al.* 2002; Xu *et al.* 2004).

ENHANCING DESIRABLE TRAITS

Currently, several influential research programs are already explicitly focussing on the development of neural engineering technologies for the purpose of enhancing human traits. Three examples of such programs are given.

NASA´s extension of the human senses program

The National Aeronautics and Space Administration (NASA) has an ``Extension of the Human Senses´´ research group that focusses on developing ``alternative methods for human-machine interaction as applied to device control and human performance augmentation´´.[2] Thus, the group endeavors to replace traditional interfaces such as keyboards, mice, joysticks, and microphones with bio-electric control and augmentation technologies. For example, a silent speech interface is being developed that works with electrodes placed upon the throat to measure muscle movements, which are then translated into a limited vocabulary. The interface allows for silent communication and speech augmentation. Another area of research focusses on developing BCIs using electroencephalography.

DARPA´s brain–machine interface program

The Defense Advanced Research Projects Agency (DARPA) of the US Department of Defense has allotted US$24 million to support the proposals for brain–machine systems research of six different laboratorie. According to Alan Rudolph, program manager of the DARPA initiative, the objective is not only to develop technologies that will restore ``but will also *augment* human capabilities´´ (Huang 2003). An important aim is to ``eventually equip soldiers, for example, to control superfast artificial limbs, pilot remote vehicles, and guide mobile robots in hazardous environments, using only the power of their thoughts. Even more remarkable, such devices could enhance decision-making, upgrade memory and cognitive skills, and even allow one person´s brain to communicate wirelessly with another´s´´ (Huang 2003).

---

[2] NASA, Extension of the Human Senses Group, http://www.nasa.gov/centers/ames/research/technology-onepagers/human_senses.html. (Accessed on March 1, 2008.)

Converging technologies for improving human performance

Another powerful research agenda focusses on the convergence of nanotechnology, biotechnology, information technology, and cognitive science and the way in which this so-called NBIC (nano-bio-info-cogno) convergence can and should be used to enhance human performance. This idea was developed in several ``NBIC workshops´´ in the USA (see Gordijn (2006) for a description and critique of this program). The first of these workshops, entitled ``Converging Technologies for Improving Human Performance´´, was organized by the National Science Foundation (NSF) and the Department of Commerce and held at the NSF in Virginia in December 2001. Many proponents of NBIC convergence intend to achieve improved human performance by technologically reshaping ourselves. They propose the use of brain-to-brain interaction and brain–machine interfaces. Furthermore, they recommend that we enhance our sensory, motor, and cognitive skills and abilities. The proponents of NBIC convergence even speculate about humanity becoming ``like a single, distributed and interconnected `brain´´´ by the end of this century (Roco & Bainbridge 2003). They expect that this will mean ``an enhancement to the productivity and independence of individuals, giving them greater opportunities to achieve personal goals´´ (Roco & Bainbridge 2003).[3]

THE FUTURE OF NEURAL ENGINEERING

Nobody knows the future development of neural engineering. After all, further scientific development cannot be predicted down to the last detail, on principle (Popper 1982). Therefore, the following scenario, based on extrapolating current trends, can only claim a certain probability.

Shift from therapy to enhancement

In the short term, most neural engineering applications will probably continue to aim at safely and effectively achieving therapeutic goals. However, developing effective and safe therapeutic neural engineering technologies is likely to indirectly contribute to the development of new enhancement options. After all, most strategies to reinstate lost

---

[3] Similar scenarios are put forward by so-called transhumanists such as Nick Bostrom.

functions might also be used to enhance normal functions. Thus, supposing a successful further development of therapeutic neural engineering, it is reasonable to expect that, in the medium or long term, research may come up with safe and effective ways to improve human abilities as well. In principle, neural engineering strategies of improvement might be developed in all the four areas of sensory, motor, and cognitive abilities, as well as mood and vegetative functions.

Improvement of sensory abilities

Enhancement of sensory abilities might focus on visual perception, for example, such as to enlarge the ability to detect electromagnetic waves to a far greater visible range. Similarly, the range of sound perception might be extended. Furthermore, the chemical senses, gustation and olfaction, would be eligible for enhancement. However, the development of therapeutic neural engineering strategies to counterbalance the inability to taste and smell does not seem to have got past its initial stages. In addition, there is great interest in developing artificial prostheses with the sense of pressure perception. This strand of research might engender ways to enhance our ability to touch.

Additionally, our set of senses might perhaps be extended with new ones such as electroception, echolocation or other ones. For example, proponents of NBIC convergence advocate the development of new senses such as the ``information-gulping sixth sense´´, which would enable us to instantaneously gulp down the information of an entire book, making it a structural part of our wetware ``ready for inferencing, reference, etc., with some residual sense of the whole, as part of the sensory gulp experience´´ (Spohrer 2003).

In addition, there are ideas about the possibility of combining the sensory abilities of various individuals. For example, neural prostheses facilitating the enhancement of particular sensory skills might be simultaneously implanted in several people and then linked up. Individuals could in this way not only perceive their own images, noises, smells and/or tastes, but also those of others (Warwick 2000).

Improvement of motor abilities

Research is being done into enhancing motor abilities so as to achieve faster running or supernatural muscle power. However, these research activities still follow a traditional approach using muscle facilitated motor output as a starting point. More revolutionary enhancements will involve brain–computer interfaces that enable operating devices by thought alone. These motor enhancement systems do not depend on human muscles with their inherent range of action depending on natural body morphology. Instead, they will enable control over an extensive range of artificial motor actions, thus hugely extending both motor power and sphere of action. The army will evidently be one of the first interested. Soldiers might operate fighting robots on far away battlefields; pilots might remote-control planes and so on. Moreover, normal citizens might also profit from brain–computer interfaces enabling them to operate all manner of gadgets in their ``smart houses´´, using only the power of their thoughts.

Improvement of cognitive abilities

It may become possible to develop ways of enhancing the memory – in the sense of being able to store and retrieve larger quantities of new information. In this way a new language could be learnt or a new area of work mastered at greater speed. Also conceivable would be invisible communication with persons in different locations – known as *cyberthink* (Maguire & McGee 1999). In time, conventional communication by telephone could even become superfluous. Cyberthink could facilitate the development of new mentally linked social communities. In addition, a chip could be implanted in the brain, which would function as a kind of reference book. Then, whenever certain questions are pondered it would be activated – as an image superimposed on the normal visual image, but without rendering it invisible. Another possibility could be in-built face recognition programs in the human brain, which would provide the name of – and maybe further information about – a person encountered. Finally, in principle the technologies carry the potential for *mind-merging*. Such an admittedly far-fetched scenario, familiar from science-fiction literature, includes the vision of connecting/integrating the minds – or parts thereof – of several individuals using different BCIs in order to achieve ``super-intelligence´´.

Improvement of mood and vegetative functions

The current high consumption of Prozac and Viagra demonstrates the market potential of enhancers of mood and vegetative functions. In 2001 an implanted device was patented in the US that stimulates nerves in the spinal cord with electrical impulses to trigger an orgasm at the push of a button. Stuart Meloy, the developer of the gadget, regards the implant as helpful for women unable to achieve orgasms naturally. This technology reveals a new horizon of neurally augmented sexual functions (Meloy & Southern 2006). But why arouse nerves when the brain can be stimulated directly to produce pleasure? A considerable amount of animal research suggests that intracranial stimulation of certain brain regions might produce pleasure or positive effects (see, for example, Wise 1996). Further research might enable subtle ways to enhance moods in humans.

Widespread use of neural engineering technologies

Once supply is growing, demand is unlikely to react indifferently. When current interest for enhancement technologies such as cosmetic surgery and dentistry, smart drugs, mood enhancers, growth hormones, and sports doping can be taken as an indication, there will probably be a viable future market for effective, safe, and affordable neural engineering enhancement technologies.

ETHICAL CHALLENGES

To discuss the ethical challenges of enhancement by neural engineering is to take part in the general controversy about enhancing human traits using modern medical technology. Several of the arguments presented below also play an important role with regard to other forms of enhancement, such as cosmetic surgery, growth hormone treatment, or enhancing cognition or mood via psychopharmacology.[4] A second group of arguments deals with features particular to neural engineering and thus is specific to these technologies.

Before we enter into the ethical enquiry of enhancement by neural engineering, we need to stress that we take a cautiously positive stance towards enhancement as such, which we will not justify in detail. We neither regard enhancement by medical means as a reprehensible violation of human nature, nor do we agree with the charge that improvement is a problematic goal for medicine or society at large (President's Council 2003; Sandel 2007; Habermas 2003). Thus, we do not argue that there is anything *inherently* wrong with enhancement as such. Yet a closer look reveals that the widespread use of neural engineering as an enhancement technology might trigger certain

---

[4] For a very good collection of essays on different forms of enhancement, see Parens (1998).

difficult problems. Responsible development and appropriate use of neural engineering will hinge on adequately dealing with the following ethical challenges.

Proportionality

A positive balance should exist between the benefits of a medical intervention and its risks. In addition, therapy is generally considered more beneficial and therefore fundamentally more valuable than enhancement (Daniels 2000). Enhancing interventions still tend to be regarded as not absolutely necessary, since the body being enhanced is already healthy. Consequently, we may assume a greater readiness to accept risks associated with therapeutic interventions than those associated with enhancing interventions.

The risks associated with new neural engineering technologies are not easy to assess in advance. If neuroimplants were involved, risks would primarily be related to the surgical interventions for purposes of implantation, as well as to the maintenance or upgrading of the implant. Furthermore, risks might result from the possibility that the human organism might not tolerate a particular implant. However, since we can assume that any experience gained with therapeutic neural engineering would also profit future enhancing interventions, the desired proportionality between benefits and risks could in time also be arrived at here. Several technologies would simply allow for a so-called double use as both a therapeutic device and an enhancer. Enhancement using these technologies would not entail any additional risk besides the risks deemed acceptable when developing promising new therapeutic interventions. A good example of such a double use would be deep brain stimulation, which has been developed slowly, with a clearly therapeutic intention, and under careful consideration of risk–benefit analyses. The surgical interventions involved in DBS could one day become absolutely standard interventions, involving calculable and minimal risks. In this case, exploring the enhancing potential of DBS would, at least in terms of risk proportionality, be unproblematic.

However, there are several applications of neural engineering that will require substantial further development of existing technology, far beyond a simple double use. Since no disease calls for rapid uploading of large chunks of specific information or for the merging of senses of several individuals, such devices would from the start be developed with a view to using them as enhancers. Developers may utilize several technical elements of established therapeutic interventions, such as the type of surgery, the type of chip/prosthesis, and the knowledge about neuroimplants gained from therapeutic applications. However, there will not be sufficient knowledge of how a human brain would react to rapid information-gulping or to sense-merging. A lot of experimental research would have to be undertaken to gain insight into these questions. It is hard to imagine that institutional review boards would easily approve surgical research protocols of this kind in healthy participants, especially when the intention is to develop, not a therapeutic device, but a predominantly enhancing one (Foster 2006). Altogether, the issue of a positive risk–benefit ratio in the short and long term is far more complicated in neural engineering technologies designed primarily for enhancement than in those originally intended for therapeutic application. Since neuroimplants are still in the initial stages of their development, it is difficult to estimate how the various risk areas will unfold in the future.

The ``neurodivide´´

Since modern society is very performance-oriented, it is easy to imagine that people might be interested in interventions to improve cognitive ability. After all, these abilities are a decisive factor in acquiring a career, material wealth, and social prestige. Parents might equip their children with safe and effective neural engineering systems to enhance their cognitive ability and then continually update them to outdo the competition and attain long-term success.

How would such a development affect social justice?[5] Social differences are not unfair per se. For example, it is often considered only fair that somebody who works harder and performs better should also earn more and be allowed to enjoy a higher standard of living. Unfair social differences only arise as a result of an ethically unjustifiable distribution of social goods such as status, prestige, money, or employment. Could the further development and application of neural engineering enhancement technologies bring about such an unjust distribution of goods?

If neural engineering enhancement technologies could, without payment, be made available to the population at large, there would be no exacerbation of existing inequalities. Anybody interested in doing so could undergo an intervention and profit accordingly. This scenario

---

[5] For an excellent discussion of this question with a focus on genetic enhancement, see Buchanan *et al.* (2000).

would therefore not promote social injustice. However, bearing in mind the present shortage of money in the health sector, it would appear far more probable that enhancement technologies might be reserved for the wealthy. After all, no country is likely to take on board the enormous costs of a population-scale improvement in cognitive abilities. Thus, only those people who already enjoy a lofty social status and considerable material wealth would profit from enhancing neural engineering technologies. Additional opportunities for social and professional improvement would be made available to precisely those people already at the top of the social hierarchy. This is problematic for two reasons. Not only would it further exacerbate the existing gap between the rich and the poor, it would also obstruct the principles of equal opportunity and solidarity with the weak.

Limitless enhancement

Once neural engineering enhancement technologies would provide not only a *restitutio ad integrum* (restitution of the integral body and its functions), but also a *transformatio ad optimum* (an improvement in human constitution so as to achieve a certain ideal beyond the purely curative), a positive feedback loop would command further developments. After all, in contrast with the restoration of health, improvement beyond therapy does not know any natural limits. Thus, abilities and functions, which have already been improved on one occasion, could be improved again once technology has progressed further, and then again and again. In addition, once a certain number of people would have undergone enhancing interventions, others would feel themselves under increasing pressure to do likewise. Without such interventions they might fear not being able to keep up with those around them. This would be especially relevant for people in certain high-pressure occupations, such as pilots, soldiers, academics, etc. In many jobs the enhancement of certain abilities and traits could be regarded as a material advantage over the competition in the field, and a lot of pressure to undergo enhancement procedures may develop. In fact, there is already a lot of anecdotal evidence that enhancement by psychopharmacology has become a widespread habit among members of the professional groups mentioned. It does not require a great stretch of imagination to assume that these people will be among the first to use neural engineering technology in order to improve specific capacities both substantially and permanently. Doubts as to the voluntariness of these decisions are warranted, and a preemptive discussion about possible regulations of neural engineering and the protection of people in certain occupations from undue pressure is necessary.

Moreover, in time, the attitude could become ingrained that in order to be successful, not only in a high-pressure occupation but in life, one has to submit one´s body to all manner of enhancing interventions available. As a result, attitudes towards conventional human abilities could change quite negatively in the long term. Average abilities could become almost akin to defects, in need of elimination. People could become afraid that their normal traits are fundamentally inadequate. As a result, neural engineering enhancement technologies could trigger a medicalization of so far absolutely ordinary and normal human abilities.

Authenticity and identity

Most enhancing technologies that involve a change of mood, sensory experience, or cognitive capacities face the charge that, by using them, people become less authentic. A popular version of this argument states that for a person to be authentic, she must be `true to herself´ and feel that her experiences and feelings are `her own´´ (Parens 2005). Critics of enhancement fear that by altering emotional or cognitive states through drugs or other interventions, people become alienated from their own feelings and experiences and separated from the world as it really is (Parens 2005; Elliott 2003). Users of enhancement who have taken a short-cut by technology may achieve a desirable state, but they can no longer be described as having achieved it *themselves*, nor can they claim the experience as *their own*. Hence they lose awareness of who they are, and what the world is truly like. This criticism applies especially to neural engineering technologies, since these would alter emotional and cognitive states substantially and permanently. Moreover, a lot of neural engineering research aims specifically at developing means of separating an agent from her actions, such as, for example, the development of thought-controlled devices.

However, the criticism employs a very particular interpretation of authenticity. There is another way of understanding what being authentic means, namely living a life of self-fulfillment and self-creation (DeGrazia 2005). In fact, many people report feeling alienated all their lives because they are unable to do certain things they want to do or to change certain features of their personality they feel do not correspond with how they see themselves. In this interpretation of authenticity, enhancement technologies can be employed to bring people closer to the way they would like to be, thus making them more instead of less authentic. Enhancement can be the means to achieve a particular state that fits the image a person has of herself, and which she otherwise would not be able to experience. If an enhancement intervention is chosen by a well-informed person in order to help her attain certain goals in her life, there is little reason to suspect that she will be alienated afterwards – it is, after all, *her* idea of how she wants to be which she is trying to fulfill. There may be other reasons to carefully monitor the decisions of people who wish to use enhancement, such as the suspicion that their desire to enhance themselves does not stem from their own idea of how they want to be, but rather from cultural or peer pressure, but these worries relate to compromised autonomy, not to a lack of authenticity.

Neural engineering is far more likely to affect the identity of people than their authenticity. DeGrazia (2005) distinguishes between numerical and narrative identity. Numerical identity is the ``relationship an entity has to itself over time in being one and the same entity´´. An account of numerical identity provides criteria – either biological or psychological – for an entity in question to continue to exist through change. In contrast, narrative identity involves people´s self-conception: their most important values, their way of defining themselves, their implicit autobiography, their relationships to particular people, their roles, and so on. It might be argued that enhancement by neural engineering could disrupt the narrative identity of a person. However and quite analogously to the argument spelled out above, if the enhancement intervention was chosen autonomously and by a well-informed agent, this would not necessarily have to be the case. Instead, she could incorporate the change into her self-conception and self-definition, thus making it part of her narrative. By contrast, a disruption of numerical identity is far more likely. It is a specific feature of some potential neural engineering technologies such as cyberthink, mind-merging, or the combination of sensory abilities of several people, that there literally could be a change in numbers. Are persons during mind-merging or cyberthink sessions distinct persons, or do they become one person? If sensory abilities are combined, whose are the resulting sensations? Technologies such as mind-merging lend themselves to a host of interesting Parfitian scenarios. Even though they may still be a long way off, their potential to challenge our concept of numerical identity should be anticipated.

The transparent society

Privacy can be understood as the power of a person or group to control information about themselves. Consequently, it involves the ability to prevent data becoming known to others than those whom one chooses to be informed. Brin (1998) argues that further developments in sur-veillance, communication, and information technology will erode privacy. In the long run this development will leave us with two options. We may decide to limit the power of surveillance to ``the authorities''. After all, monopolizing surveillance might still offer the illusion of privacy, although true privacy will obviously have vanished. Alterna-tively, we might settle on a society that offers everyone equal access to technologies of surveillance. As a result, the illusion of privacy would be destroyed, but we would at least be able to watch the watchers in turn. Considering that the worst abuses of power might result from lack of transparency and liability, Brin prefers a society in which the public has the same access to surveillance options as those in power.

Brin is basically right in his stance against monopolizing surveil-lance. However, in his analysis he does not take into account the development and widespread use of neural engineering technologies, which would likely severely aggravate the danger of loss of privacy and thus reinforce his argument. After all, standard use of neural engin-eering technologies to improve all manner of human abilities would further intensify links between humans and computers. BCIs, for example, might permanently link up brains to computers for all manner of purposes. Contact to diverse databases for information retrieval would be made directly via the brain. Similarly, neural engineering might facilitate more intensive links between human beings. Commu-nication with geographically remote people would then be permanently given – using the cyberthink communication system, for example – via a direct link from brain to brain. All these applications might facilitate the possibility of retracing and registering the exact location, actions, and thoughts of any ``linked-up'' or ``plugged-in'' human being.

If widespread use of neural engineering technologies is indeed inherently associated with severe restrictions of privacy, this brings up the question of what limitations of privacy can still be justified in the light of the advantages that the neural engineering technologies gen-erate for their users. For example, what trade-offs between privacy and enhancement can still be regarded as proportional? In addition, studies should be made of how surveillance monopolies might be prevented.

Mind control

In 2002, Talwar and Chapin at the State University of New York Downstate Medical Center developed remote-controlled rats that have electrodes implanted in their brains and wear a small radio receiver and electrical stimulator in a backpack. Remote stimulation in the sensorimotor cortex causes a sensation in their left or right whiskers, and stimulation in the medial forebrain bundle (MFB) is interpreted as pleasure. Using remote MFB stimulation as a reward the rats can be directed to move left, right, and forward as a reaction to whisker signals (Talwar *et al.* 2002). This fascinating achievement demonstrates a worrying potential of neural engineering research.

Mind control involves deliberate manipulation by certain agents of a person´s or a group´s thinking, behavior, emotions, or decisions. As such it establishes an infringement of the manipulated subjects´ autonomy. Could someone ever be interested in exploring the possibilities of neural engineering technologies to control human minds? If you extrapolate historical developments, the answer would be affirmative. In the 1950s and 1960s, for example, the CIA ran a mind control research program code-named Project MKULTRA. Different strategies to develop methods of mind and behavior control were studied within this program. However, at that time the use of electronic signals to alter brain functioning was still too rudimentary to achieve effective control over the mind (US Senate 1977).

Currently, this situation might change very rapidly. Further development of neural engineering technologies will likely facilitate new and more effective methods of mind control. For example, powerful and highly targeted transcranial magnetic stimulation might perhaps be used to influence certain thought processes. In addition, BCIs might be exploited to send subliminal information, i.e. signals or messages designed to pass below the normal limits of perception, thus subconsciously influencing users of these BCIs without their even noticing it. Thus, effective means will have to be developed to prevent these and comparable scenarios, preferably better than today´s methods, to prevent computer viruses, worms, Trojan horses, spyware, adware, and other malicious and unwanted software infiltrating, damaging or controlling a computer system without the owner´s informed consent.

The experience machine

Owing to technical limitations, it is at present impossible to create truly convincing virtual reality experiences. They are predominantly visual experiences that occasionally include additional auditory information and only rarely haptic force feedback. A technical device such as a keyboard or a mouse facilitates interaction with the virtual environment. Thus, current computer-generated virtual environments are easily distinguishable from reality. In the long term, however, neural engineering might enable an improvement of virtual reality technologies to the extent that it would become nearly impossible to distinguish a virtual from a real environment. Highly sophisticated BCIs, powerful supercomputers programmed with the rules of a highly detailed virtual world, might provide users with all of their sensory input, thus creating artificial experiences indistinguishable from real ones. Thus, in the long term neural engineering might develop something very similar to what Nozick (1974) calls an ``experience machine´´, i.e. a machine that would give you any experience you desired by direct stimulation of the brain.

Nozick examines the question of whether you should ``plug into´´ this machine for the rest of your life and presents three counter-arguments. First, we do not just want to have the experience of doing certain things. Instead, we want to do the things themselves. Second, we want to be a certain way and a certain sort of person. However, when plugged into the experience machine a person´s character gradually dissolves. Third, we want to be able to interact with a reality that is deeper than that which people can construct. Thus, we believe that there is a reality that might not be amenable to human computer-generated reproduction. Nozick uses his argument to demonstrate that desirable experiences and feelings of pleasure are not the only things that have value in themselves.

The choice given to us in Nozick´s scenario is whether to plug in *for the rest of our life*. What would change, one might ask, if we could plug in for any chosen period of time? In this more realistic scenario Nozick´s original arguments become less convincing. However, there are still arguments that might urge us to be cautious. For example, frequent use of the experience machine might lead to a virtual reality addiction, causing neglect of important duties and responsibilities. Hence, addicts would increasingly be at risk of facing problems in their social surroundings, at school or at the workplace. The growing problem of people becoming addicted to role-playing computer games provides ample warning in this respect.

Furthermore, frequent immersion in computer-generated virtual reality environments, instantly providing us with all manner of desired experiences, might change our attitudes negatively. The experience of instant gratification might, for example, corrode the virtue of patience to an extent that it makes us significantly less well adapted to real life.

Finally, regular immersion in virtual reality environments might cause difficulties in distinguishing between real and artificial experiences. As virtual reality environments become progressively more real, how is one to determine whether one is plugged in? It might become excessively difficult to tell, on the basis of one's perceptions alone, whether one is interacting with an artificial or with a real environment. This may cause quite some existential confusion.

CONCLUSION

Neural engineering has a huge potential for restoring the health and functionality of the nervous system. Furthermore, it might improve all manner of human abilities. However, in order to guarantee responsible development and appropriate use of neural engineering technologies, several ethical problems will have to be tackled. Immediately problematic are the risks that are potentially involved in connection with the required surgical interventions and with the tolerance of the body towards neuroimplants. Furthermore, several undesirable effects could surface in connection with neural engineering enhancement technologies in the long term. Firstly, privacy, autonomy, and numerical identity could be violated. In addition, the application of enhancing neural engineering technologies would be in danger of promoting social injustice. Besides, widespread use of neural engineering for the purpose of enhancement could fan the flames of medicalization. Finally, intensive use of virtual environments might cause addiction, trigger negative personality changes, and blur the difference between artificial and real environments. Taken overall, these ethical problems appear substantial. Anticipative debate is needed to avoid these pitfalls and facilitate responsible further development and appropriate use of neural engineering technologies.

REFERENCES

Avery, D. H. *et al.* 2006. A controlled study of repetitive transcranial magnetic stimulation in medication-resistant major depression. *Biological Psychiatry* **59** (2): 187–94.

Brin, D. 1998. *The Transparent Society: Will Technology Force Us to Choose Between Privacy and Freedom?* New York: Addison-Wesley.

Buchanan, A. E., Brock, D. W., Daniels, N. & Wikler, D. 2000. *From Chance to Choice. Genetics and Justice.* Cambridge: Cambridge University Press.

Daniels, N. 2000. Normal functioning and the treatment-enhancement distinction. *Cambridge Quarterly of Healthcare Ethics* **9**: 309–22.

DeGrazia, D. 2005. Enhancement technologies and human identity. *Journal of Medicine and Philosophy* **30**: 261–83.

Elliott, C. 2003. *Better Than Well: American Medicine Meets the American Dream*. New York: Norton.

Foster, K. R. 2006. Engineering the brain. In Illes, (ed.) *Neuroethics. Defining the Issues in Theory, Practice, and Policy*. New York/Oxford: Oxford University Press, pp. 185–200.

Gilula, M. F. & Kirsch, D. L. 2005. Cranial electrotherapy stimulation review: a safer alternative to psychopharmaceuticals in the treatment of depression. *Journal of Neurotherapy* **9**(2): 7–26.

Gordijn, B. 2006. Converging NBIC technologies for improving human performance: a critical assessment of the novelty and the prospects of the project. *Journal of Law, Medicine & Ethics* **34**(4): 726–32.

Graham-Rowe, D. 2003. World´s first brain prosthesis revealed. *New Scientist Online Edition*, 15 March: http://www.newscientist.com/article.ns?id=dn3488. (Accessed on March 1, 2008.)

Greenberg, B. D., Gabriels, L. A., Malone, D. A. Jr. *et al*. 2008. Deep brain stimulation of the ventral internal capsule/ventral striatum for obsessive-compulsive disorder: worldwide experience. *Molecular Psychiatry*, May 20. [Epub ahead of print.]

Habermas, J. 2003. *The Future of Human Nature*. Cambridge, MA: Polity Press.

Huang, G. T. 2003. Mind Machine Merger. *Technology Review* May 2003: http://viterbi.usc.edu/pdfs/structured/in_the_news_4333.pdf. (Accessed on March 1, 2008.)

Kennedy, P. R. & Bakay, R. A. 1998. Restoration of neural output from a paralysed patient by a direct brain connection. *Neuroreport* **9**(8): 1707–11.

Leigh, R. *et al*. 2006. Neuronal ensemble control of prosthetic devices by a human with tetraplegia. *Nature* **442**: 164–71.

Maguire, G. Q. Jr. & McGee, E. M. 1999. Implantable brain chips? Time for debate. *Hastings Center Report* **7**: 7–13.

Mayberg, H. *et al*. 2005. Deep brain stimulation for treatment-resistant depression. *Neuron* **45**(5): 651–60.

Meloy, T. S. & Southern, J. P. 2006. Neurally augmented sexual function in human females: a preliminary investigation. *Neuromodulation* **9**(1): 34–40.

Nozick, R. 1974. *Anarchy, State, and Utopia*. New York: Basic Books.

Parens, E. (ed.) 1998. *Enhancing Human Traits*. Washington, D. C.: Georgetown University Press.

Parens, E. 2005. Authenticity and ambivalence. Toward understanding the enhancement debate. *Hastings Center Report* **35**(3): 34–41.

Popper, K. 1982. *The Open Universe: An Argument for Indeterminism*. London: Hutchinson.

Poulet, E. *et al*. 2005. Slow transcranial magnetic stimulation can rapidly reduce resistant auditory hallucinations in schizophrenia. *Biological Psychiatry* **57**(2): 188–91.

The President´s Council on Bioethics. 2003. *Beyond Therapy. Biotechnology and the Pursuit of Happiness*. New York: Dana Press.

Prochazka, A., Mushahwar, V. K. & McCreery, D. B. 2001. Neural prostheses. *Journal of Physiology* **533**(1): 99–109.

Roco, C. & Bainbridge, W. S. 2003. Overview. Converging technologies for improving human performance. Nanotechnology, biotechnology, information technology and cognitive science (NBIC). In Roco, M. C. & Bainbridge, W. S. (eds.) *NBIC Convergence for Improving Human Performance. Nanotechnology, Biotechnology, Information Technology and Cognitive Science*. Dordrecht/Boston/London: Kluwer Academic Publishers, pp. 1–27.

Sandel, M. J. 2007. *The Case Against Perfection: Ethics in the Age of Genetic Engineering.* Cambridge, MA: Harvard University Press.

Spohrer, J. 2003. NBICS (nano-bio-info-cogno-socio) convergence to improve human performance: opportunities and challenges. In Roco, M. C. & Bainbridge, W. S. (eds.) *NBIC Convergence for Improving Human Performance. Nanotechnology, Biotechnology, Information Technology and Cognitive Science.* Dordrecht/Boston/London: Kluwer Academic Publishers, pp. 101–17.

Talwar, S. *et al.* 2002. Behavioral neuroscience: rat navigation guided by remote control. *Nature* **417**: 37–8.

US Senate. 1977. *Joint Hearing before The Select Committee on Intelligence and The Subcommittee on Health and Scientific Research of the Committee on Human Resources,* 95th Congress, 1st Session, August 3, 1977: http://www.scribd.com/doc/919815/Project-MKULTRA-the-CIAs-Program-of-Research-and-Behavioral-Modificationjoint-hearing-before-the-U-S-Senate-1977-transcript. (Accessed on March 1, 2008.)

Warwick, K. 2000. Cyborg 1.0. Kevin Warwick outlines his plan to become one with his computer. *Wired* **8**(2): http://www.wired.com/wired/archive/8.02/warwick.html. (Accessed on March 1, 2008.)

Weiland, J. D. & Humayun, M. S. 2006. Intraocular retinal prosthesis: big steps to sight restoration. *IEEE Engineering in Medicine and Biology* **25**(5): 60–6.

Wise, R. A. 1996. Addictive drugs and brain stimulation reward. *Annual Review of Neuroscience* **19**: 319–40.

Xu, S. *et al.* 2004. A multi-channel telemetry system for brain micro-stimulation in freely roaming animals. *Journal of Neuroscience Methods* **133**: 57–63.

15

Neurotechnology as a public good
Probity, policy, and how to get there from here

A. M. JEANNOTTE, K. N. SCHILLER, L. M. REEVES,
E. G. DERENZO & D. K. MCBRIDE

NEUROTECHNOLOGY: A FOCUS FOR PUBLIC POLICY

The field of neuroscience draws together many disciplines in the study of the nervous system and the properties of mind. Although understanding the basic structure and physiology of the brain and its processes has led to high-impact findings, it is typically the manipulation or application of this knowledge that is most interesting to individuals outside the scientific community. The development and use of neurotechnologies, those tools and devices that interact with and modulate the nervous system, is a fast-emerging area of technical achievement that has vast potential to impact our understanding of, and interaction with the brain. The rapidly growing field of neurotechnology research and development employs knowledge and tools from diverse fields. It is through interdisciplinary, collaborative thinking that great advances have been made to develop, research, and transfer neurotechnology to the clinic and beyond. Such technologies include functional magnetic resonance imaging (fMRI), electroencephalography (EEG), functional near-infrared spectroscopy (fNIRS), deep brain stimulation (DBS), and neural prosthetics. Investigation into the mechanisms and functions of the brain is leading to a vastly improved understanding of brain disease, injuries, human cognition, and behavior, and will give us an unprecedented ability to heal, enhance, and manipulate the nervous system.

Scientific and Philosophical Perspectives in Neuroethics, ed. J. J. Giordano & B. Gordijn. Published by Cambridge University Press. © Cambridge University Press 2010.

Many ethical, legal, and social implications (ELSI) of these technologies and their identified and potential uses have emerged, with
others still to surface, as the scientific community and general public
have increasing access to medical and commercial neurotechnologies
(Eaton & Illes 2007). As the field of neuroscience evolves, neurotechnologies will continue to advance in parallel, and their applications
will demand an analysis of the relevant ELSI. Several neurotechnologies
already evoke ELSI concerns, and will require immediate consideration.
Other issues may not emerge for many years, yet this time course
remains unpredictable, given the rapidity of scientific advance and
technological development. Given this incalculable pace, it is critical
that discussions of the ethical, legal, and social issues be engaged, and
that a thoughtful process for evaluation and guidance be logically
applied as the developments and uses of neurotechnology progress,
and new issues, questions, and concerns emerge. Ultimately, it is
envisioned that such a process will lead to sound public policy to
assure the safe and respectful creation and application of neurotechnologies that can be employed in a variety of settings, including
healthcare, national security, and even daily life. Although it may be
argued that we are far from actually enacting such policies, it is clear
that there is both the need, and viable forums, for educated and
socially conscious discussions to ensure the responsible conduct,
studies, and applications of technology.

GETTING TO POLICY

The road to widely supported public policy is neither straight, short, nor
clear, particularly when the issues are those that prompt contemplation
about the quality of life, social and judicial systems, and the nature of
our ``selves'' and minds. Such issues arising from the use and impact(s)
of existing or potential neurotechnologies range from the more mun-
dane aspects of daily activities and entertainment, to the treatment of
disease and maintenance of public health, to more abstract domains,
such as the definition of what it means to be human, and consideration
of personal rights. Achieving public policy that addresses the needs
of every stakeholder would aid consumers, developers, researchers,
and practitioners in safely and confidently using neurotechnologies.
Although not all aspects of use and applications need to (or should) be
regulated at the federal or state level, oversight (e.g. via professional
society guidelines) would aid responsible development and increase
public confidence in these technologies.

One mechanism by which broad public and scientific acceptance of public policy regarding an emerging technology can be built is through grassroots efforts (Joss 1999). In the beginning stages, such efforts are advanced by simply bringing the discussion to new audiences and by initiating a forum for reasoned, informed discussion about new technologies. As technologies become more widely available and public awareness of them increases, a more formal, coordinated process among public groups or institutions should be fostered.

Toward this end, the Center for Neurotechnology Studies (CNS) at the Potomac Institute for Policy Studies in Arlington, Virginia (USA) implemented a series of workshops to bring together experts from various (scientific and humanties') disciplines to identify and discuss the existing and potential issues focal to neurotechnological advancements. This endeavor led to much discovery, in part through trial and error, which will be discussed in this chapter. Yet this is not a process that is unique or without precedent; other organizations have started similar discussions on several focus areas within neuroscience (Marcus 2002; Illes *et al.* 2006). The results of these independent efforts must be communicated to both professional and public audiences and used to build a formalized dialog toward constructing guidelines and policy. These large groups have the ability to govern acceptable practices within a field, and lobby for safe and respectful regulation of neurotechnologies at the congressional and executive level, eventually leading to public policy that has both social acceptance, and state and federal endorsement.

This process cannot, nor should not occur in haste, but rather must entail critical reflection, analysis, and thoroughly vetted intention and action(s). However, engaging the process must occur sooner, rather than later, as it is vital to preempt decisions about neurotechnology, rather than lament them. As evidenced by this book (and others in the field) there is currently a growing public interest in neuroethics. This is a critical aspect to any discourse on neurotechnology, as a range of potentially positive and/or negative uses, applications, and implications must be anticipated. Although it is likely that science will seek some path of self-regulation, there is still considerable benefit to be gained from a formal process through which to establish guidelines for research, and for the use of available techniques and technologies. Scientists are often concerned that their work will be seen for its positive contributions and efficient advancement of their field. A notable product of such successes is the wide adoption of scientific and technological breakthroughs by both the scientific community and target consumers. Still, efficiency can prove to be contentious, if the moral value of any research or technology is, or becomes, questionable. Thus, ELSI and safety concerns must be addressed throughout, rather than subsequent to research, development, testing, and evaluation (RDTE).

To be sure, the most accepted and appropriate scientific guidelines and regulations are those that emerge from the field itself. Thus, any effort to establish ELSI-related guidelines for the application and use of neurotechnologies must be careful to consider the involvement of neurotechnology scientists and engineers. The goal is to facilitate the creation of guidelines and a formal process (or framework) for discussing ELSI issues in a balanced forum, with the ultimate objective of establishing public policy for the application and use of neurotechnologies. These are ambitious goals and objectives, to say the least, but they must be attempted, and it is hoped that some form of general agreement that forms the groundwork for a Neurotechnology Code of Ethics will emerge from these pursuits.

Steps to develop a formal framework and replicable process could serve as a model to address other (neuro)ethical, legal, and social debates. A formalized process to address these concerns was part of the Human Genome Project and the National Nanotechnology Initiative. The Human Genome Project set aside approximately 5% of total spending for ELSI research, as it was anticipated that the advent of genetic manipulation would affect many aspects of the human condition (Collins *et al.* 1998). Similarly, the National Nanotechnology Initiative, established to coordinate nanotechnology R&D across the federal government, included a specific focus area to address ethical, legal, and social issues germane to both the development and the use of nanotechnologies (Mnyusiwalla *et al.* 2003; NSET 2007). Neurotechnology developers, researchers, and clinicians must learn from the issues and discussions that have faced other scientific fields and look to the ``lessons learned´´ from such issues for guidance.

THE WORKSHOP

The ``Developing Ethics Guidelines for Research and Use of Neurotechnologies´´ workshop was convened by the Center for Neurotechnology Studies of the Potomac Institute in April 2008 as a first step toward building a dialog between researchers, scientists, ethicists, legal scholars, philosophers, and others concerned with ELSI as relevant to policy associated with neuroscience and emerging technologies. The workshop culminated with a discussion-based working group to test a process to identify ELSI and build consensus around the best approach to adequately address these concerns. The long-term goals of this project were to:

(1)   Develop a methodology for addressing and prioritizing neurotechnology-related ELSI for the purposes of informing and supporting sound public policy;

(2)   Test the reproducibility of the analysis of ELSI in a wide variety of settings and audiences to produce comparable data sets of well-organized public moral discourse on specific ELSI regarding the development, research, and/or use of neurotechnology;

(3)   Build these data sets so that they can be studied to identify a nexus of public moral consensus and points where consensus has yet to emerge for purposes of guiding policy formulation.

This workshop, and others planned in the series, as well as the conjoined efforts of the Decade of the Mind Project, and associated Neuroethics, Legal, and Social Issues (NELSI) initiative, are aimed at creating venues for elucidating and analyzing evidence- and safety-gaps, guiding research, and informing public policy, guidelines, and federal regulations that can be employed and continuously adapted for the future, as neuroscience evolves and new neurotechnologies are created.

DEVELOPING A FRAMEWORK

To move forward in developing a framework, several critical questions will need to be addressed. Who will develop and use such a process? What technologies or components of use will the process address? How will the framework be structured so that it can evolve in parallel with both scientific and technological advancements? The CNS-sponsored workshop sought to generate at least initial responses to these questions, and attempted to devise an analytic methodology that could sort ELS issues on the basis of identifying points of consensus and potential dissention. In this way, the critical components needed to sustain an authentic dialectic focussed upon neurotechnology-related ELSI became evident. Thus, while this workshop can be seen as an overview of the state of several neurotechnologies, their potential impact(s), and the creation of a nascent ELSI analytic methodology, future discussion must delve more deeply into the uses and implications of specific, next-generation neurotechnologies, how the values and needs of particular user groups and stakeholders affect the scope and conduct of neurotechnology research, and how to ensure that neurotechnology is studied and implemented in ways that uphold ethical integrity and moral good.

If an initial goal for the workshop was to shape the debate on neurotechnology ELSI, a second was to convene a working group of scholars from varied backgrounds who were expert and interested in these issues, and who were sensitive to the concerns of all representatives, without alienating any individuals or groups. This organizational approach helped to develop useful discussion, and fostered a more dialectical interaction that focused upon six key tasks:

(1)   Development of common terminology and facilitation of multidisciplinary discussions among neurotechnology and ELSI researchers;

(2)   Identification of current and future challenges faced by neurotechnology developers, researchers, and clinicians;

(3)   Development of a set of best practices, and/ or recommendation of guidelines for the responsible development and appropriate use of neurotechnologies, if deemed appropriate;

(4)   Formulation of an algorithm for identifying, studying, and addressing existing theoretical, scientific, and technical challenges;

(5)   Planning for public education, communication, and involvement of selected future discussions; and

(6)   Development of a widely applicable, reproducible process for addressing ELSI in varied applications of neurotechnologies.

Piloted process 1: creating ELSI thought bank accounts

Figure 15.1 illustrates a potential mechanism proposed to elucidate and discuss ELSI issues as related to neurotechnology. The first step was to identify ELSI issues from the literature; the next was to identify a specific component of a neurotechnology or its application to examine. Then specific issues were categorized into ethical, legal, or social areas. From this point, a question was shaped with the intention of assessing consensus on an issue. We posit that this method could be used to collect data on ELSI, analyze opinions and values, and provide information to other working groups for subsequent discussion, evaluation, and action.

How do we build consensus?

Consensus: (Webster's Dictionary)
1. Majority of opinion
2. General agreement or concord; harmony

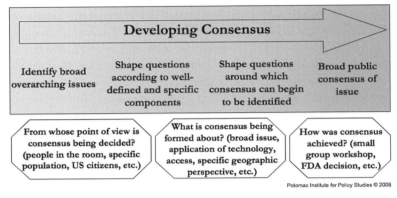

Figure 15.1 Framework for building public moral consensus.

In testing the proposed process, it was clear from the outset that it was first important to decide upon the particular neurotechnology to be evaluated. That is, although there were both generic and specific ELSI, only after deciding on a particular neurotechnology on which to focus can any group train useful attention and analysis on the relevant ELS issues.

List of neurotechnologies

The Working Group quickly generated a list of significant neurotechnologies, in order to select one for in-depth discussion and analysis of extant and potential ELS issues. The list of possible technologies to address included: brain–machine interfaces; memory alteration; neurotherapies/enhancement; neurogenetics; ``brain-reading´´ technologies (intended to include all brain imaging and other data collection tools, i.e. EEG, fMRI, fNIR, etc.); and transcranial magnetic stimulation/electrostimulation.

The neurotechnology for analysis

Neurogenetics was selected by general group agreement as a pilot topic because all participants had a basic familiarity with the topic, and this seemed to be relatively straightforward in the light of the existing body

Table 15.1 *List of ELSI to rank each neurotechnology*
Scoring scale: 1, least critical to discuss immediately; 5, most critical to address immediately.

ELSI	Technology X Score
Common definitions, lexicon, at the intersection of multiple disciplines	
Privacy	
Regulation/oversight	
Quality of data, techniques, interpretation, great variance; sound science is not being uniformly used or applied; accuracy of data	
Stereotyping, stigma, or discrimination based on neuroscience/use of neurotechnologies	
IRB process and concerns; research ethics	
Access; issues of justice, equity	
Consent: informed, voluntary	
Personhood	
Approved vs. off-label use	

of ELSI-related information pertaining to genetic research and therapies. The following examples illustrate potential neurogenetics ELS issues: (1) a certain genetic anomaly may prevent an individual from getting a job (because of a perceived link to neural function or behavior); and (2) genetic variation (e.g. in 5-HTTLPR, specifically, two copies of the short allele of the serotonin transporter) has been linked to predisposition and expression of certain mental disorder(s).

Ranking of ELS issues for selected neurotechnology

A ranking worksheet listing ten common ELSI for analysis was given to participants (see Table 15.1). ``Technology 1´´ was delineated as neurogenetics. ``Technology X´´ in the table above is a placeholder for whichever technology the group chooses to discuss; in this workshop, neurogenetics was selected.

Participants anonymously scored each ELS issue for neurogenetics. The scoring ranged from 1 to 5, 1 being least important to consider

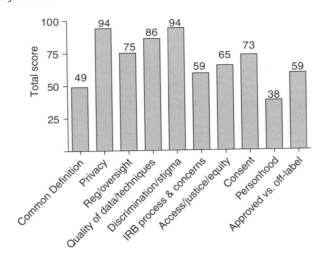

Figure 15.2 Breakdown of scoring of ELSI for neurogenetics.

immediately, and 5 being most important to consider immediately. The group recommended that these criteria be further refined and more precise definitions be formulated. These suggestions were subsequently addressed, and led to the development of a contingency quad chart (see Table 15.3).

Group responses to the first ranking exercise are shown in Figure 15.2. The issues with the highest scores were: (1) discrimination/stigma and (2) privacy, each receiving a total numerical score of 94 (22 responders). Quality of data/techniques received the next highest score of 86, followed by regulation and oversight (75) and consent (73). The group focussed upon the issue of discrimination/stigma, reasoning that in neurogenetics, privacy and discrimination are closely related and often reciprocal; any neurogenetic information could potentially lead to discrimination and stigma, and so privacy concerns would be paramount.

Categorization of discrimination/stigma ELSI related to neurogenetics

For the issue of discrimination/stigma related to neurogenetics, the group addressed specific ethical, legal, and social issues, making separate lists for each. It was recognized that many issues would tend to overlap in other areas (for example, an ethics issue would likely have some legal and social aspects), and therefore it might not be productive to try to separate ethical, legal, and social issues, as an agreement on the categorizations may never be fully be reached. However, it was

Table 15.2 *ELSI divided list for stigma and discrimination related to neurogenetics*

Technology 1: neurogenetics
Issue: stigma and discrimination

E, Ethics Issues (3rd)	L, Legal Issues (2nd)	S, Social Issues (1st)
Reproductive genetics	Invasion of privacy	Eugenics: economic, political, financial, cultural
Autonomy: individual vs. communitarian (i.e. military applications)	Evidence admissibility of science	Shame
Selfness	Legal culpability	Insurance
Personhood (definition) Dignity	Legislation Surreptitious sampling (passive consent)	Employment Family relationships
Economics	EEOC, hiring discrimination	Social contacts
Distributive justice	Genotyping and sentencing	Genetic determinism
Compensatory justice	Inheritance, parental rights, retroactive responsibility	Prejudice/bias
Commutative justice (who gets what, on what basis)	Reproductive issues	Social misanthropy (e.g. phrenology)
Addiction/treatment	Mandated/ coerced testing licensing, hiring	Public health
Veracity/paternalism	Confidentiality	Responsibility
Personal responsibility	Gene laws (eugenics)	Education
Corporate and/or social responsibility	Workmen´s compensation, military	Self-fulfilling prophecy/behavior
Survival of society	Intellectual property	Media communication of science
Utilitarianism/social utility	Addiction/treatment	Identity: social, ethnic, national, cultural, and links to biology (genetic basis?) Birth rates

clear that the issues could be divided into respective primary categories, and later be cross-referenced. Table 15.2 presents the ethical,
legal, and/or social factors categorized as a discrimination/stigma issue
in the area of neurogenetics (NB: issues are listed in the order they
were generated; no horizontal relationship is implied).

Conclusions on piloted process 1

An important outcome of this exercise was the discussion of anonymity and its usefulness in analyzing neurotechnology-related ELS
issues. It was noted that anonymity in voting on these kinds of sensitive issues is critical to developing moral discourse at a depth of
analysis that will be truly meaningful to the development of optimal
public policy. The problems of power differentials within a discussion
group (e.g. dyads of employers and employees, or discussion groups
involving military personnel, where rank is a respected component of
group dynamics) along with standard discussion group dynamic pitfalls (e.g. group think), and the important symbolism of the privacy of
the ballot box, assure that participant opinions on the critical ELS
issues are represented as independently and faithfully as possible.
Feedback was that session participants agreed that anonymity was
important.

Despite the apparent efficacy of this process, it was still lacking a
solid methodological strategy. That is, a process needed to be devised
for answering the following criterion-setting questions.

(1)   What neurotechnologies most require analysis of relevant ELS
      issues?
(2)   How does a group/population/community select which neuro-
      technology upon which to focus?
(3)   Ought the focus for ELSI analysis be based on whether a par-
      ticular neurotechnology is already or soon to be available, or the
      putative impact that the neurotechnology in question is antici-
      pated to incur?

Piloted process 2: quad chart for classifying the immediacy and novelty of neurotechnologies

To evaluate the importance of a neurotechnology or its application,
and the immediacy required in addressing its related ELS issues, a
matrix was created that could be used to organize the ELSI, as seen in

Table 15.3 *Issue categorization: quad chart to delineate critical issues and their immediacy*

	New/ novel	Old/non-novel
Pressing	Brain implants for therapy	Neurogenetics: stigma/ discrimination
Not pressing	Brain implants for cognitive enhancement	Use of fMRI for research

Table 15.3. The classification schema was organized by factors of immediacy of concern, and novelty of the technology or its application, as presented below.

(1)   Classifications of novelty as: (A) a new technology or a novel use of an existing technology, versus (B) a technology or issue that is old, or a use that has long been approved.

(2)   Determinations of immediacy and impact: (A) a technology, application, or issue is pressing to address, versus (B) not pressing to address.

Each of these categories requires further clarification and delineation. It was suggested that both sets of criteria were contingent upon both a timeline of when a technology would emerge, and the impact it might be expected to have. These variables would not only assist classification, but would help to focus policymakers on those neuro-technologies that are most relevant and critical within a certain time frame.

New/novel/old: classifying the technology

This stratification identified technologies and related ELS issues that were immediately applicable or that represented near-future con-cerns. There was much debate about defining this category. It was suggested that novel/new versus old could be classified by deter-mining what type of neurotechnology is available, what technology will soon be developed, and when such progress will occur. In addition, it was noted that novel uses of old technologies, such as EEG, could raise new ELS issues. The novel/new vs. old classification should also assess any existing ELSI literature or guidelines that may exist for older technologies or applications, and identify how and why a novel technology would or would not be covered under any extant policy.

Pressing/not pressing: immediacy

Whether a particular technology or circumstance arising from the development or use of technology incurred rapid and/or large-scale impact and effects was considered to be the "pressing factor" with regard to the need for ELSI discussion. Accordingly the operational definition of the "pressing factor" (versus non-pressing factor) classification was suggested as:

(1) Any technology coming online in a 1–5 year time frame;

(2) A matter of urgent social importance that is time-critical;

(3) A disruptive technology for which no significant applicable legislation, regulation, guidelines, or model practices exist;

(4) Neurotechnologies that may result in expansive quantitative or qualitative changes in important domains of society (e.g. health, security, etc.);

(5) Time urgency and magnitude of potential benefits versus harms as regards the rapidity and number of persons potentially affected;

(6) The existence of, or potential for faulty practices, flaws in technologies and algorithms, etc., especially as relates to technologies that are in current clinical/research use, and the criticality of methods/approaches for accountability or responsibility for such issues.

Conclusions regarding piloted process 2: quad chart development

The resulting quad chart, as developed, could be used in a range of contexts to organize technologies, application areas, ELSI, and the immediacy with which these issues need to be addressed. Neuro-technology-related ELS issues may be specific to the quadrant in which a technology is conceptually situated. A classification process could list technologies and applications, and (1) identify whether a technology meets the new/old or pressing/non-pressing criteria, and then (2) prioritize the relevant ELSI within each quadrant. The new/novel/pressing categories should be considered first, as these are the temporal and magnitude domains in which issues for policy debate will most likely arise. It is critical that when employing this (type of) quad chart, users must (1) remain aware of the perspectives and values of information providers (i.e. agentic bias), and (2) substantiate categorizations and criteria organization with data and reasoning. This information will help to define and shape priorities and communicate how and why particular technologies and ELS issues are targeted, and in this way facilitate more accurate analysis, and better inform public discourse on these issues across diverse populations of users.

Lessons learned

Undeniably, developing a classification process for categorizing and ranking ELSI related to neurotechnologies and their applications will be critical for timeline generation of guidelines and policy formulation. However, this system must also incorporate some fluidity and flexibility. As science evolves, the critical ELS issues of neurotechnology research and use will advance; it is likely that this progress may proceed in unforeseen directions and generate unanticipated questions, problems and issues. In light of this, continued involvement of a working group will be necessary to allow iterative identification, interpretation, analysis, and potential resolution of these scenarios.

It must be emphasized that sound public policy cannot be developed without some form (and/or extent) of public moral consensus. Care must be taken to ensure that (1) consensus of whatever group of experts is discussing the issues should not be assumed to represent consensus among other groups, and (2) policy should not be solely based upon small group consensus. To facilitate time- and resource-conservative discussions between different groups, it might be appropriate to develop additional tools that could be used by different groups to enhance or sustain context- or concept-mapping, thereby making inter-group discourse somewhat easier and more transparent.

One of the conclusions drawn by the CNS working group was that two-part methodology (that first identifies ELSI, then engages an analytic algorithm similar to that characteristically used in bioethical case analyses) can be adapted and consistently applied when evaluating neurotechnology-related ELSI. The first phase is focal to the technology in question. The steps in this phase are (1) to identify what technologies are new and different, (2) identify those issues that can be resolved using existing frameworks, and (3) focus time and effort on the technologies and the specific ELS issues relevant to each particular neurotechnology that are truly new and challenging. This process can be integrated into use of the quad chart detailed above. There are some existing tools for dealing with these issues in frameworks developed for other technologies, such as genetics and nanotechnology (Collins *et al.* 1998; Mnyusiwalla *et al.* 2003). The second phase is focussed on evaluating the ELSI impact on various circumstances and agents. These steps include: (1) establishing the relevant facts of the science and circumstances of use and application; (2) identifying the agents/stakeholders involved; (3) defining relative values and perspectives of stakeholder groups; (4) identifying and evaluating evidence gaps; (5) proposing what actions could be implemented; and (6) using a dialectical approach to determine what actions should be implemented (and why and how). This two-phase process can be used to inform and formulate guidelines, codes of ethics, lists of best practices, policies, or regulations that will be useful in clinical, research, and public policy settings, and that can be applied to new technologies, across various populations.

Still, several fundamental concerns persist. The first is whether the timelines proposed for developing policies or guidelines to address neurotechnology-related ELSI considerations are reasonable (and prudent). For sure, there remains contention as to whether the field is ready for policy and/or regulatory development, or whether the field is already tardy in formulating guidelines and policies for technologies that are already in use, and which may have broad social impact. We maintain that the answer to such questions is dependent on the specific neurotechnology or application. Specific sub-disciplines may not accept, or be prepared, for regulation; thus, the process must be based upon discussions within the field, and must occur through a capable understanding of both technical and ELSI perspectives (rather than being developed and imposed by some external governing body). The development and application of neurotechnologies in the academic, industrial, governmental, and public sector will raise distinct ELSI and may require different regulatory approaches. This prompts the question of the ``unique nature'' of neuroscience and neurotechnologies: is there something about research in areas of brain, mind, and self (or in technologies that interact with them) that makes these fields and applications qualitatively different than research, and use in other fields (and the regulations necessary to guide these endeavors)? As noted elsewhere in this volume, this is a point of some debate, but if it is indeed the case that this work sustains some fundamentally distinct import, then it may be that a unique type and area of policy formulation (i.e. ``neuropolicy´´) might be needed, and this too will require serious discussion and consensus.

OTHER EFFORTS

The CNS workshops are not the first effort to facilitate dialogue about the ethical, legal, and social issues arising from the field of neuroscience. In 2002 the Dana Foundation held a a now well-known conference, ``Neuroethics: Mapping the Field´´ (Marcus 2002), which essentially introduced the term to an American audience, defined what a neuroethics could and should seek to achieve, and provided a template upon which the current construct(s) of the field are based, at least in part. The American Academy for the Advancement of Sciences has also recognized this issue and in 2004 and 2005 held symposia on ``Neuroscience and Law´´ and ``Neuroethics and Religion´´, respectively. Several other meetings have occurred that have brought these concerns to a community of neuroscientists, psychologists, engineers, clinicians, ethicists, legal scholars, and representatives of specific social interests. For over 35 years the Society for Neuroscience has maintained a Social Issues Committee, and has recently incorporated bioethical issues into its mission statement. In response to this activity, a professional organization, The Neuroethics Society, was formed to formalize such a multidisciplinary dialogue. However, few of these efforts have focussed specifically on neurotechnology and the issues it could incur. Sandia National Laboratories has recognized this, and in response has developed ethical guidelines and surety methods for use in cognitive systems research and applications (Shaneyfelt 2006). This is an important step that needs to be expanded and diversified for other areas and contexts of neurotechnology research and use. In this light it is important that discussion regarding the ELSI unique to neurotechnologies occurs across a variety of institutions, professional societies, and publics on an international scale. Clearly the scope of neurotechnology effects will impact the world stage. For this reason, the discourse must entail global participation, and conjoin the international community as a viable forum (Illes *et al.* 2005).

MAPPING THE PATH FORWARD

Our hope is that the efforts and process discussed herein might provide framework for others to initiate similar discussion and analysis of ELSI related to the use of neurotechnologies. Such efforts are critical if neurotechnology is to be responsibly developed and used in ways that achieve social good and respect the concerns of public citizens and scientists. Furthermore, to be genuine in this pusuit, the dialog must directly involve stakeholders from both inside and outside the scientific community. Neurotechnology has the potential to impact daily activities, health and well-being, and national (if not global) security; such wide reach necessitates discussion that is broadly inclusive across groups, interests, publics, and nations.

If we are to responsibly develop best practices and a working ethics for neurotechnology, we must recognize a number of key tasks that lie ahead, including:

(1) Identification of all neurotechnologies, their applications, and use, and possible/potential future uses or applications;

(2) Formulating ways and means for keeping such a list current and sustainable;

(3) Developing common (``neurally relevant´´) vocabulary and definitions that will facilitate an interdisciplinary discussion;

(4) Developing and testing a process for analysis of neurotechnology-related ELSI, and creating key points of consensus in these regards;

(5) Determining what research needs to be done to inform and guide discussions regarding the existing and potential applications of neurotechnologies; and

(6) Defining what guidelines and/or policies may be needed, and how these can/should be developed within each user group (developer, researcher, clinician, etc.) to best address relevant stakeholder needs.

We believe that a strong educational infrastructure could facilitate discussion, understanding, and acceptance of neurotechnologies and related fields. Such broad-stance educational programs (ranging from formal education to specific types of public information and discourse) can be currently developed and implemented, employing tools and expertise gained from research to date. One critical facet of such educational enterprise is public outreach programs that can improve awareness and understanding of the uses of neurotechnologies, potential issues that may be raised, and how these might impact the social milieu. These types of public sessions could also be used to recruit participants for focus groups in which new issues are identified, and/or scientific perspectives are discussed with a lay audience. Undergraduate, graduate, professional, and continuing educational programs should entail sound analyses of neurotechnology and related ELSI in a well-rounded curriculum of not only science and technology, but also ethical, legal, and social foci; such programs would, by necessity and design, be both inter- and trans-disciplinary, and should seek to train individuals with diverse interests.

Finally, any hope of achieving acceptable regulation and oversight of neurotechnology is incontrovertibly reliant upon funding. Just as the Human Genome Project and the National Nanotechnology Initiative had financial support that was dedicated for ELSI research, it will be critical for federal, state, and even local government(s) (as well as private foundations) to devote funds to subsidize and sustain neurotechnology-focussed ELSI research. Legislation, termed the National Neurotechnology Initiative (NNTI), has been proposed to establish and support federal-level economic efforts, in coordination with the larger effort known as the Decade of the Mind (DoM) project. This latter endeavor seeks to generate up to US$4 billion in federal fiscal support for basic and applied studies of brain–mind function and consciousness, and the use(s) of neurotechnology in both research and practical applications (e.g. medicine, public safety, etc.). A major component of this legislation is that a portion of the funding will be allocated for the study of ELSI.

SUMMARY

A template and/or framework based upon the workshop described in this chapter could be used to organize, prioritize, and formalize a process to address neurotechnology ELSI, and build consensus about the most advantageous means to make safety, privacy, and health of the public an inherent property of all neurotechnological progress. Neurotechnology is already revolutionizing our understanding of the nervous system, and providing the ability to treat diseases with previously unimaginable efficacy. Moreover, the information and knowledge gained through the use of neurotechnology may revolutionize our understanding of what it means to be human and our relationship to the world around us, and could improve the quality of our lives. However, with every new technology and capability, and perhaps especially when considering the epistemic, ontological, and sociopolitical lability of our concepts of brain, mind, and self, there is a need to thoroughly consider the potential issues, unanticipated outcomes, and possible misuse(s) of these technologies and/or the information they deliver. Thus, it is important that there is a formalized dialog that evolves in parallel with neurotechnological progress, to address the opportunities, possibilities, and challenges such advancement will inevitably incur.

This chapter summarized the initial efforts undertaken by the Center for Neurotechnology Studies for beginning a dialog and attempting to formalize a process for future discussions regarding existing and emerging neurotechnologies and relevant ELSI. Forthcoming CNS-sponsored ELSI workshops will be aimed at continuing these discussions and refining the process with appropriate representatives from the public, private, and government sectors. It is hoped that this process will allow us to reap the benefits of neurotechnologies and provide safeguards for the researchers and public as new capabilities continue to emerge.

ACKNOWLEDGMENTS

The authors thank the participants in the workshop and those who provided inputs during the development of the framework, and hope that they will continue to participate in the process.

REFERENCES

Collins, F. S., Patrinos, A., Jordan, E. *et al.* 1998. New goals for the U.S. Human Genome Project: 1998–2003. *Science* **282**: 682–9.

Eaton, M. L. & Illes, J. 2007. Commercializing cognitive neurotechnology – the ethical terrain. *Nature Biotechnology* **25**: 393–7.

Illes, J., Blakemore, C., Hansson, M. G. *et al.* 2005. Science and society: international perspectives on engaging the public in neuroethics. *Nature Review Neuroscience* **6**: 977–82.

Illes, J., De Vries, R., Cho, M. K. & Schraedley-Desmond, P. 2006. ELSI priorities for brain imaging. *American Journal of Bioethics* **6**: W24–W31.

Joss, S. 1999. Public participation in science and technology policy- and decision-making – ephemeral phenomenon or lasting change? *Science and Public Policy* **26**: 290–3.

Marcus, S. J. (ed.) 2002. *Neuroethics: Mapping the Field.* San Francisco, CA: Dana Press.

Mnyusiwalla, A., Daar, A. & Singer, P. 2003. `Mind the gap´: science and ethics in nanotechnology. *Nanotechnology* **14**: R9–R13.

Nanoscale Science, Engineering and Technology Subcommittee (NSET) of the National Science, and Technology Council. 2007. *The National Nanotechnology Initiative: Strategic Plan December 2007.* Executive Office of the President. http://www.nano.gov/NNI_Strategic_Plan_2007.pdf. [Accessed June 12, 2008.]

Shaneyfelt, W. L. 2006. *Ethical Principles and Guidelines for the Development of Cognitive Systems.* SAND2006–0608. Albuquerque, NM: Sandia National Laboratories.

16

Globalization: pluralist concerns and contexts

Shaping international policy in neuroethics

R. H. BLANK

INTRODUCTION

This chapter shifts attention to the public policy context of neuroscience and examines the possibilities and problems inherent in attempts to shape an international policy agenda in neuroethics. The line between neuroethics and neuropolicy is a porous one and ultimately all of the most important neuroethics issues will find themselves embroiled in the policy arena. Like genetics and stem cell research, neuroscience promises to be a highly controversial political issue in and across countries. It, too, raises political and cultural red flags that arise whenever we deal with human cells, selves, and societal values. However, although the political ramifications of human genetic research have been well documented and widely analyzed over the past decade, and the social, legal, and ethical dimensions funded as part of the human genome project, there has been no methodical scrutiny given to neuroscience. In light of the rapid advances in our knowledge of the structure and functions of the central nervous system (CNS), it is timely to examine the impact of this new understanding and the vast array of applications that accompany it on human behavior, social institutions, and our perceptions of the human condition.

The array of techniques and strategies for intervention in and imaging of the brain are expanding rapidly and are certain to be joined in the future by even more remarkable capabilities. In addition to

Scientific and Philosophical Perspectives in Neuroethics, ed. J. J. Giordano & B. Gordijn. Published by Cambridge University Press. © Cambridge University Press 2010.

treating neural diseases and disorders, these innovations promise increasingly precise and effective means of predicting, modifying, and controlling behavior. Moreover, although advances in neuroscience and technology are impressive, much of the popular literature tends to over simplify and exaggerate the claims of presumed efficacy, thus heightening the fears of those persons who see it as a threat and creating unsubstantiated hope in those persons who expect to benefit from it. Although this helps to bring attention to neuroscience, it also intensifies the debate and hardens contrasting predispositions on what should be done.

As one of the most dynamic and consequential areas of biomedical research, neuroscience must be analyzed in a broader policy context. Research initiatives, individual use, and aggregate social consequences of unfolding knowledge about the brain and the accompanying applications require particularly close scrutiny because of the centrality of the brain itself to human behavior and thoughts. As one of the last frontiers of medicine, intervention in neuroscience has strong support because it promises benefits to many patients suffering from an array of behavioral, neurological, and mental disorders and injuries. Given the inevitability of expanded strategies for exploration and therapy of the brain, however, it is important that the policy issues surrounding their application be clarified and debated before such techniques fall into routine use.

Historically, experimental and clinical interventions in the brain have elicited controversy from many directions. Most illuminating are the issues surrounding past innovations of frontal lobotomies, electroshock therapy, and abuses of psychotropic drugs. Although new advances promise considerable benefits, such as genetic technologies, the transformation in neuroscience challenges social values concerning personal autonomy and rights and for some observers raises the specter of mind control and a *Clockwork Orange*-type society. Neuroscience represents an important new policy area that must be studied much like genetics, reproductive techniques, and organ transplantation. In fact, given its centrality to human existence, it is argued that neuroscience policy might well be considered a prototype for analysis of the social impacts of future biomedical intervention. As such, neuroscience policy and politics is a critical area of study for neuroscientists, social scientists, and ethicists.

This chapter first looks at the linkages between neuroethics and neuropolicy and overviews emerging policy issues. It then examines three policy dimensions relevant to neuroscience: research and development of the technologies; individual use of technologies; and the aggregate societal consequences of a technology. Next, it discusses the wide array of potential governmental involvement in neuroscience and presents the range of opinions regarding such options. Following this, the policy process is examined with emphasis on the agenda-setting stage and on the role of experts. Finally, using the emergence of gen-ethics as comparison, the chapter concludes by analyzing the potential for establishing an international neuroethics policy. It argues that divergent value systems, pluralist social structures, and cultural differences not often appreciated by western ethics are powerful impediments to the development of an international consensus on neuroethics and neuropolicy.

NEUROETHICS AND NEUROPOLICY

Roskies makes an important distinction in delineating two main divisions of neuroethics: the *ethics of neuroscience* and the *neuroscience of ethics* (Roskies 2002). In turn, the ethics of neuroscience comprises (1) the ethical issues raised in the course of designing and executing neuroscientific studies (*the ethics of practice*) and (2) the evaluation of the ethical and social impact that the results of those studies might have on existing social, ethical, and legal structures (*the ethical implications of neuroscience*). The second major division for Roskies is the *neuroscience of ethics*. Traditional ethical theory has centered on philosophical notions such as free will, self-control, personal identity, and intention, which can now can be investigated from the perspective of brain function through imaging studies (Roskies 2002). While the *ethics of neuroscience* has clear public policy implications, the *neuroscience of ethics* is likely to remain the domain of philosophers and academicians for some time to come. See, for example, Farah (2005) and Illes and Bird (2006). Attention here, therefore, is focussed on the former category where neuroethics most evidently intersects with public policy.

The move of neuroethics to policy domain alters the context by bringing to the forefront political considerations and divisions. In most countries, this risks placing the resolution of these issues in the milieu of interest group politics. With the high economic, social, and personal stakes surrounding neuroscience, this is unavoidable. Moreover, because neuroethics is laden with moral overtones that defy easy resolution, although ad hoc working rules might be developed, achieving consensus and building policy is considerably more problematic than other policy areas (Bonnicksen 1992). The issues raised in neuroethics are reflected in the almost daily announcements of new findings in neuroscience and related scientific fields and in the development of innovative technological applications. Intervention in the brain is a particularly controversial policy area because of the rapid succession of advances in knowledge and the shortened lead time between basic research and application. As noted by Hyman, the potential use of brain imaging ``to reconstruct a person's recent experience or investigate his or her veracity'' not only raises traditional bioethical questions of privacy but also engages broader communities who are not often represented in discussions of bioethics (Hyman 2007).

POLICY ISSUES OF BRAIN INTERVENTION

With our every intervention and every observation in every human brain, we face a multitude of ethical issues. Even electroconvulsive therapy, used more or less successfully since the 1930s, is still ``one of the most controversial treatments in medicine'' (Carney & Geddes 2003). The reasons are familiar. Less widely appreciated, though, is how easily traditional topics in clinical and research ethics merge into new topics in political ethics and, therefore, policy. The following are but a sample of the many issues that broach both ethics and policy.

First, however conscientiously elicited, consent is unlikely to be informed fully for any first intervention and may be less competently offered, albeit better ``informed'', for subsequent interventions. Consent is a concern prior to any medical procedure, but consent in this case has to come from the very organ that needs evaluation, assistance, or repair or that presents itself, once or repeatedly, for experimentation. On the one hand, the question arises as to whether fully informed consent is possible; on the other, paternalistic imputation of consent may seem sufficiently sensible to weaken safeguards and trigger fears of potential abuse.

Second, while often a fine one in medicine generally, the line dividing experimentation and therapy disappears here in the sense that each person's brain is unique in ways affecting identity, memories, judgments, and preferences. As the brain defines the person, even minor alterations might shade a definition of self or, more observably, an assessment of character. Moreover, the complexity of the human brain assures side effects that can never be fully predictable. As in other areas of medicine there has been a tendency to move quickly from experimental to therapeutic status in developing these innovations. Although this is understandable given the vulnerability of patients who normally undergo these techniques, their very vulnerability warrants a cautious approach.

This concern over risks and uncertainties is especially critical when the techniques themselves are used in non-medical, commercial settings. Caution is especially vital when an intervention is irreversible, as is the case of psychosurgery, but caution is also important when short- or long-term consequences may be too subtle to notice, too idiosyncratic to define, or too safely within the range of normal to be called adverse. Concern is deepened when treating behavioral disorders without clear organic origin or when modifying questionably disordered behaviors troublesome principally to families, societies, governments, or insurers.

Third, any form of intrusion in the brain conjures the image of mind control, unsettling assumptions of individual responsibility and widening the scope of culpability. In parallel fashion, the incremental elucidation of neurological factors in human behaviors, especially aberrant behaviors, may greatly complicate moral, civil, and jurisprudential argument (Spence *et al.* 2002; Gazzaniga 2005).

Fourth, to whatever extent judgments of character are supplanted by judgments of genetics or neurons, stigmatization will adapt, moving from an evaluative realm in which intuition serves imperfectly to one in which it serves only to harm. People with mental disorders are treated differently from those with somatic diseases; discrimination against the mentally ill, including discrimination in budgeting for their care, is widespread even among the well-meaning. In a coming era of neuroscience insight, such discrimination might lessen in old ways while worsening in new ones, the balance of the two trends being hard to predict. The potential to pigeonhole and discriminate on the basis of test results could lead to negative consequences, including the development of a ``neuroscientific underclass´´ denied access to societal benefits on the basis of their neuroscience test results (Garland 2004).

Fifth, intervention in the brain raises questions of distributive justice, mainly involving access to services, many of which are costly and are likely to become even more so. Although resource allocation questions, to date, have been rare in neuroethics discussions, they are critical because, whereas resources are finite, demands and expectations fueled by new technologies have few bounds. It might be premature to speculate about the relative costs and benefits of yet undeveloped procedures, but it is logical to assume that cumulatively their cost will be high. As such, these interventions also raise questions as to who should have priority for use of these procedures, whether insurance companies must pay for what are at best experimental treatments, and to what extent a government can or should regulate their use. Will access be equitable and coverage universal, and, if so, how will it be funded? Or will it be available to the affluent, but largely denied to persons who lack sufficient resources?

This question of access becomes of critical importance when we move into an era in which endowment of social advantage becomes possible through enhancement of brain function (Wolpe 2003). Could such endowment ever be fair if not available on an equitable basis? Here the comments of Mehlman and Botkin regarding genetic technology are highly relevant. They make a persuasive case that access to the benefits of these technologies is bound to be inequitable, particularly in the US, because the traditional market-oriented, third-party payer system leaves out many people (Mehlman & Botkin 1998).

Sixth, and more broadly, what priority should the search for knowledge about the brain and ever expanding uses of this knowledge have vis-à-vis other strategies and health care areas? What benefits will it hold for the population as a whole, compared with other spending options? Over the past several decades, there has been a proclivity to develop and widely diffuse expensive curative techniques without first critically assessing their overall contribution to health outcomes. In contrast, the availability of effective and inexpensive imaging tests could provide valuable information for disease prevention and health promotion by targeting individuals who are at heightened risk for diseases that could be reduced by early intervention. What priority should these interventions have, particularly when used to treat behavioral problems?

Any of the aforementioned issues may be accompanied by others peculiar to specific applications. Examples are numerous, their settings various. Drugs used to treat attention-deficit hyperactivity disorder (ADHD) are widely thought to be over-used in children and may be surprisingly risky, even when indicated, in adults. Despite their ubiquity, or perhaps because of it, drugs used to treat mood disorders are highly controversial especially when prescribed to children (Perring 1997; President's Council 2003). Likewise, the profusion of imaging techniques for research on human behavior has recast a perennial clinical epistemological problem: the incidental finding linked in published research to a behavioral tendency out of character, literally, with the individual under examination (Illes *et al.* 2004).

The policy implications of the new neuroscience, then, are expansive and touch upon most areas of the human existence. Because of the availability of sensitive knowledge about the brains of individuals that accompanies diffusion of the applications outlined here, major issues will center on what type of information should be collected and what to do with it once we have it. Because of the issues inherent in brain intervention (consent, stigmatization, privacy, autonomy, and so forth), these techniques also should be scrutinized as to their impact on the basic democratic concepts of freedom and equality. "Researchers are delving into the most intimate details of who we are, including such things as our personality traits, moral reasoning and tendency to violence. While their aims are commendable, many of their results raise big questions" (Editorial 2004).

One set of concerns centers on the commercial uses of cognitive neuroscience. Relatively innocuous applications of brain imaging such as the rapidly growing area of neuromarketing strike many observers as dangerous (Singer 2004). Other even more contentious commercial applications such as lie detection (Wolpe *et al.* 2005) are already with us and there most likely will be pressures to utilize brain scans as a screening device for job and school applicants and other non-medical uses in the near future. Phillips (2004) is particularly concerned with the potential use of brain scans to make predictions about a behavior or illness: "who might be a paedophile (sic), who might be violent, who might develop a mental illness or prion disease . . . ?" Like knowledge of human genetics, neuroscience is a double-edged sword.

Complicating the problem of how we handle our new knowledge of the brain is a tendency to exaggerate the significance of this research. In most imaging studies even the statistically significant differences in brain structure and function are often very subtle and limited, but extrapolation is alluring and commonplace in media headlines because its subject (the human brain and behavior) is so important and innately dramatic. However, as Garland (2004, p.1) suitably warns: "the use of flawed or incomplete science, or the reliance on scientific predictions beyond what the science is prepared to support, are exactly the kinds of concerns that should be foremost in the public mind when contemplating the potential impact of predictive technologies or techniques".

POLICY DIMENSIONS OF NEUROSCIENCE

Although many of the specific issues raised by neuroscience applications are unique, fundamentally the policy dimensions are similar to other areas of biomedical research. At their base, there are three policy dimensions relevant to neuroscience. First, decisions must be made concerning the research and development of the technologies. Because a considerable proportion of neuroscience research is funded either directly or indirectly with public funds, it is important that public input be included at this stage. The growing prominence given forecasting and assessing the social as well as technical consequences of biomedical technologies early in their research and development represents one means of incorporating broader public interests. One problem is how to best design assessment processes so as to evaluate efficacy, long- and short-term safety, and social impact of neuroscience. The need for anticipatory policy making is crucial here but, until now, largely absent.

The second policy dimension relates to the individual use of technologies once they are available. Although direct government intrusion into individual decision making in health care has, until recently, been limited, governments do have at their disposal an array of more or less explicit devices to encourage or discourage individual use. They include tax incentives, provision of free services, and education programs. Although conventional regulatory mechanisms may generally be effective in protecting potential users or targets of new neuroscience applications, it is critical that their effectiveness be assessed and they be modified accordingly. Neuroscience policy, like genetic policy, has distinctive importance in contemporary politics because it challenges intensely held societal values relating to the self, privacy, discovery, justice, health, and rights.

The third dimension of biomedical policy centers on the aggregate societal consequences of widespread application of a technology. For instance, how might using neural imaging to type personalities affect our concept of equality of opportunity or equality of respect between individuals? How might neural imaging techniques be used in employment and what social and economic impacts would this have? What impact would the diffusion of neural grafting have on the provision of health care? Policy-making here requires a clear conception of goals, extensive data to predict the consequences of each possible course of action, an accurate means of monitoring these consequences, and mechanisms to cope with the consequences if they are deemed undesirable. Moreover, the government has a responsibility of ensuring quality control standards and fair marketing practices.

As Figure 16.1 shows, the governmental response to neuroscience developments can take many forms. Moreover, governmental intervention can occur anytime from the earliest stages of research to

Ban or block technology	Regulate technology	Discourse individual use	Take no action	Encourage individual use	Mandate use of technology

Figure 16.1 Types of government involvement in neuroscience.

the application of specific techniques. Neuropolicy, then, can be permissive, affirmative, regulatory, or prohibitive. The government always has the option of taking no action, thus permitting any actions by the private sector. It can also make affirmative policies that promote or encourage certain activities, for example, government funding of research or provision of services to facilitate more widespread use of a particular technique or application. The question of whether the government ought to be providing such encouragement, and if so by what means, is a subject of debate. Should public funds be used to pay for expensive interventions when patients cannot afford them? Should private insurers be required by law to cover these expenses? Affirmative policies are often redistributive; thus there is potential conflict between the negative rights of individuals to use their resources as they see fit and the positive rights of recipients of government support who require it to maintain a decent level of existence. Also, in some instances, the line between encouraging and coercing or mandating use can be crossed.

Although regulatory policy can be framed to apply only to government-supported activities, it usually consists of sweeping rules governing all activities, both in the public and private sectors. Regulation can be used to ensure that standards of safety, efficacy, and liability are adhered to, and unlike professional association guidelines, which also set minimum standards, regulations have the force of law and usually include legal sanctions for violations. Martin and Ashcroft (2005) present useful distinctions regarding the regulation of neurotechnology. The **institutions** of regulation range from local ethics committees, to the courts, to sub-national and national bodies, both private and public. The **functions** of regulation can focus on safety, restriction of access to a specific class of users, deterring abuse or misuse, and so forth. The **impacts** of regulation can be desired and expected, desired and unexpected, undesired but expected, and undesired and unexpected. Importantly, they will affect different segments of society differently. The **subjects** of regulation focus on who is regulated and who is affected by such regulation; the **principles** of regulation relate to the extent to which regulatory policy is designed with specific moral or social principles of regulation in mind. Finally, there are various **styles of regulation:** centralist or democratic, formal or informal, egalitarian or libertarian in respect of distributive justice, libertarian or communitarian in respect of criminal justice, and so forth.

Lastly, although far less common than regulation, prohibitive policies can be implemented that reduce the options available in neuroscience applications. The most straightforward form is to create laws that impose criminal sanctions on a particular research activity such as human cloning or a specific application such as surrogate motherhood. Another type of prohibitive policy is to preclude public funding of specific areas of research and development (e.g. certain types of human fetal or embryo research). It remains to be seen whether any areas of neuroscience are candidates for prohibition, but governments do have that option. Such policies often reflect political motives or are a response to interest groups´ demands.

Figure 16.2 illustrates the range of policy options available. Many of these options have been used by various countries with regards either to stem cell research, reproductive technologies, genetic technologies or past brain interventions. They clearly demonstrate the wide divergence of policy responses available as well as the diametrically opposed positions on the role of the government that are found among various segments of society. Given the record in these related fields, there appears very little likelihood of anything approaching a consensus emerging either on the role of government in neuroscience or the preferred policies regarding specific applications.

SETTING A NEUROETHICS AGENDA

The difficulties of international neuropolicy making can be best understood if analyzed as part of the broader policy process that occurs in every country. There have been many useful analyses of this process by political scientists, most of whom devise a series of stages or types of action. For example, James Anderson views the process as consisting of five stages:

1. Problem identification and agenda setting
2. Policy formulation
3. Policy adoption
4. Policy implementation
5. Policy evaluation

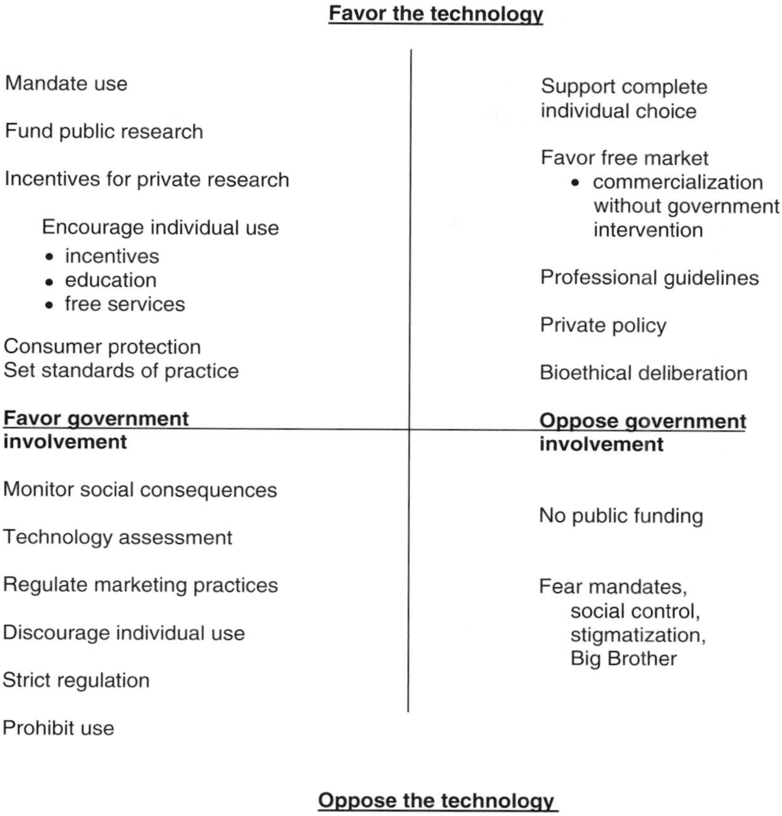

Favor the technology

Mandate use	Support complete individual choice
Fund public research	
	Favor free market
Incentives for private research	• commercialization without government intervention
Encourage individual use	
• incentives	
• education	Professional guidelines
• free services	
	Private policy
Consumer protection	
Set standards of practice	Bioethical deliberation
Favor government involvement	**Oppose government involvement**
Monitor social consequences	
	No public funding
Technology assessment	
Regulate marketing practices	Fear mandates, social control, stigmatization, Big Brother
Discourage individual use	
Strict regulation	
Prohibit use	

Oppose the technology

Figure 16.2 The role of government in neuroscience.

In the problem identification and agenda setting stage, an issue becomes a matter of public concern (Anderson 1990). Of the multitude of problems faced by society, only a small number receive public recognition, with even some issues that are salient matters of public debate failing to trigger governmental action. To explain why this happens, Cobb and Elder (1983) identify two agendas. The systemic agenda consists of ``all issues that are commonly perceived by members of the political community as meriting public attention and as involving matters within the legitimate jurisdiction of existing government authority''. In contrast, the institutional or formal agenda is ``that set of items explicitly up for active and serious consideration of authoritative decision makers''. The systemic agenda consists of general categories that define which legitimate priorities may be considered by government while the institutional agenda consists of those problems perceived by decision makers as warranting serious attention resulting in an effort to develop a course of action.

After an issue has been placed on the government´s formal agenda, policy formulation begins. This is a complex process involving a range of actors inside and outside government. Interest groups push for particular policies and attempt to influence priorities. Formulation usually includes analysis of various policy options, including inaction. Although policy adoption, which typically includes a legislative enactment or an executive directive, is usually the most salient stage of policy-making, policy formulation is the stage where the boundaries of government action are defined.

After a policy is adopted, the focus shifts to the executive branch, which is responsible for implementation. Agencies make rules (which explain how the legislation is to be applied), adjudicate (apply the rules to specific situations and settle disputes), use their discretion to enforce the rules and laws, and maintain program operations. Policy formulation, adoption, and implementation are often closely related, since the policy process is generally one of continual, incremental change.

Once a policy has been implemented, it is important to evaluate its impact. What change, if any, has taken place, and has that change been positive or negative? Evaluation consists of the comparison of the expected and the actual performance levels to determine whether the goals have been met. It is also the stage where the impact of new technologies on the existing policy can be assessed and adjustments in policy made to accommodate them. Are new policies needed or can existing policies simply be adapted? Anderson (1990, p. 223) makes a useful distinction between policy outputs, which ``are the things actually done by agencies in pursuance of policy decisions and statements´´, and policy outcomes, which ``are the consequences, for society, intended and unintended, that stem from governmental action or inaction´´.

To be effective, a neuropolicy must progress through all five stages. But the newness of many neuroscience issues means that most urgent attention must be focussed on the initial stage, agenda setting. Simply because an issue is a matter of public concern does not guarantee that policy makers will recognize it, consider it a legitimate priority, and put it on the formal agenda. There are a multitude of issues competing for placement on the formal agenda. Dorothy Nelkin (1977) points out that the policy importance of a technological innovation depends on both the degree to which it provokes a public response and how it is perceived by organized economic and political interests. Only those issues that are "commonly perceived by members of the political community as meriting public attention and involving matters within the legitimate jurisdiction of existing government authority" are placed on the systemic agenda (Cobb & Elder 1983, p. 85).

There is a vast literature on agenda setting that is relevant to getting neuroethics on the policy agenda of the various countries. Cobb *et al.* (1976) suggest there are four phases of agenda setting. Issues are initiated, their solutions are specified, support for the issue is expanded, and if successful, only then the issue enters the institutional agenda. Initiation can come either from the outside through non-governmental groups, mobilization by decision makers themselves, or from the inside by influential groups with special access. Cobb and Ross (1997) focus on agenda denial, that is, "the political process by which issues that one would expect to get meaningful consideration from the political institutions in a society fail to get taken seriously".

Most prominent in the field of agenda setting is the work of John Kingdon (1995), who stresses the importance of timing and suggests that moving an issue on to or higher up on the agenda involves three processes: problems, proposals, and politics. **Problems** refer to the process of persuading policy makers to pay attention to one problem over others. A problem's chances of rising on the agenda are heightened if it is perceived as serious by policy makers. **Proposals** refer to the process by which they are generated, debated, and adopted, and typically it takes patience, persistence, and a willingness to use many tactics by supporters. Framing a proposal in such a way that it is seen as technically feasible, compatible with policy maker values, reasonable in cost, and enjoying wide public support increases the chance of success. Finally, **politics** here refers to political factors that influence agendas, such as the political climate and the voices of advocacy or opposition groups. While these three elements operate independently, the actors can overlap. For Kingdon, successful agenda setting requires that at least two elements come together at a critical time, thus opening up a **policy window**. Policy windows, however, are not just chance opportunities; they also can be nurtured. Furthermore, under the right circumstances, they can be seized upon by key players in the political process to put an issue on the agenda (Kingdon 1995). Baumgartner and Jones (1991) argue that the image of the policy problem is crucial: "When they are portrayed as technical problems rather than as social questions, experts can dominate the decision-making process. When the ethical, social or political implications of such policies assume center stage, a much broader range of participants can suddenly become involved".

Agenda setting in federal systems like the US and Germany is complicated because policy-making can take place at the federal, state, and local level, with multiple agendas existing in various institutions at each level. A particular problem might be perceived and acted on by decision makers in one institution at one level of government in one state but not be perceived at all, or be perceived differently, in others. Developments that would cause a particular issue to be placed on the government agenda, such as technological change, interest group demands, or a widely publicized event, might take place only in certain geographical areas. In contrast, in highly centralized unitary systems like Britain and New Zealand, movement to the national agenda can be more rapid when the conditions are favorable (Timmermans 2001).

A complicating factor for neuroethics is the continual interaction among the myriad professional associations, business enterprises, and individual practitioners in the private sector which are active participants in neuroscience and can thus influence neuropolicy. The agendas of the wide range of institutions and organizations in the public and private sectors may be in parallel or even overlap. The mass media can also play a significant role in getting issues recognized by policy makers and, under the right circumstances, be decisive in pressuring them to act quickly in response to a perceived ``crisis''.

Although attention here focusses on public policy-making, Bonnicksen (1992) presents a private-sector policy model that defines ``regularized rules and procedures in the medical setting as the desired end of decision-making''. She favors increased emphasis on this model because she believes that governmental action has been ``unlikely, premature, and unwise'' in many areas of biomedicine.

> Private policies have weaknesses, but these can be partly remedied by political strategies. Public policies, in contrast, are difficult to refine or revamp if found to be erroneous or misguided. Traditional values of self-determination are perhaps more easily protected in the medical than in the political setting. At the very least, a private policy alternative warrants consideration for contentious biomedical issues.
>
> Bonnicksen 1992, p. 55

It is argued here, however, that although it remains important that private-sector solutions be pursued, the wide scope of issues emerging from neuroscience and their broad implications for many societal groups make them a matter of public concern and, thus, public policy.

It warrants caution to those who are in a rush to see public action regarding neuroethics issues that policy design is principally an incremental process not manifested in quick, decisive action. The emergence of neuropolicy, like the genetic and reproductive policy that preceded it, is most likely to come in fits and starts in a fragmented, unsystematic manner. Most policy analysts now agree that policy-making is not the textbook rational process, but at best an incremental one where, among other constraints, analysis is limited to a small number of alternatives at best; the emphasis is on ills to be remedied rather than positive goals to be met; and any analysis of the long-term consequences is sparse. Moreover, under the incremental model, new policies do not usually vary substantially from past decisions, meaning that novel areas like neuroethics have a difficult time penetrating the process inertia. Policy as a product of bargaining, compromise, and accommodation favors status quo both because standard bureaucratic operating procedures tend to promote continuation of existing practices and because decision makers avoid even considering choices that vary significantly from existing practices for fear they would make agreement difficult. Therefore, while genetic and reproductive issues have been on national and international policy agendas for several decades, they remain at best patchwork and often unsettled even among developed western countries. Although scientific knowledge in the genetic and reproductive areas spread fast across the international scientific community, considerable policy disparities remain in these countries, and only a handful have anything approaching a comprehensive policy.

ROLE OF EXPERT INPUT

Governments have at their disposal many mechanisms for facilitating expert input, although they usually function only after an issue is already on the political radar scope. Permanent mechanisms include the use of internal bureaucratic expertise, science advisors, offices of science and technology, and science advisory councils; while temporary mechanisms include task forces, ad hoc committees, commissions, consultants, conferences, hearings, issues papers, and white papers, among others. These mechanisms can be specific to a particular application of neuroscience, wider in scope across the range of policy implications flowing from it, or, as illustrated by the President's Council on Bioethics in the US, cover a wide swathe of bioethics issues.

Although neuroscience issues, cumulatively, might be termed neuroethics, they are in fact social issues of considerable policy importance. For this reason, they also epitomize very sensitive political issues, thus demonstrating the difficulty of creating dispassionate panels of diversely trained individuals at the national, much less the international level. There is an unstated assumption among some ethicists that consensus can be reached on broad principles within which the specific issues can then be resolved. However, in multicultural societies with sensitivity to diversity, this kind of consensus seems unlikely. Therefore, although it might be tempting to call for national (or international) neuroethics advisory bodies, there are pitfalls to centralization where a capture by political interests might be accompanied by the capture by a small cadre of experts who are presumed to speak for a more diverse community of persons with valuable expertise and experience who are, deliberately or not, left out of the influence loop.

The strength of the current informal and decentralized system of neuroethics (as illustrated by the proceedings of the major meetings so far held on this topic under the auspices of the Dana Foundation, the Wellcome Trust, and others; the Asilomar meeting; as well as special issues of the *American Journal of Bioethics*, the *Journal of Medical Ethics, Nature Reviews Neuroscience*, and so forth), is that it does allow for a broad airing of ideas, including those that might be ignored or minimized in a more centralized forum. If policy makers in a country create a national neuroethics advisory body, for instance, they might well view it as *the* authoritative voice of neuroethics. There is little evidence in the short history of bioethics to inspire confidence that a national commission or analogous body would deal more effectively with the issues of neuroscience than the current decentralized approach. Moreover, how can such a body be guaranteed sufficient autonomy to insulate it from political pressures, both in defining its mandate and agenda and presenting its outcomes? Moreover, as evidenced from many bioethicists' responses to the President's Council on Bioethics, one must question how enthusiastically its findings would be received even by the broader neuroethics community.

Although international organizations often contribute to the debate over regulation of new technologies or deal with the problems these innovations raise through reports, conferences, conventions, and opinions, there is little evidence they commonly have decisive influence on policy-making at the national level. For instance, Bleiklie *et al.* conclude that with ``respect to the supranational level, there has been little pressure from the European Union and international organizations for unifying policies'' on regulating reproductive technologies (Bleiklie *et al.* 2003). Moreover, while countries often study how the issues have been dealt with in other countries, again there is little evidence they rush to adopt policies already in place elsewhere. Lesson drawing is of limited explanatory relevance in policy design though it might have influence at the agenda-setting stage.

In recent years, there has been considerable theorizing over the concept of policy convergence which contends that as countries industrialize they will converge towards the same policy mix (Bennett 1992). For instance, some policy scholars argue that there are global trends in the formation of health policies, and that the objectives and activities of health systems internationally are becoming more alike (Chernichovsky 1995; Field 1999). Convergence is further bolstered by globalization and by the development of an international health forum through the Internet where people from all countries can comparison shop (Stone 1999). In addition, explicit efforts by international organizations such as the OECD, WHO, and the EU help prepare the foundation for what Harrison *et al.* (2002) refer to as ``ideational convergence''. Convergence is intuitively attractive because similar problems potentially make for similar solutions. This assumption is also supported by the fact that ultimately there are only a limited number of policy instruments available to address a particular policy problem.

On the other hand, critics of convergence theories argue that it oversimplifies the process of development and underestimates significant divergence across countries (Howlett & Ramish 1995; Pollitt 2002). Convergence, they argue, downplays the importance of country-specific factors other than economic development. Moreover, a cross-national study of the health systems of nine developed nations found some convergence of ideas but considerable variation in policy (Blank & Burau 2007). While health care goals and priorities demonstrate convergence in some areas, by and large countries continue to adopt diverse and often culture-bound strategies to deal with the similar problems facing them.

Even in the area of bioethics per se there continues to be wide divergence across countries. As noted by Darryl Macer and others,[1] bioethics has had a distinct western bias and focusses on concepts that may have little relevance to other countries. Three-quarters of the world's population is not linked to concepts assumed by the conventional western bioethics community as critical in medicine. Illes, Blakemore and associates (2005) well summarize the recent expansion of interest in and activities surrounding neuroethics in a variety of countries. With few exceptions, however, activity is most pronounced

---

[1] See the *Eubios Journal of Asian and International Bioethics*, published by the Eubios Ethics Institute, Christchurch, New Zealand.

in western countries. Only in Japan among the Asian countries has there been notice of the ethical considerations of neuroscience and even there it has been muted (Fukushi *et al.* 2007).

Similarly, in a study of 12 countries regarding end of life decision making, Blank and Merrick (2004) found that concepts of brain death, advance directives, and the withholding of life support technologies have little relevance in most less developed countries. For example, in some African and Asian cultures advance directives are viewed as inviting death and in most poor countries the notion of passive euthanasia is meaningless since there are no technologies to withhold or withdraw. Similarly, a recent comparative study of reproduction-assisting technologies in the US and European countries found wide variation in policy response in terms of both access and autonomy (Bleiklie *et al.* 2003). Moreover, in many countries, even the presence of these issues on the public agenda has lagged, and in some cases they are considered taboo subjects. Despite globalization and other forces that promote convergence of policies, cultural and other country-specific variables are quite persistent and resistant to technological change. Cultural and religious differences are of a magnitude often not appreciated by western bioethicists and will be powerful impediments to development of an international consensus on neuroethics and neuropolicy.

LESSONS FROM GENETHICS AND GENETIC POLICY

Because of the large overlap between the two fields, those scholars advocating an international neuroethics might learn from the experience of genethics. Despite its solid grounding in ELSI and wide visibility, debate continues over whether the establishment of genethics is advisable. While Suzuki and Knudtson (1989) and others were arguing for a genethics to deal with the problems raised by the new genetics in the early 1990s, Maddox (1993) downplayed the notion that the sequencing of the genome and related developments in molecular biology created ethical problems that are intrinsically unique: "this new knowledge has not created novel ethical problems, only ethical simplifications". Macer (1993), in a follow-up letter in *Nature*, agreed that there is no inherent value clash between genetics and human values as some would like to have us believe. He argued that the concept of genethics "should be stopped" and that what instead is needed is "a revival and renewed discussion of ethical values as society interacts with technology, and reassurance that scientists are responsible. ...". Society, then, does not need a new ethics to cope with the impact of genetic technology.

On the broader level, one criticism of genetic policy-making is that it has been largely reactive in scope, offering little in the way of anticipatory solutions. Although national commissions or similar bodies have studied these issues and made recommendations in many countries and the ELSI program has produced innumerable academic studies, most governments have either chosen to take an affirmative stance (often based purely on economic grounds) through funding genome research and encouraging diagnostic and therapeutic applications, or attempted to avoid the issues. Furthermore, genethics has been criticized as the almost exclusive domain of ethicists and journalists, who in some cases make little effort to communicate with the genetic science and research community and often take a combative stance on the issues (Maddox 1993). As a result, the broader public is often left on the sidelines. Although enlightened public debate over goals and priorities related to the issues is warranted, it can be argued that genethics has not gone beyond providing a framework for action by clarifying the ethical and moral issues surrounding the science and technology of genetics. While this might be a start, Knoppers (2000) sees the ``general failure to develop and include the ethics of public interest, public health, and the notion of civic participation in genetic research for the welfare of the community or for the advancement of science˝ as discouraging.

CONCLUSIONS

Since the May 2002 conference on neuroethics in San Francisco a few short years ago, neuroethics has made swift and impressive progress in achieving a high visibility in the neuroscience and bioethics communities through symposia, forums and workshops, newsletters, articles, and books, all of which are well documented elsewhere (Farah 2005; Illes & Bird 2006; Illes *et al.* 2005). This solid base of activity, culminating in the creation of the Neuroethics Society in Asilomar in May 2006, bodes well for building an international presence. Despite this auspicious start, however, the task of putting neuroethics on national and international policy agendas will proceed considerably more slowly. As demonstrated here, potential roadblocks to building an international neuroethics policy include the vagaries of entering the policy realm, where things proceed at a much slower pace, and the many social, cultural, and religious dimensions of neuroscience issues, which undermine efforts at consensus building. Heterogeneous value systems, pluralist societal structures, and the polyglot ethics of the global community combine to make it very unlikely that an international neuropolicy agenda will evolve. This, however, does not mean that the current efforts and activities are for naught, only that much more of the same is needed.

The emerging attention given to neuroscience has raised awareness of its importance to all aspects of human life, but it has not yet placed it high on the policy agenda even within the health care arena. Given the vastness of neuroscience ramifications for society, however, this will change. The political debate surrounding the emerging knowledge about the brain and new intervention techniques promises to be intense. The wide array of new intervention capacities and the tremendous costs of CNS-related health care problems, along with the emergence of the view of inseparability of the mental and physical dimensions of health, will demand considerably more attention by policy makers in the coming decades. This analysis, if anything, demonstrates the pressing need for more systematic, anticipatory analysis of the social consequences of the rapid diffusion of these impressive, often dramatic, innovations. This requires a broadening of the scope of neuroethics to include policy analysts and social scientists as well as continued efforts to raise a heightened awareness of its ramifications among attentive publics and opinion leaders.

REFERENCES

Anderson, J. E. 1990. *Public Policy-Making: An Introduction*. Boston, MA: Houghton Mifflin.

Baumgartner, F. R. & Jones, B. D. 1991. Agenda dynamics and policy subsystems. *Journal of Politics* **53**: 1047.

Bennett, C. J. 1992. What is policy convergence and what causes it? *British Journal of Political Science* **21**(2): 215–33.

Blank, R. H. & Burau, V. 2007. *Comparative Health Policy*, 2nd edn. Basingstoke: Palgrave.

Blank, R. H. & Merrick, J. C. (eds.) 2004. *End of Life Decision Making: A Comparative Study*. Cambridge, MA: MIT Press.

Bleiklie, I., Goggin, M. L. & Rothmayr, C. (eds.) 2003. *Comparative Biomedical Policy: Governing Assisted Reproductive Technologies*. London: Routledge Press.

Bonnicksen, A. L. 1992. Human embryos and genetic testing: a private policy model. *Politics and the Life Sciences* **11**(1): 53–62.

Carney, S. & Geddes, J. 2003. Electroconvulsive therapy. *British Medical Journal* **326**: 43.

Chernichovsky, D. 1995. Health system reforms in industrialized democracies: an emerging paradigm. *The Milbank Quarterly* **73**(3): 339–56.

Cobb, R. W. & Elder, C. D. 1983. *Participation in American Politics: Dynamics of Agenda-Building*, 2nd edn. Baltimore, MD: Johns Hopkins University Press.

Cobb, R. W. & Ross, M. H. 1997. *Cultural Strategies of Agenda Denial*. Lawrence, KS: University Press of Kansas.

Cobb, R. W., Ross, J.-K. & Ross, M. H. 1976. Agenda building as a comparative political process. *American Political Science Review* **70**(1): 126–38.

Editorial. 2004. Misplaced faith in 'Mind Reading' scans is sure route to injustice. *New Scientist* 31 July: 3.

Farah, M. J. 2005. Neuroethics: the practical and the philosophical. *Trends in Cognitive Sciences* **9**(1): 34–40.

Field, M. G. 1999. Comparative health systems and the convergence hypothesis: the dialectics of universalism and particularism. In F. D. Powell & A. F. Wessen (eds.) *Health Care Systems in Transition: An International Perspective*. Sage: Thousand Oaks.

Fukushi, T., Sakura, O. & Koizumi, H. 2007. Ethical considerations of neuroscience research: the perspectives on neuroethics in Japan. *Neuroscience Research* **57**: 10–16.

Garland, B. 2004. Neuroscience and the law. *Professional Ethics Report* **17**(1): 1–3.

Gazzaniga, M. S. 2005. *The Ethical Brain*. New York: Dana Press.

Harrison, S., Moran, M. & Wood, B. 2002. Policy emergence and policy convergence: the case of 'Scientific-Bureaucratic Medicine' in the United States and United Kingdom. *British Journal of Politics and International Relations* **4**(1): 1–24.

Howlett, M. & Ramish, M. 1995. *Studying Public Policy: Policy Cycles and Policy Subsystems*. New York: Oxford University Press.

Hyman, S. E. 2007. Neuroethics: at age 5, the field continues to evolve. The Dana Foundation, www.dana.org.

Illes, J., Blakemore, C., Hansson, M. G. *et al.* 2005. International perspectives on engaging the public in neuroethics. *Nature Reviews Neuroscience* **6**: 977–81.

Illes, J., Rosen, A. C., Huang, L. *et al.* (2004). Ethical consideration of incidental findings on adult brain MRI in research. *Neurology* **62**: 888–90.

Illes, J. & Bird, S. J. 2006. Neuroethics: a modern context for ethics in neuroscience. *Trends in Neurosciences* **30**(10): 1–7.

Kingdon, J. W. 1995. *Agendas, Alternatives, and Public Policies*, 2nd edn. New York: Longman.

Knoppers, B. M. 2000. From medical ethics to 'Genethics.' *Lancet* **356**: s38.

Macer, D. 1993. No to 'Genethics'. *Nature* **365** (9 September): 102.

Maddox, J. 1993. New genetics means no ethics. *Nature* **364**(8 July): 97.

Martin, P. & Ashcroft, R. 2005. Background paper prepared for the 2005 Wellcome Trust Summer School on 'Neuroethics'.

Mehlman, M. J. & Botkin, J. R. 1998. *Access to the Genome: The Challenge to Equality*. Washington, D.C.: Georgetown University Press.

Nelkin, D. 1977. Technology and public policy. In I. Spiegal-Rosing & D. DeSolla Price (eds.) *Science, Technology and Society*. Beverly Hills, CA: Sage.

Perring, C. 1997. Medicating children: the case of ritalin. *Bioethics* **11**(3–4): 228–40.

Phillips, H. 2004. Private thought, public property. *New Scientist* 31 July: 38–41.

Pollitt, C. 2002. Clarifying convergence. Striking similarities and durable differences in public management reform. *Public Management Review* **4**(1): 471–92.

President's Council on Bioethics. 2003. *Beyond Therapy: Biotechnology and the Pursuit of Happiness*. Washington, D.C.: Government Printing Office.

Roskies, A. 2002. Neuroethics for the New Millennium, Commentary. *Neuron* **35**: 21–3.

Singer, E. 2004. They know what you want. *New Scientist* 31 July: 36–7.

Spence, S. A., Hunter, M. D. & Harpin, G. 2002. Neuroscience and the will. *Current Opinion in Psychiatry* **15**(5): 519–26.

Stone, D. 1999. Learning lessons and transferring policy across time, space and disciplines. *Politics* **19**(1): 51–9.

Suzuki, D. & Knudtson, P. 1989. *Genethics: The Clash between the New Genetics and Human Values.* Cambridge, MA: Harvard University Press.

Timmermans, A. 2001. Arenas as institutional sites for policymaking: patterns and effects in comparative perspective. *Journal of Comparative Policy Analysis* **3**: 311–37.

Wolpe, P. R. 2003. Neuroethics of enhancement. *Brain and Cognition* **50**: 387–95.

Wolpe, P. R., Foster, K. R. & Langleben, D. D. 2005. Emerging neurotechnologies for lie-detection: promises and perils. *American Journal of Bioethics* **5**(2 March): 39–49.

17

The human condition and strivings to flourish

Treatments, enhancements, science, and society

A. GINI & J. J. GIORDANO

THE HUMAN CONDITION: STRIVINGS TO FLOURISH

From a naturalistic perspective, humans, like any species, are defined both by their biology and by how this biology has established certain capabilities and limitations. In inhabiting diverse environments, the human species has been forced to confront such limitations (of form and function), and develop resourcefulness to survive in the niche(s) we occupy. And, as in other species, our survival is dependent, at least in part, upon the ability to maximally adapt to, and/or compensate for, both biological and environmental constraint(s). Yet, as evidenced by history, human beings are achievers. This is shown by the artifacts of our existence: social structures, tools, and implements that represent a striving to overcome our (self-apparent and/or self-declared) frailties and shortcomings. In short, humans show a trend toward not merely surviving, but flourishing (Gow 2002).

We propose that one neuroanthropologic view of human history could depict a species specific tendency toward enhancing our function, so as to occupy and subordinate increasingly broader niche(s) (Havercamp & Reiss 2003). Thus, human history is punctuated by our attempts to break the bonds of biological restrictions, and ``be more than we are´´; our relative dependence has been overcome by forming sociocultural cooperatives, our fears appeased by myth and assuaged

Scientific and Philosophical Perspectives in Neuroethics, ed. J. J. Giordano & B. Gordijn. Published by Cambridge University Press. © Cambridge University Press 2010.

by knowledge, and our weakness(es) compensated by intellect and invention. In this way, we can (and perhaps should) view our history as defined by its artifacts of biology, society, and machination (BioSoMa), in interaction.

These developments have afforded some sense of protection against the impact(s) of the natural world (e.g. hunger, predation, disease, and death), and impart a utopian ideal of humanity. Yet, at the same time, each and all have dystopian potential, as initially unforeseen consequences become apparent and/or irreconcilable (Gordijn 2005). The extent, scope, and pace of such changes has become more broad and rapid, respectively, as a consequence of the (first and second) industrial revolution(s), the integration of chemistry and machinization into almost all phases of society, the nuclear age, and the advent of computational technology and biotechnology. In many ways, we strive to be more physically adept, cognitively capable, emotionally resilient, socially adroit, and resistant and/or recuperative to the ravages of disease, injury, time, and environment (Illich 1976).

It may be that the longing for (and attempts at) enhancement are, in fact, inherent in human nature (Caplan & McHugh 2004). We opine that this is so, and believe that, through ongoing interactions of genotype, phenotype, and environment, the human brain has developed to be intuitive and analytic, and that these qualities of human cognition compel the desire and need for ever-expanding capability (Deacon 1997), making progress something of a demiurge (Habermas 1970). To some extent, even what is accepted to be bona fide ``medical treatment´´ is, in reality, an enhancement of physiological capabilities, in compensation for (an actual or perceived) deficit in some aspect of function, adaption, and/or thriving. In this chapter, we argue that the treatment–enhancement debate is, at the core, reducible to an academic issue of semantics and/or taxonomy, in one way or another. In other words, treatment–enhancement distinctions are of a practical kind that are reliant upon definitions of normality, abnormality, disease, and illness, and in this way based at least partly upon social constructs that dictate what such terms ``mean´´, relative to the provision of certain resources as public good.

In light of this, any neuroethics – in the traditions of both the neuroscience of moral thought, and ethical analyses of neurological research and applications – must acknowledge the ``natural tendencies´´ to seek such enhancement(s), and thus be less concerned about the face value of treatment–enhancement distinctions, and somewhat more focussed upon (1) an understanding of the social values and contexts that define constructs of illness (as relates to psychiatric function in particular), (2) how such constructs give rise to legal and public issues and practices (inclusive of methods and allocation of treatment and justification of enhancement(s), and (3) the establishment of morally sound guidelines for, and reflective governance of, these intentions and practices. This is not to imply that social distinctions are moot, or not worthwhile. To the contrary; we opine that neuroethics entails a human ecology that reflects the interaction of embodied brain-minds that are embedded within sociotemporal environments.

Neuroethics is not divorced from social and legal issues; hence (neuroethical) discussion of what represents a treatment is contingent upon, and must be aware (if not critical) of, the contemporary qualification(s) of what constitutes ``normality´´. As these qualifications change over time and across culture, we believe that so too do distinctions of treatment(s) and enhancement(s). The pattern of acceptance, use, and utility are all woven into the social fabric and *Weltanschauung*. As Paul Root Wolpe has noted, the question at hand is not whether to draw the line, but ``. . . where, and what kind of line do we draw´´ (Wolpe 2008).

Therefore, we argue that any neuroethical consideration of treatment–enhancement (perhaps more intuitively called ``flourishing´´) must first and foremost relate to the epistemic and anthropologic domains of (a neuro)philosophy, to gain deeper appreciation for the nature of the human condition and what it ``means´´ to be human. Thus, this chapter operates from a basic premise: enhancement – in some form or another – is a basic human striving. From this point, we do not wish to belabor a discussion of neuropharmacologic or biotechnologic implementations and their possible use(s) in medical, social, military or even recreational settings. There are prodigious writings that address each and all of these issues elegantly, and in great detail. Perhaps we can offer little more to that discourse, other than the suggestion that any consideration of treatment or enhancement rests upon how we define disease. Given (1) the consilient focus of the Decade of the Mind project that attempts to reconcile neural, cognitive, and psychological studies, (2) the potential for reconciling neurology and psychiatry, (3) the relative ambiguity of neuropsychiatric disease classification, (4) development of new codification for the next edition of the Diagnostic and Statistical Manual (V) of the American Psychiatric Association, and (5) call for diagnostic criteria that could be relevant on a more international scale, we feel that a neuroethics of enhancement (and treatment) will need to embrace the tenuousness of social constructs, values, and implications.

TREATMENT OR ENHANCEMENT: ON COFFEE, CULTURE, AND SOCIAL CONVENTION(S)

Given the aforementioned premises, what could the tradition of coffee drinking teach us about neural treatment or enhancement? Dependent upon frame of reference, one could make the case that a cup of coffee and neuroenhancing agents (i.e. ``smart drugs``) may be either qualitatively different, or similar, as regards both specific effect(s) and more general social meaning. But how valid are such distinctions, or perhaps more accurately, how persistently valid will such distinctions continue to be as science advances, and social valuation(s) of scientifically relevant ``facts`` change?

In the first case, we can look to distinctions in pharmacologic structure, mechanisms of effect, side- and adverse-effect profiles, and even perhaps intent of development and/or use (so called ``on- or off-label`` utilization). Or perhaps we can claim difference because unlike many of the new(er) neuroenhancing (i.e. nootropic) agents and techniques, caffeine has a long history that provides some security by virtue (or illusion) of a ``folk empiricism`` (not unlike opium). Is our comfort with caffeine justified according to the ``Western medical dogma`` of believing that an agent exerts particular function(s) only when its mechanism is known and evidenced (Giordano *et al.* 2003)? This raises several interesting points, namely how much do we need to know before this comfort level is reached, what (levels of) information, knowledge, and evidence must be obtained, and how (and by whom) is this ``evidence`` judged? (Rosenberg & Donald 1995; Boswell & Giordano 2009; Giordano & Pedroni 2007)? Certainly, safety is a paramount factor, but this is operative in the evaluation of any product, technique or technology, and although we might weigh benefit, burden, and risk ratio(s) relative to the necessity versus (mere) desire for a particular agent, technique or technology, this alone does not explicitly support or sustain categorizations of treatment or enhancement.

In the second case, we must consider that many of these categories and premises are irrelevant to the criteria we employ to determine use and utility – there are a lot of things that are mechanistically different that produce similar or identical outcomes. Much social decision and action is dependent upon consequentialist goals; often it is only outcome(s) that are accorded, particularly if such outcomes achieve positive individual status within the social hierarchy (Pettit 1993; Baron 2006). At least as regards the use of pharmacological agents to facilitate ``flourishing``, it must be remembered that any drug can only augment or diminish the physiological activity inherent in the biological system (s) that it affects (Gilman *et al.* 1975). At least at this point in time, we cannot take a drug that makes us fly, extract oxygen from water, or photosynthesize. Moreover, our speed and efficiency of cognitive capacity can only be increased to a particular extent. Is it "wrong" or unethical to strive toward that limit? Is it wrong to pursue higher education, and earn multiple degrees, etc.? Whereas these pursuits might be regarded as "natural", the use of certain agents to achieve (or facilitate our striving toward) these goals could be seen as artificial. But if a cup of coffee makes us somewhat more energetic, alert, attentive, and perhaps engaging, is this not "artificial"? Is this "unethical"? And what if a person is socially uncomfortable, easily bored, or reads at a slow pace? If coffee mitigates these difficulties, is it a treatment or an enhancement?

Indubitably, coffee is routinely used as a nutriceutical, given that its active ingredient, caffeine, exerts predictable pharmacologic effect (s) (Nehlig *et al.* 1992; Fredholm 1995). So too do many nootropic drugs (Mondadori 1993). Can we discriminate a treatment or enhancement based upon a specific mechanism, or perhaps even the specificity (i.e. "cleanness") of effect, and if so, what criteria, and who decides? Maybe treatment–enhancement distinctions are dose-dependent. But given that new information on pharmacogenetic variability, the respective amplitude of effects, and left- or rightward shifts in individual dose-response profiles, are likely to differ, thus any dose-related categorization might still be relative and/or arbitrary (if not invalid) (Anderson 2005). Along these same lines, classification according to side- and/or adverse effect(s) profile(s) would also be seen as inappropriate, as these too are frequently dose-dependent (e.g. high-dose caffeine-induced arrhythmia and/or psychosis), and may individually vary (based upon pharmacogenetically different patterns of metabolism, excretion, and ligand–substrate interactions) (Spear *et al.* 2001).

To be sure, much has been written on the topic of psychological enhancement, and this discussion is indeed rich (Glannon 2006, 2008). Simply, we argue that intrinsic characteristics of a substance, technique, or technology are not sufficient to determine whether it is a treatment or an enhancement. Rather, such distinctions rest upon intent and use – is an agent intended to remedy and/or correct a clinically relevant flaw or dysfunction – and the definitions that underlie clinical criteria. Leon Kass has claimed that "... .therapy ... is the use of biotechnical power to treat individuals with known diseases, disabilities or impairments, in an attempt to restore ... normal health and fitness. Enhancement ... is the ... use of biotechnical power to alter, by direct intervention ... the `normal` workings of the human" (Kass 2003). Still, if we state that treatment represents amelioration toward a normalized baseline, whereas ``enhancement´´ is the betterment or augmentation of capability in the absence of dysfunction, what can be said about prophylaxis? How alert should one be before driving home late at night through pouring rain? What about before an important interview? And what of the naturalness of fatigue, or even cognitive capacity – by not accepting the ``fact´´ of one's physiological condition, are we not in some way seeking enhancement, even if such enhancement only elevates (i.e. ``returns´´) us to some arbitrary baseline level of performance or ability? Here an argument can be levied that such baselines have already been achieved and maintained, and a treatment re-establishes such normalcy of function or form. But what are we to make of the aging process? (Langreth 2002; Lane *et al.* 2004.) Is gonadal hormone replacement treatment or enhancement, given that the (implicit) goal is to retain or return some characteristic(s) of youth that (``natural´´) aging has altered or purloined? (Lyerly *et al.* 2001.) Are these justifications equally applicable for (1) men as well as women; (2) pharmacologic compensation for age-induced changes in other neuroendocrine systems, and according to what or whose criteria, and to what extent?

Although Kass's definitions could be regarded as valid, at least prima facie, he rightly notes – as do others – that face-value discriminations become problematic when applied to subjective states, and various cultural circumstances. In concordance, we believe that this begs the question of what is meant by normality, disease, and illness. There is an abundant literature addressing this topic that illustrates varying opinions, arguments, and a persistent lack of consensus (Sisti *et al.* 2004; Nordenfeldt 1995). Yet if we are going to attempt some operationally objective definition of treatment and enhancement, then some metric(s) of normality, abnormality, and the meaning of these terms and constructs is required. Given (1) the focus upon neuro-enhancement and (2) the use of the ``neuro´´ prefix to denote contexts relevant to brain structure and function (i.e. ``mind´´), then the discussion axiomatically engages the debate surrounding the nature of neuropsychological normality, disease, and illness.

NORMALITY, NORMS, AND NEUROETHICS

In this regard, we are confronted with the use of the medical model in psychiatry, and must therefore engage the controversy about what constitutes a psychiatric disorder. Cassell's definition of disease as an ``event of tissue(s)´´ and illness as the subjective experience of disease or disorder in an embodied patient is somewhat colloquial, but nevertheless important and erudite (Cassell 2004). But how do we genuinely evaluate psychiatric ``disease´´ (Sadler 2005; Haslam 2003)? Is it a process or a state (or both)? Are there absolute criteria that dictate what type and extent of variance from a functional norm is significant enough to uniformly compel and sustain nosology? Is there some durable ``disease reality´´ manifested at greater than two negative standard deviations from some mean? And what population(s) shall or should be used to identify the mean? Does current information about genomic and phenotypic variability sustain the use of broad-based population models?

And what of the experience of illness and pain? To date, universally objective measures of pain are lacking and subjective report remains the deciding variable in both assessment, and the nature and trajectory of intervention (see Chapter 8, this volume). How much – and in what dimensions and domains – must a person (or other organism, e.g. a racehorse) experience pain (discomfort or suffering) in order to reach a clinically relevant point at which treatment is appropriate? If a patient is suffering but does not meet this clinical criterion, do ministrations of comfort constitute enhancement? Of course, this then generates discussion about the relative meaning of pain, suffering, and fortitude versus the merit(s) of care, and opens the debate surrounding existential loss versus existential gain (Parens 2005).

But let us not forget that almost all of these criteria can change (e.g. socio-religious ideas about the virtues of suffering, and taxonomic variability of successive editions of the DSM). What core criteria validate disease? What if years of social discomfort are now diagnosed – under a new classification scheme – as ``social phobia´´? Of course, one of the prototypic examples of such changing criteria is that of ADD/ADHD in both children and adults (Tait 2005). This speaks to the need to work to establish normative, yet pragmatic standards for identifying the presence of (neuropsychiatric) diseases/disorders, as consistent with current epistemic models. Working in our group, Rachel Wurzman and Tejas Patil have focussed upon the hierarchical levels of dynamical neural networks that function non-linearly to adapt to various (internal and external) constraints and attractors (Giordano & Wurzman 2008a, b; Wurzman et al. 2008). Within this model, progressive loss of non-linearity (i.e. summative linearity) imparts dysfunction at successive tiers or levels in the networked hierarchy. The stability or instability of the system(s) is dependent upon ongoing genotypic, phenotypic, and environmental reciprocity, and is expressed as a spectrum of traits, functions/dysfunctions, and characteristics that may vary in extent, severity, and manifestation over time. This model reflects current understanding of neural systems (and the organisms in which these systems are embodied) as dynamic and complex (Kelso 1995). Of course, we recognize that this too may be a contingency that is based upon, and therefore reflective of, the contemporary scientific models that are *en vogue*.

But while we may seek an eidetic approach to, and norm(s) for, (neuropsychiatric) normality, abnormality, and disorder, such an eidos does not axiomatically define the threshold at which progressive linear disruption represents a clinically relevant (disease or illness) entity. Such clinical thresholds are decided by consensus, using aggregate statistics or descriptors of qualities that are indicative of dysfunction at a level that is quantifiably meaningful (Morris 2000). In other words, the threshold of normality and abnormality, disease and health, at some level, must be publically relevant. This establishes the point at which the responsibility to provide treatment becomes recognizable, compelling the obligation not to abandon those that are acknowledged as "more vulnerable" than others in the community (Kant 1998; Giordano 2006a). Yet, this too is speculative, and reflects the current *Zeitgeist* of medical morality and bioethics.[1]

Despite the investment in scientific research, it remains unclear whether we are committed to evaluate normality, abnormality, disease, and illness in these ways, or whether diagnostic approaches based

---

[1] Maturing from the Belmont Report, contemporary bioethics asserts a strong patient-centered stance. Obviously a number of ethical systems and theories can be employed to navigate the moral terrain of the clinician–patient relationship, and sustain the primacy of patients' best interests. Perhaps most well-known is the use of mid-level principles (i.e. beneficence, non-maleficence, justice, and respect for autonomy) as proposed by Tom Beauchamp and James Childress. The patient-centered focus of the principlist approach aligns an overarching maxim of non-harm with the good of upholding patient integrity and autonomy. Alfred Tauber has advocated an "other-based" approach that is reliant upon the philosophy of Levinas, and acknowledges intrinsic relational asymmetries imparted by patienthood (and is somewhat reflective of a Kantian orientation in this regard). Consideration for the marginalizing effect of disease and illness as a fundamental factor that instantiates the patient as the subject of the physician's moral responsibility is paramount to an ethics of care, as derived from feminist philosophy, and advocated by such scholars as Annette Baier, Donna Gillespie, and Margaret Little. Primacy of patients' best interest is also a central tenet of virtue ethics in medicine, perhaps most strongly advocated by Edmund Pellegrino and David Thomasma, who have called for a reconstitution of beneficence as a cardinal virtue in upholding the moral responsibility of physician to patient.

upon such models are too complicated, esoteric, and/or expensive to be of any practical use. In the absence of some objective scheme for discriminating these domains, are we prepared to judge whether something is a treatment or enhancement simply upon subjective grounds? Clearly, the libertarian movement has increasingly rejected state or medical parentalism, both in reaction to renown impropriety (e.g. state-run eugenics programs, etc.), and owing to anxieties about possible social inequity, and duplicitous governmental control of healthcare subsidies (Campbell 1995). The commercial impact and broad effect(s) of technology (most recently and notably of the Internet) have led to a decentralized model of medical resource provisions, in which direct access to goods and services is becoming *de rigueur* (Giordano & Neale 2007). This has generated a consumer culture, commoditized much of society including healthcare, and instantiated a market ethos in which personal agency is equated with autonomy, and autonomy is regarded as ``free choice'' (Giordano 2006b).

Thus, our concern is that any and all such substances, techniques and technologies, irrespective of distinction, will become easily available, seen as a public and individual ``right'', and such free choice will become the norm, owing to demand. To be sure, this could incur supply-side restriction (so as to preserve market values), which would lead to issues of distributive justice. To counter this possible scenario, guidelines and regulation(s) must be developed and imposed to prevent over-acquisition (i.e. ``demand frenzy''), and potential danger(s) of over- and/or inapt use. Obviously, this brings us back to the notion of establishing a clinical threshold, and the obligations to adhere, assess, and act responsibly to respond to such threshold criteria and their implications for the development, use, and provision of care (i.e. treatment) as public good (May 1975).

CONCLUSION

So, in sum, we see that the aforementioned criteria, while factual in their own right, can be selectively used or disavowed to support the postulated identities of what constitutes treatment or enhancement (and the undergirding concepts of normality, abnormality, disease, and illness). It is important to recall that such ``facts'' remain tentative, and contingent not only upon scientific knowledge, but also upon the social climate that dictates thresholds of practicality, utility, patterns, and boundaries of use. Ultimately, this reinforces the fiduciary of science and medicine to conduct research and practice(s) in ways that are technically right and morally sound, so as to avoid misinformation, misconception, and misuse. It may be that all treatments are forms of enhancement, and that all enhancements might be viewed as treatment – if only subjectively. Humanity seeks to flourish, and the status quo entails progress (Lenk 1973). Given the proposed relationship between the moral and therapeutic nature of medicine (Pellegrino 1987), and a regard for ethics as human ecology (Flanagan 2002), there are those that advocate that any attempts at cognitive augmentation must be accompanied by parallel devotion to moral enhancement (Persson & Savulescu 2008). Perhaps this is so; but we argue that such moral facility need not be dependent upon applications of some new drug or technology. Rather we hold that it arises as a function of human deliberation, reflection, and communication. The neuroethical goal is to adopt a discursive approach that not only works in the normative realm, but also translates into application through dialectic that is sensitive and responsive to the interactions of moral, legal, and social domains.

It may be that the problems we are trying to solve (through both neuroenhancement and treatments) are often ones we have created ourselves, through the artifacts of our biology, social institutions, use of technology, and pervasiveness of the market. In light of this, we posit that any comprehensive ethical approach to the treatment–enhancement issue cannot exclude equal consideration of the multiplicity of influences that shape society, and the operational definitions of normality, disease, and illness. A simple, somewhat intuitive reflection upon the analogy between a cup of coffee and a brain-enhancing drug or technology may take us closer to viewing the essence of human beings as complex, multidimensional, and relational creatures, whose needs and aspirations are difficult to satisfy because of an innate capacity for overcoming our limitations, continuous improvement, and facilitating social stature. Thus, authentic neuroethical analysis requires insight to the evolutionary neuroscience of the human brain, the anthropology and historicity of human nature, and regard for the interaction of these variables in creating, experiencing, and enacting the human condition. Without attention to these difficult factors and questions, any attempt at resolving the neuroenhancement debate will remain incomplete and unsatisfactory.

REFERENCES

Anderson, G. 2005. Sex and racial differences in pharmacological response: where is the evidence? Pharmacogenetics, pharmacokinetics, and pharmacodynamics. *Journal of Women's Health* **14**(1): 19–29.

Baron, J. 2006. *Against Bioethics*. Cambridge, MA: MIT Press.

Boswell, M. V. & Giordano, J. 2009. Evidence-based or evidence-biased: the need to re-appraise and re-align levels of information with stakeholder values. *Pain Physician* **12**: 9–12.

Campbell, A. 1995. *Health as Liberation. Cleveland, OH: Pilgrim Press.*

Caplan, A. L. & McHugh, P. R. 2004. Shall we enhance? A debate. *Cerebrum* **6**: 13–29.

Cassell, E. 2004. *The Nature of Suffering and the Goals of Medicine.* Oxford: Oxford University Press.

Deacon, T. 1997. *The Symbolic Species: The Co-Evolution of Language and the Brain.* New York, NY: WW Norton & Company.

Flanagan, O. 2002. *The Problem of the Soul: Two Visions of Mind and How to Reconcile Them.* New York, NY: Basic Books.

Fredholm, B. 1995. Adenosine, adenosine receptors and the actions of caffeine. *Pharmacology and Toxicology* **76**(2): 93–101.

Gilman, A., Goodman, L. & Gilman, A. 1975. *The Pharmacological Basis of Therapeutics.* New York: Macmillan.

Giordano, J. 2006a. The moral community of the clinical pain medicine encounter. *Practical Pain Management* **6**(5): 60–3.

Giordano, J. 2006b. Pain medicine, morality, and the marketplace: time for a change. *Practical Pain Management* **6**(1): 88–9.

Giordano, J. & Neale, A. 2007. Daniel Callahan redux – business and medicine, ``can this marriage work?´´ *Delaware Medical Journal* **79**(5): 185–7.

Giordano, J. & Pedroni, J. 2007. Pain research: the relationship of knowing and doing. *Practical Pain Management* **7**(5): 28–30.

Giordano, J. & Wurzman, R. 2008a. Neurological disease and depression: the possibility and plausibility of putative neuropsychiatric spectrum disorders. *Depression: Mind and Body* **4**(1): 2–5.

Giordano, J. & Wurzman, R. 2008b. Chronic pain and substance abuse: spectrum disorder and implications for ethical care. *Practical Pain Management* **8**(6): 53–8.

Giordano, J., Garcia, M. K., Boatwright, D. & Klein, K. 2003. Complementary and alternative medicine in mainstream public health: a role for research in fostering integration. *Journal of Alternative and Complementary Medicine* **9**(3): 441–5.

Glannon, W. 2006. *Bioethics and the Brain.* Oxford: Oxford University Press.

Glannon, W. 2008. Psychopharmacological enhancement. *Neuroethics* **1**(1): 45–54.

Gordijn, B. 2005. Nanoethics: From utopian dreams and apocalyptic nightmares towards a more balanced view. *Science and Engineering Ethics* **11**(4): 521–33.

Gow, D. 2002. Anthropology and development: evil twin or moral narrative? *Human Organization* **61**(4): 299–313.

Habermas, J. 1970. Technology and science as ideology. In J. J. Shapiro (transl.) *Toward a Rational Society.* Boston, MA: Beacon, pp. 81–122.

Haslam, N. 2003. Categorical versus dimensional models of mental disorder: the taxometric evidence. *Australian and New Zealand Journal of Psychiatry* **37**(6): 696–704.

Havercamp, S. & Reiss, S. 2003. A comprehensive assessment of human strivings: test-retest reliability and validity of the Reiss profile. *Journal of Personality Assessment* **81**(2): 123–32.

Illich, I. 1976. *Limits to Medicine: Medical Nemesis, the Expropriation of Health.* New York, NY: Marion Boyars Publishers.

Kant, I. (ed.) 1998. *Groundwork for the Metaphysics of Morals.* Cambridge: Cambridge University Press.

Kass, L. 2003. *Beyond Therapy: Biotechnology and the Pursuit of Happiness.* Washington, D.C.: President´s Council on Bioethics.

Kelso, J. 1995. *Dynamic Patterns: The Self-Organization of Brain and Behavior.* Cambridge, MA: MIT Press.

Lane, M., Ingram, D. & Roth, G. 2004. The serious search for an antiaging pill. *Scientific American* **14** (3): 36–41.

Langreth, R. 2002. Viagra for the brain. www. forbes.com/forbes/2002/0204/046. html

Lenk, H. 1973. *Technokratie als Ideologie: Sozialphilosophische Beitrage zu einem Politischen Dilemma.* Stuttgart: Kohlhammer.

Lyerly, A., Myers, E. & Faden, R. 2001. The ethics of aggregation and hormone replacement therapy. *Health Care Analysis* **9**(2): 187–211.

May, W. F. 1975. Code, covenant, contract, or philanthropy. *Hastings Center Report* **5**(6): 29–38.

Mondadori, C. 1993. The pharmacology of the nootropics; new insights and new questions. *Behavioral Brain Research* **59**(1–2): 1–9.

Morris, D. 2000. *Illness and Culture in the Postmodern Age.* Berkeley, CA: University of California Press.

Nehlig, A., Daval, J. & Debry, G. 1992. Caffeine and the central nervous system: mechanisms of action, biochemical, metabolic and psychostimulant effects. *Brain Research Review* **17**(2): 139–70.

Nordenfelt, L. 1995. *On the Nature of Health.* Dordrecht: Kluwer.

Parens, E. 2005. Authenticity and ambivalence: toward understanding the enhancement debate. *Hastings Center Report* **35**(3): 34–41.

Pellegrino, E. 1987. Toward a reconstruction of medical morality. *Journal of Medical Humanities* **8**(1): 7–18.

Persson, I. & Savulescu, J. 2008. The perils of cognitive enhancement and the urgent imperative to enhance the moral character of humanity. *Journal of Applied Philosophy* **25**(3): 162–77.

Pettit, P. 1993. *Consequentialism.* Hanover: Dartmouth Publishing Company.

Rosenberg, W. & Donald, A. 1995. Evidence based medicine: an approach to clinical problem-solving. *British Medical Journal* **310**: 1122–6.

Sadler, J. 2005. *Values and Psychiatric Diagnosis.* Oxford: Oxford University Press.

Sisti, D, Caplan, A. & McCartney, J. 2004. *Health, Disease, and Illness: Concepts in Medicine.* Washington, D.C.: Georgetown University Press.

Spear, B., Heath-Chiozzi, M. & Huff, J. 2001. Clinical application of pharmacogenetics. *Trends in Molecular Medicine* **7**(5): 201–4.

Tait, G. 2005. The ADHD debate and the philosophy of truth. *International Journal of Inclusive Education* **9**(1): 17–38.

Wolpe, P. 2008. Introductory remarks to the panel. *First Meeting of Neuroethics Society.* Washington, D.C.

Wurzman, R., Jonas, W. & Giordano, J. 2008. Pain and depression: potential and possibility for putative spectrum disorders. *Pain Practitioner* **17**(3).

18

The limits of neuro-talk

M. B. CRAWFORD

> If he be a man engaged in any important inquiry, he must have a method, and he will be under a strong and constant temptation to make a metaphysics out of his method, that is, to suppose the universe ultimately of such a sort that his method must be appropriate and successful.
>
> E. A. Burtt, *The Metaphysical Foundations of Modern Science* (1925)

In this nascent age of ``neurolaw´´, ``neuromarketing´´, ``neuropolicy´´, ``neuroethics´´, ``neurophilosophy´´, ``neuroeconomics´´, and even ``neurotheology´´, it becomes necessary to disentangle the science from the scientism. There is a host of cultural entrepreneurs currently grasping at various forms of authority through appropriations of neuroscience, presented to us in the corresponding dialects of neuro-talk. Such talk is often accompanied by a picture of a brain scan, that fast-acting solvent of critical faculties.

Elsewhere in this issue, O. Carter Snead offers a critique of the use of brain scans in the courtroom in which he alludes to, but ultimately brackets, questions about the scientific rigor of such use. For the sake of argument, he proceeds on the assumption that neuroimaging is competent to do what it is often claimed to do, namely, provide a picture of human cognition.

But there are some basic conceptual problems hovering about the interpretation of brain scans as pictures of mentation. In parsing these problems, it becomes apparent that the current ``neuro´´ enthusiasm

Matthew B. Crawford, ``The Limits of NeuroTalk´´, *The New Atlantis*, Number 19, Winter 2008, pp. 65–78. Reprinted with permission. For more information visit www.TheNewAtlantis.com.

Scientific and Philosophical Perspectives in Neuroethics, ed. J. J. Giordano & B. Gordijn. Published by Cambridge University Press. © Cambridge University Press 2010.

should be understood in the larger context of scientism, a pervasive cultural tendency with its own logic. A prominent feature of this logic is the over-extension of some mode of scientific explanation, or model, to domains in which it has little predictive or explanatory power. Such a lack of intrinsic fit is often no barrier to the model nonetheless achieving great authority in those domains, through a kind of histrionics. As Alasdair MacIntyre has shown in another context (that of social science), all that is required is a certain kind of performance by those who foist the model upon us, a dramatic *imitation* of explanatory competence that wows us and cows us with its self-confidence. At such junctures, the heckler performs an important public service.

TAXONOMIES OF MIND

As applied to medical diagnosis (for example, in diagnosing a brain tumor), a brain scan is similar in principle to a mammogram: it is a way of seeing inside the body. Its success at doing so is straightforward and indubitable. However, the use of neuroimaging in psychology is a fundamentally different kind of enterprise: it is a research method, the validity of which depends on a premise. That premise is that mental processes can be analyzed into separate and distinct faculties, components, or modules, and further that these modules are instantiated, or realized, in localized brain regions. Jerry Fodor, the Rutgers University philosopher of mind, begins his classic 1983 monograph *The Modularity of Mind* thus:

> Faculty psychology is getting to be respectable again after centuries of hanging around with phrenologists and other dubious types. By faculty psychology I mean, roughly, the view that many fundamentally different kinds of psychological mechanisms must be postulated in order to explain the facts of mental life. Faculty psychology takes seriously the apparent heterogeneity of the mental and is impressed by such prima facie differences as between, say, sensation and perception, volition and cognition, learning and remembering, or language and thought.

With its due regard for the heterogeneity of our mental experience, this modularity thesis is indeed attractive as a working hypothesis. The difficulty lies in arriving at a specific taxonomy of the mental. The list of faculties Fodor gives in the paragraph above could be replaced with an indefinite number of competing taxonomies – and indeed, Fodor gives a taxonomy of taxonomies. The discipline of psychology exhibits a lack of agreement on the most basic elements of the mental.

The problem of classifying the mental is one that infects the neuroimaging enterprise at its very roots. Some observers argue this problem is fatal to the interpretation of brain images as representing well-defined cognitive processes. One such critic is William Uttal, a psychologist at Arizona State University. In his 2001 book *The New Phrenology: The Limits of Localizing Cognitive Processes in the Brain*, Uttal shows that there has been no convergence of mental taxonomies over time, as one might expect in a mature science. ``Rather´´, he writes, ``a more or less expedient and highly transitory system of definitions has been developed in each generation as new phenomena are observed or hypothetical entities created´´.

Uttal suggests that the perennial need to divide psychology textbooks into topic chapters – ``pattern recognition´´, ``focal attention´´, ``visual memory´´, ``speech perception´´, and the like – has repeatedly induced an unwitting reification of such terms, whereby they come to be understood as separable, independent modules of mental function. The ad hoc origin of such mental modules subsides from the collective memory of investigators, who then set out to search for their specific loci in the brain.

Ideally, the phenomenological work of arriving at a taxonomy of the mental would be accomplished *prior* to the effort to tie mental functions to brain regions, because without such a taxonomy in hand, there is a real risk that arbitrary features of the imaging technology will yield artifacts that may then, like textbook categories, get reified as mental modules. Such artifacts are just the tip of a metaphysical iceberg of the sort Burtt warned of in the epigraph above.

Moreover, an even more fundamental problem haunts the modular theory of mind assumed in cognitive neuroscience: it may be that neither mental functions, nor the physical systems that realize them, are decomposable into independent modules. Uttal argues that rather than distinct *entities*, the various features of cognition are likely to be *properties* of a more general mental activity that is distributed throughout the brain. For example, is it possible neatly to distinguish perception from attention?

Uttal asks of attention,

> Is it a ``stuff´´ that can be divided, allocated, and focused and that is available only in limited amounts, and thus can be localized in a particular part of the brain? Or, to the contrary, is it an attribute or characteristic of perception … inseparable as the diameter or whiteness of a golf ball is from the physical ball itself ? … It seems plausible that many of the psychological components or modules we seek to locate in a

particular region of the brain should be thought of as properties of a
unified mental ``object'' rather than as analyzable and isolatable entities.

This argument is, perhaps, a bit tendentious – who in the neuroimaging
literature suggests attention is a ``stuff''? Rather, attention is thought to
be a *function* realized in some brain region. But this correction does not
vacate the force of Uttal's criticism, because functions, like properties, are
distributed (they require a whole system or mechanism to be realized),
and one must pause to ask: what are the boundaries of the pertinent
system? A danger inherent in the localization thesis may be illuminated
by analogy to an internal combustion engine. In describing an engine,
one might be tempted to say, ``the opening of the intake valve is caused by
the movement of the rocker arm''. Except that the rocker is, in turn, set in
motion by the camshaft, the camshaft by the crankshaft, the crank by a
connecting rod, the rod by the piston. But of course, the piston won't
move unless the intake valve opens to let the air–fuel mixture in. This
logic is finally circular because, really, it is the *entire* mechanism that
``causes'' the opening of the intake valve; any less holistic view truncates
the causal picture and issues in statements that are, at best, partially true.
Given that the human brain is more complexly interconnected than a
motor by untold orders of magnitude, it is a dubious undertaking to say
that any localized organic structure is the sufficient cause and exclusive
locus of something like ``reason'' or ``emotion''.

Such dichotomous mental categories are regularly employed by
social scientists who have taken up neuro-talk, and in the popular
press: the amygdala is said to be the seat of emotion, the prefrontal
cortex of reason. Yet when I become angry, for example, I generally do
so for a *reason*; typically I judge myself or another wronged. To cleanly
separate emotion from reason-giving makes a hash of human experience, and seems to be attractive mainly as a way of rendering the mind
methodologically tractable, even if at the cost of realism.

Such naïve psychological modularity can get installed in institutional practices that have real coercive power, such as lie detection.
There are now at least two companies, No Lie MRI, based in San Diego,
and Cephos, based in Boston, that are actively commercializing the
application of neuroimaging to lie detection. Margaret Talbot, writing
in *The New Yorker* in 2007, described the neuroimaging studies of
deception conducted by Daniel Langleben, a psychiatrist at the University of Pennsylvania, that undergird the claims of No Lie MRI:

> These allegedly seminal studies look exclusively at ... people who
> were instructed to lie about trivial matters in which they had little stake.

> An incentive of twenty dollars can hardly compare with, say, your
> freedom, reputation, children, or marriage – any or all of which might
> be at risk in an actual lie-detection scenario.

This is to treat lying as a ``cognitive´´ process in the narrowest sense, as
opposed to a mental act with inherent ethical content and pragmatic
consequences.

Here cognitive science reveals its roots in ``the linguistic turn´´ in
philosophy that began with the rise of logical positivism a century ago.
The logical positivists were preoccupied with consistency of sentences,
and conceived reason to be syntactical or rule-like. It is what computers
do. Such a view takes no account of what Henri Bergson called ``the
tension of consciousness´´, that feature of an embodied being who has
interests and finds himself situated in a *world*. Talbot nicely elaborates the
richness of the phenomena we gather under the term ``lie´´, and the
problem it poses for any narrowly cognitive scheme of lie detection:

> small, polite lies; big, brazen, self-aggrandizing lies; lies to protect or
> enchant our children; lies that we don´t really acknowledge to ourselves
> as lies; complicated alibis that we spend days rehearsing. Certainly, it´s
> hard to imagine that all these lies will bear the identical neural signature.
> In their degrees of sophistication and detail, their moral weight, their
> emotional valence, lies are as varied as the people who tell them. As
> Montaigne wrote, ``The reverse side of the truth has a hundred thousand
> shapes and no defined limits´´.

Trying to identify a universal, merely formal element of real-life lying
and disentangle it from emotional capacities, moral dispositions, and
worldly situations, on the supposition that the function ``lie´´ has its
own distinct ontology, may make as much sense as trying to separate
the whiteness of a golf ball from the ball, to use Uttal´s analogy. The
thesis of mental modularity seems to be attractive mainly because it is
convenient for talking about thinking and, as we shall see, for
designing experiments. But notice that it can also undergird technologies such as brain-scan lie detection that may come to have real
consequences in the world – affecting ``your freedom, reputation,
children, or marriage´´, as Talbot reminds us. Just because such technologies aren´t adequate to our mental reality doesn´t mean they won´t
be deployed; the checkered history of past lie-detection technologies
shows this. It is significant that No Lie MRI solicits inquiries from
corporate customers on its website. Even if the technology doesn´t pass
the bar of public trust for use by civil authorities, it may satisfy corporate managers looking for new ways to intimidate employees.

Those who would use science to solve real human problems often must first translate those human problems into narrowly technical problems, framed in terms of some theoretically tractable model and a corresponding method. Such tractability offers a collateral benefit: the intellectual pleasure that comes with constructing and tinkering with the model. But there is then an almost irresistible temptation to, as E. A. Burtt said, turn one's method into a metaphysics – that is, to suppose the world such that one's method is appropriate to it. When this procedure is applied to human beings, the inevitable result is that the human is defined downward. Thus, for example, thinking becomes ``information processing''. We are confronted with the striking reversal wherein cognitive science looks to the computer to understand what human thinking is.

DEEP PROBLEMS OF INSTRUMENTATION

If the critique of mental modularity is valid, how can one account for the fact that brain scans do, in fact, reveal well-defined areas that ``light up'' in response to various cognitive tasks? In the case of functional (as opposed to structural) neuroimaging, what you are seeing when you look at a brain scan is the result of a subtraction. Functional magnetic resonance imaging (fMRI), for example, produces a map of the rate of oxygen use in different parts of the brain, which stands as a measure of metabolic activity. Or rather, it depicts the *differential* rate of oxygen use: one first takes a baseline measurement in the control condition, then a second measurement while the subject is performing some cognitive task. The baseline measurement is then subtracted from the on-task measurement. The reasoning, seemingly plausible, is that whatever shows up in the subtraction represents the metabolic activity associated solely with the cognitive task in question.

One immediately obvious (but usually unremarked) problem is that this method eliminates from the picture the more massive fact, which is that the entire brain is active in both conditions. A false impression of neat functional localization is given by the presentation of differential brain scans which subtract out all the distributed functions. This subtractive method is ideally suited to the imaging technology, and deeply consistent with the modular theory of mind. But is this modular theory of mind perhaps attractive in part *because* it lends itself to the subtractive method?

In the late 1990s and early 2000s, some of the more critical cognitive neuroscientists complained that researchers were simply sticking people in the magnet to see what ``lights up´´, with no real theory in hand, and such studies would get published in prominent scientific journals. These critiques had some effect, and the discipline has mostly moved beyond looking for ``the spot for X´´. Indeed, cognitive neuroscientists deserve credit for the methodological finesse they have developed in response to the complexity of mind. In a 1999 article in *Behavioral and Brain Sciences*, Cambridge neuroscientist Friedemann Pulvermuller offered a thorough account of the difficulties that arise in the effort to localize linguistic functions. The problem with the subtractive method, he wrote, is that ``in many experiments there are [not one, but] several differences between critical and control conditions´´, on such dimensions as perception (a word is seen or not on a screen), attention, classification (the word may be a noun or verb or meaningless pseudo-word, for example), motor response (the subject may be required to hit a button as part of his or her response), search processes (the subject may need to recall the word), and semantic inferences. Given that ``an area is found to `light up´ ... it is not clear which of the many different cognitive processes relates to the difference in brain activity´´. Similarly, Michele T. Diaz and Gregory McCarthy write in the November 2007 issue of the *Journal of Cognitive Neuroscience* that ``the coactivation of cognitive processes unrelated to word processing *per se* ... likely influence[s] the pattern of activation obtained in even the simplest word processing tasks´´.

University of Chicago ``social neuroscientist´´ John T. Cacioppo and colleagues offered a philosophically sophisticated treatment of these methodological hazards of neuroimaging in a 2003 article in the *Journal of Personality and Social Psychology*. They describe as a ``category error´´ the

> intuitively appealing notion that the organization of cognitive phenomena maps in a 1:1 fashion into the organization of the underlying neural substrates. Memories, emotions, and beliefs, for instance, were each once thought to be localized in a single site in the brain. Current evidence, however, now suggests that most complex psychological or behavioral concepts do not map into a single center in the brain. What appears at one point in time to be a singular construct (e.g. memory), when examined in conjunction with evidence from the brain (e.g. lesions) reveals a more complex and interesting organization at both levels (e.g. declarative vs. procedural memory processes). Even if there is localization, it will likely be elusive until there are coherent links between psychological–behavioral constructs and neural operations.

As these articles indicate, the problem of distributed, mutually intertwined mental functions is very much at issue in the trenches of neuroscience, however much grand theorists may find it expedient to ignore such difficulties and insist, as Steven Pinker does in *How the Mind Works*, that ``the mind is organized into modules or mental organs, each with a specialized design that makes it an expert in one arena of interaction with the world''. Simplifications like this are not culturally innocent, as they provide the indispensable pretext for the grab at authority by entrepreneurs such as No Lie MRI, which in turn may come to justify the exercise of coercive power by civil authorities.

Perhaps the most fundamental limitation of functional imaging, vis-à-vis the claim that it allows us to ``peer inside the mind'', is that there is a basic disconnect of time scale. Brain scans are emphatically *not* images of cognition in process, as the neural activity of interest occurs on a time scale orders of magnitude faster than hemodynamic response (the proxy for neural activity measured by fMRI). Uttal writes,

> This raises, once again, a profoundly disconcerting problem for the users of imaging procedures: the cumulative measure of brain metabolism is neither theoretically nor empirically linked to the momentary details of the neural network at the micro level – the essential level of information processing that is really the psychoneural equivalent of mentation. From this point of view, the ``signs'' of brain activity obtained from the scanning system are no more ``codes'' of what is going on than any other physiological correlate, such as the electrodermal response or an electromyogram.

I take Uttal to mean that a brain image provided by fMRI may serve as a *sign* of mentation, but because of the time-scale difference, it does not preserve the machine states that (on the computational theory of mind) *encode* mentation. With such signs, we do not have a picture *of* a mechanism. We have a sign *that there is* a mechanism. But the discovery that there is a mechanism is no discovery at all, unless one was previously a dualist.

RESPECT THE MACHINE

But suppose imaging technology were one day to achieve both the spatial and temporal resolution to give us a precise picture, down to the neuronal level, of the physical correlates of mentation as it occurs. What then? To fully understand even a simple mechanism can be a surprisingly elusive undertaking, as is known by anyone who has – to use another engineering example – tried to set up a train of beveled gears that transmit a rotary motion through a right angle (as in the Ducati motorcycle engines of a few decades ago). In such a gear train there are forces acting in directions that do not correspond to any of the observed motions. There are thrust and side forces that are *intellectually* manageable (they can be expressed mathematically) but *practically* far from trivial. An experienced engine builder may require an entire day playing with shims and tolerances to get it right.

Though beveled gears are only barely more complex than the simple machines of Archimedes (the lever, the pulley, etc.), the human race had to await the genius of Leonardo to receive them, like some revelation. At a much higher level of sophistication, mechanisms can be intractably complex things – famously, the most subtle applications of science and engineering have as yet been unable to fully reproduce the prized characteristics of Stradivari's violins, for example. The human brain, everyone agrees, presents complexity that is simply colossal by comparison – by one estimate, the number of possible neuronal pathways is larger than the number of particles in the universe.

But for a certain kind of intellectual, the mere act of *positing* that some mystery has a mechanical basis gives satisfaction. A heady feeling of mastery rushes in prematurely with the idea that *in principle* nothing lies beyond our powers of comprehension. But to be knowable in principle is quite different from being known in fact. Hands-on mechanical experience frequently induces an experience of perplexity in formally trained engineers. We may be emboldened to speculate, in a sociological mode, whether a lack of such mechanical experience ``enables'' a certain intellectual comportment which doesn't give the machine its due, and isn't sufficiently impressed with this difference between the knowable and the known.

A species of metaphysical enthusiast can often be seen skipping gaily across this gap between the knowable and the known, acting in the capacity of publicist for some research program which, on cooler analysis, is seen to be in its infancy. One such is Paul Churchland of the University of California, San Diego, who writes in his 1995 book *The Engine of Reason, the Seat of the Soul* that ``we are now in a position to explain how our vivid sensory experience arises in the sensory cortex of our brains ... [and is] embodied in a vast chorus of neural activity.... [W]e can now understand how the infant brain slowly develops a framework of concepts ... and how the matured brain deploys that framework almost instantaneously: to recognize similarities, to grasp analogies, and to anticipate both the immediate and the distant future''. As Jerry Fodor succinctly put it in a review of Churchland's book, ``none of this is true''; it is ``the idiom of grant proposals''. The critical element of Churchland's hype lies in the distinction between knowing *that* ``our vivid sensory experience arises in the sensory cortex" and explaining *how* it does so, which latter, he claims, is now accomplished. We surely know *that* "the infant brain slowly develops a framework of concepts" and "the matured brain deploys that framework almost instantaneously", but *how*? Not even to a first glimmer, as Fodor says.

OF DOGS AND PROTONS

The conceit that brain scans present an image of human cognition laid out before us for full inspection holds obvious attraction. This positive appeal is backed up by a horror at what is thought to be the only alternative to a thoroughly reductive materialism: some form of spiritualism or, more broadly, something "anti-scientific".

But one must make a distinction between ontological reduction and explanatory reduction. This distinction is a commonplace in the philosophy of science, but it is routinely ignored in the hype surrounding cognitive neuroscience. The error goes like this: from the fact that some phenomenon is composed of and dependent upon more fundamental parts, it is thought to follow that any explanation of the higher-level phenomenon can be replaced by, or translated without residue into, an explanation at the lower level of its parts. Once this reduction is (putatively) accomplished, the ontological status of the higher-level phenomenon is demoted to that of *mere* phenomenon: appearance versus reality. Our gaze is shifted away from the thing we initially wanted to understand, to some underlying substrate. This procedure is thought to be enjoined by the conviction we all share with the natural scientist: there is only one universe, and it is made up of physical particles.

Yet the natural scientist knows just as surely that our best account of that universe is, in many cases, not forthcoming from physics. We turn instead to chemistry or biology. The need for such "special" sciences that take higher-level structures as given does not compromise the bedrock ontological supposition that there is a single universe, made up of physical particles. One can have one's materialism while admitting the autonomy of higher-level disciplines. There is much confusion on this point, and it seems to be bolstered by a fear that to be less than completely reductive in one's explanatory posture somehow commits one to "spiritualism".

The explanatory independence of biology, its irreducibility to physics, is consistent with biological entities being composed of and dependent upon physical entities. The biologist believes that the dog is made up of nothing but protons, neutrons, and electrons, but he does not try to give an account of the dog at that level. Is this merely due to the limitations of our current state of knowledge? Would it be possible *in principle* to construct a comprehensive understanding of the dog starting from particle physics? The consensus view appears to be that it is not possible even in principle, due to considerations of complexity and non-linearity, or thermodynamic irreversibility (take your pick). Even within physics, lower-level accounts sometimes presuppose structure that is identifiable only at a higher level, or depend upon boundary conditions that cannot be generated from within the lower-level account. Even something as simple as a volume of gas displays ``emergent properties″ (here, an irreversible tendency toward equilibrium) that cannot be derived from the collisions between individual gas molecules (which are symmetric with respect to time).

It seems to be not scientists, but rather publicists of science, who are haunted by a sense of metaphysical hazard when confronted with phenomena that can′t be fully understood reductively. But how sincere is this horror? Is it rather a pose struck by such publicists, a histrionic display intended to cow others into submission? ``You′re not a *dualist*, are you?″ For their part, many humanists aren′t sufficiently acquainted with the principles of scientific explanation to be able to see that this kind of bullying is fraudulent in its claim to speak for science, and end up feeling resentful towards science. This is bad for humanists, and bad for science.

THE HISTRIONICS OF THE NEURO-METAPHYSICIAN

A paper recently published in the *Journal of Cognitive Neuroscience*, of all places, shines a light on the magical, totemic effect of brain scans on those viewing them. The authors of ``The Seductive Allure of Neuroscience Explanations″, a team of Yale scholars, offered their subjects various explanations for certain psychological phenomena that are familiar to everyday experience. Some of these explanations were contrived to be pointedly *bad* explanations. Their subjects consisted of three groups: neuroscientists, neuroscience students, and lay adults. The study found that all three groups did well at identifying the bad explanations as bad, except when those explanations were preceded with the words, ``Brain scans indicate″. Then the students and lay adults tended to accept the bad explanation. A complementary set of experiments by David P. McCabe and Alan D. Castel, currently in press in the journal *Cognition*, found that ``readers infer more scientific value for articles including brain images than those that do not, regardless of whether the article included reasoning errors or not".

These findings suggest that we are culturally predisposed to surrender our own judgment in the face of brain scans. More generally, we defer to the mere *trappings* of "science". This ready alienation of judgment presents an opportunity for all manner of cultural entrepreneurs who seek, not quite authority over others, perhaps, but rather to be the oracular *source* of such authority, whether in law, policy, psychiatry, or management. There is no arguing with a picture of a brain. Further, there is a ready market for the explanations offered by such entrepreneurs. Among those charged with the administration of human beings, there is a great hunger for scientific-looking accounts that can justify their interventions, as the aura of science imparts legitimacy to their efforts.

For example, professors of public policy dream of being able to use brain scans to predict a propensity, not only for violence, but also for tendencies like racial bias, as Jeffrey Rosen reported in the *New York Times Magazine* in 2007. This would open a vista of social control previously only imagined, and expand the dominion of criminologists: if human behavior is electrochemically preordained, there remains no discernible ground on which to object to preemptive interventions directed against those identified as "hard-wired" malfeasants. Such interventions might take the form of surveillance, incarceration, or alteration (through drugs, surgery, or implants).

But neurolawyers and neurocriminologists are not exactly neuroscientists. The irony is that "we have no evidence whatsoever that activity in the brain is more predictive of things we care about in the courtroom than the behaviors that we correlate with brain function", according to Elizabeth Phelps, a cognitive neuroscientist at New York University, as quoted by Rosen. In other words, if you want to predict whether someone is going to break the law in the future, a picture of his brain is no better than a record of his past behavior. Indeed it is quite a bit worse, as the correlation of future behavior with brain abnormalities is weaker than it is with past behavior. Neuroscientist Michael Gazzaniga writes in his book *The Ethical Brain* that "most patients who suffer from ... lesions involving the inferior orbital frontal lobe do not exhibit antisocial behavior of the type that would be noticed by the law". It is merely that people with such lesions have a higher incidence of such behavior than those without. So for the pragmatic purpose of predicting behavior, the story of neurological *causation* that is told by pointing to an image of a brain merely adds a layer of metaphysics, gratuitously inserted between past behavior and future behavior despite its lack of predictive power.

Rosen quotes Paul Root Wolpe, a professor of social psychiatry and psychiatric ethics at the University of Pennsylvania, as saying, ``I work for NASA, and imagine how helpful it might be for NASA if it could scan your brain to discover whether you have a good enough spatial sense to be a pilot´´. But consider: NASA currently tests your spatial reasoning directly – the intellectual capacity itself, not a neurological *correlate* of it. This is done by putting you in a flight simulator and observing your performance in a pragmatic context similar to the one you would face as a pilot. But such a pragmatic orientation doesn´t offer the excitement that comes with accessing a hidden realm of causation.

It may be worth recounting an episode from the history of science when hidden causes similarly had people excited. In the seventeenth century, one of the grand problems of science was to explain why things fall down. Descartes had developed a strictly mechanical, billiard-ball model wherein imperceptible particles impinging from above push things downward. There were other, competing mechanical models. The problem was that no such mechanical picture could account for the findings of Galileo – namely, that bodies fall with a uniformly accelerated motion and the acceleration for all bodies is identical, regardless of size. This impasse surrounding what we now call gravity could be resolved by positing a force of attraction between bodies. Newton did just this, but in doing so he was attacked by the more doctrinaire ``mechanicists´´, for whom it was a matter of principle that there could be no action at a distance. Newton was accused of re-introducing scholastic ``occult qualities´´ into nature, precisely the kind of explanation that the mechanical philosophy set out to banish, just as the current reductionism in psychology wants to banish spooky notions like ``soul´´.

While the mechanical philosophy confidently posited hidden mechanisms, on the assumption that there must be some cause that is similar to the ones we can see operating in the world, Newton was content to leave causes mysterious. He then proceeded to give a mathematical *description* of how bodies move under the mysterious attractive force: the inverse square law of gravity. Accepting the obscurity of gravity´s causes seems to have freed Newton up to attend to the phenomena, and thus to accomplish his mathematization of the phenomena. The intransigently reductive position adopted by the mechanical philosophers was abandoned. It is worth noting that our understanding of gravity, though transformed by Einstein, remains agnostic on causes. Instead of spooky action at a distance, now we have even spookier distortions of space–time. Physicists seem to be less easily spooked than cognitive scientists.

THE AUTONOMY OF THE MENTAL

Where does this leave us? I would like to make the case for giving due deference to ordinary human experience as the proper guide for understanding human beings. Such deference may be contrasted with the field of ``neurophilosophy'' (most famously, the work of Paul and Patricia Churchland), which is intent on replacing ``folk terms'' – such as ``reflection'' and ``deliberation'' – with terms that describe brain states. Needless to say, brain states are objective facts, whereas our introspective experience of our own mental life is inherently subjective. But this divide between the objective and subjective, between the brain and the mind, does not map neatly onto cause and effect, nor onto any clear distinction between a layer of reality that is somehow more fundamental and one that is merely epiphenomenal. For example, if you are told your mother has died, your dismayed comprehension of the fact, which is a subjective mental event, will cause an objective physiological change in your brain.

In light of this causal power of the mental over the physical, we begin to wonder whether it is right to think of these two types of reality as layered, in the sense that one is more causally effective than the other. It would follow from this doubt that re-describing our introspective experience of our own mental life in terms of brain states is optional, in this sense: the choice of description ought to depend on what you're trying to explain. Each description answers to a different sort of ``explanatory request'', issuing from different realms of practice. The ``folk'' description answers to the realm of everyday human experience, and the brain description answers to the realm of physiological investigation.

To insist that the brain description is superior to the mental one in a more comprehensive way, such that it may subsume the mental one and render it obsolete, there must be points of contact where the two descriptions conflict, so the better one can show itself as superior. This is what happened when, for example, the Copernican theory prevailed over the preceding view that the earth is the center of the universe. The problem with the neurological re-description of our mental life would seem to be that there is no such contact, hence no competition. Hence there is no reason for preferring one over the other, on any grounds other than pragmatic ones. There is an explanatory gap between our knowledge of the brain and what we know first-hand of ourselves, and it is difficult to imagine what kind of finding would bridge the gap. That there should be a neurological basis for our mental life is not controversial. But that beginning insight also seems to exhaust the contribution of brain scans to our self-understanding.

Bracketing the questions of the mind–body problem is unsatisfying. But such a lack of metaphysical satisfaction may be something we need to live with. To do so is a form of sobriety, as against the zeal of those who rush off to reform law, public policy, and ethics as though these ultimate questions had been settled, and always in such a way as to overturn what we know first-hand of our own agency.

Afterword

WALTER GLANNON

The past twenty years have seen remarkable progress in theoretical and clinical neuroscience. Functional neuroimaging can display real-time activation in brain regions correlating with cognitive and affective processes. Brain scans have improved the diagnosis of a range of neurological and psychiatric disorders. They can also be used to monitor the progression of these disorders and the metabolic effects of drugs used to treat them. Psychopharmacology has developed generally safer and more effective therapeutic agents for diseases of the brain and mind. Some of these agents can be used to enhance normal cognitive functions. Electrical and magnetic stimulation of the brain can control symptoms of neurological and psychiatric disorders that have not responded to other treatments. Stem-cell-based neuro-transplantation in the field of restorative neurosurgery holds promise for reversing damage from neurodegenerative diseases, stroke, and spinal cord injury. Neural prostheses may enable people immobilized by paralysis to translate their intentions into actions. All of these measures and interventions in the brain have great potential to benefit a significant number of people, enabling them to become more independent and have better quality of life.

There is also a dark side to these drugs and techniques. Atypical antipsychotics can increase the risk of patients dying from sudden heart failure. Brain scans are visualizations of statistical analyses based on a large number of images and are inaccurately described as pictures of what actually occurs in the brain. There is considerable ambiguity in interpreting information from neuroimaging and the potential for bias and abuse that could lead to discrimination by insurers and employers.

Scientific and Philosophical Perspectives in Neuroethics, ed. J. J. Giordano & B. Gordijn. Published by Cambridge University Press. © Cambridge University Press 2010.

Images of the brain have a seductive allure that could unduly influence juries deciding cases in the criminal law. In these and other respects, imaging may threaten the privacy and confidentiality of information about our brains. Deep-brain stimulation may control motor symptoms of Parkinson's disease and affective symptoms of major depression but may have adverse effects on personality and other aspects of the psyche. Transplanting stem cells into neural networks might result in uncontrolled proliferation of growth factors that could damage healthy tissue beyond areas of the brain targeted for neuroregeneration. Researchers and clinicians developing and applying these techniques have to strike a delicate balance between maximizing benefit and minimizing harm.

On a more theoretical level, research in cognitive neuroscience has yielded important insights into the brain–mind relation. While this has resulted in a better understanding of the neurobiological underpinning of mentality, it also challenges our deep-seated convictions about free will, moral reasoning, and the self. As Neil Levy points out in the Preface, ``it is our minds that make us the individuals we are''. Yet if our minds are a function of our brains, then it appears that much of our thought and behavior occurs outside of our conscious control. This raises the question of how we can plausibly retain our practices of praising, blaming, and attributing responsibility if everything we think and do can be reduced to collections of neurons, synapses, and neurotransmitters. How genes are expressed in phenotypic traits is not a function of DNA sequences alone but the result of interaction among genes, human organisms, and the environment in which they are situated. We are not just our genes. But in the light of what neuroscience has revealed about the brain–mind relation, it seems that, in D. F. Swaab's words, ``we are our brains''.

There is, however, a normative as well as an empirical dimension of human thought and behavior. Although our desires, beliefs, emotions, and decisions depend on the brain, judgments about freedom and responsibility depend to a great extent on social expectations about how we can and should act. The reasons to which we appeal in claiming that we can or cannot act freely and responsibly are shaped by the social environment in which we live. These reasons need to be informed by our knowledge of how the brain generates and sustains the mind. But they are not just a function of neuroscience and thus cannot satisfactorily be discussed solely in neuroscientific terms.

In his critical survey of mental modularity in Chapter 18, Matthew Crawford notes that there is an explanatory gap between the knowledge *that* our experience is grounded in different regions of the brain and our explaining *how* or *why* our experience arises from brain processes. James Giordano's discussion of the phenomenology of pain and Ralph Ellis' discussion of the persistent "hard" problem of consciousness suggest that there is indeed such a gap. For some, this consideration alone may not be sufficient to completely neutralize the neuroscientific challenge to subjectivity and associated metaphysical and ethical convictions. Yet for others it may be enough to defuse the threat of neuroscience explaining away mentality as a mere epiphenomenon. It may be sufficient for us to retain our concepts of the will and the self and our normative practices and institutions. Nevertheless, this debate requires a model in which empirical claims about the brain and normative claims about the mind are not mutually exclusive but complementary. Dualism is not a tenable theory; nor is reductive materialism.

This complementarity can be achieved through interdisciplinary collaboration. Giordano cites C.P. Snow's famous discussion of the rift between the two cultures of the sciences and humanities and endorses E. O. Wilson's idea of consilience, which involves working across disciplines "to create a common groundwork for explanation". Despite claims underscoring the importance of collaborative work between scientists and humanists, the most productive work on the ethical and social implications of brain science has been between neuroscientists and social scientists. Thus far, humanists have played a comparatively minor role in this collective enterprise.

On at least two theoretical issues, neuroscientists and humanists have largely been talking past rather than engaging with each other. Many neuroscientists and cognitive psychologists claim that our knowledge of the brain implies that our belief in free will is an illusion (Wegner 2002; Greene & Cohen 2004; Farah 2005). In contrast, many philosophers who have discussed the brain–mind relation argue that any plausible concept of free will is compatible with neuroscience (Mele 2009). Relying on brain imaging and other empirical measures, neuroscientists and cognitive psychologists also claim that our knowledge of the brain challenges the view that we can give objective moral justification for actions in cases of moral conflict. Philosophers argue that brain imaging reflects only our *intuitive* judgments about these cases. It does not show that we cannot form reason-based *considered* judgments as part of moral justification (Singer 2005; Kamm 2007). In one brain imaging study, a majority of healthy volunteers believed that it would be permissible to redirect a runaway trolley from one track to another in order to save five people, even though this action would kill one person. They did not believe that it would be permissible to push an innocent bystander onto the track and thereby kill him in order to stop the trolley and save the five. The activation of brain regions mediating emotions presumably explained the different intuitions about the two scenarios (Greene & Haidt 2002). Yet appeal to intuitions alone will not explain why the first action but not the second is permissible. Reasons and principles reflecting considered judgments are necessary for moral justification of actions, and there have been no convincing arguments for the claim that neuroscience rules out our ability to make these judgments. Brain scans showing activation in cortical and subcortical regions when individuals are presented with moral dilemmas provide only a first approximation to a moral justification. They are more in the domain of descriptive than normative ethics. Philosophers need to be more attuned to empirical factors describing how people form intuitions that some actions are permissible or impermissible. At the same time, neuroscientists and cognitive psychologists need to be more attuned to how normative factors explain why these actions are permissible or impermissible. Each group needs to inform and be informed by the other.

In a landmark paper cited by several authors in this volume, Adina Roskies distinguished two branches of neuroethics: the ethics of neuroscience; and the neuroscience of ethics (Roskies 2002). While the first involves questions such as how to weigh the benefits and risks of different interventions in the brain, the second involves questions about how the neural substrate grounds moral psychology. To date, there has been more consensus-building in the first, applied, branch of neuroethics than in the second, theoretical, branch. Just as mental processes are best understood not as realizations of localized brain functions but as emergent features of an interconnected set of neural networks, so too will a better understanding of neuroscience and neurophilosophy emerge from professionals of different disciplines working together rather than independently. This model has a medical analog in the field of psychoneuroimmunology, which studies how the brain is influenced by interaction among the mind and the central nervous, endocrine, and immune systems.

As Alexis Jeannotte *et al.* and Robert Blank emphasize, interdisciplinary collaboration should lead to the formulation and implementation of international policies guiding applications of neurotechnology. These policies would go some way toward ensuring the safety and efficacy of this technology in a range of therapeutic uses. Regarding the use of techniques for cognitive enhancement, policies should be formulated in a way that would promote individual liberty without exacerbating social inequality. The international debate should be modeled after the ELSI program (ethical, legal, and social implications) of the Human Genome Project. A valuable product of this debate could be a neuro-ethical analog of the US Genomic Information Nondiscrimination Act (GINA) of 2008. By thinking downstream about the potential effects of neurotechnology, all stakeholders can constructively debate the benefits and risks and reach consensus on how different interventions in the brain can or should be used. We may also speculate on the longer-term possibilities of neurotechnology. Neural prostheses do not just enable people to regain motor control but integrate into their brains. This and other technologies directly affecting the brain may push us to rethink our concept of ourselves as persons or humans and consider whether they are part of an evolution from a human to a posthuman world (Gordijn & Chadwick 2008).

The chapters in this richly textured volume offer fascinating perspectives on multiple dimensions of basic and applied neuroscience. They explore the full range of philosophical, ethical, and social implications of the field and its intersection with radiology, biomedical engineering, and nanotechnology. They capture the excitement and significance of historical, actual, and emerging research in and applications of techniques in brain science, showing how great progress can be made in discussing the key questions along interdisciplinary lines.

REFERENCES

Farah, M. 2005. Neuroethics: the practical and the philosophical. *Trends in Cognitive Sciences* **9**: 34–40.

Gordijn, B. & Chadwick, R. (eds.) 2008. *Medical Enhancement and Posthumanity*. Berlin: Springer.

Greene, J. & Cohen, J. 2004. For the law, neuroscience changes nothing and everything. *Philosophical Transactions of the Royal Society of London* **359**: 1775–85.

Greene, J. & Haidt, J. 2002. How (and where) does moral judgment work? *Trends in Cognitive Sciences* **6**: 517–523.

Kamm, F. M. 2007. *Intricate Ethics*. Oxford: Oxford University Press.

Mele, A. 2009. *Effective Intentions: The Power of Conscious Will*. New York: Oxford University Press.

Roskies, A. 2002. Neuroethics for the new millennium. *Neuron* **35**: 21–3.

Singer, P. 2005. Ethics and intuitions. *The Journal of Ethics* **9**: 331–52.

Wegner, D. 2002. *The Illusion of Conscious Will*. Cambridge, MA: MIT Press.

Index

abortion, cell donation for
    neurotransplantation 194–5
adult stem cells *see* somatic stem cells
    (SSCs)
afterlife, arguments for 15–18
Age of Enlightenment 37–8
AIDS dementia 19
Alzheimer's disease (AD)
    cell therapy 191, 197, 208
    gene therapy 28
    loss of autonomy 141–4
    molecular treatment trial 193
    reactivation of atrophic neurons
        23–5
    use of fMRI 246
amygdala 9, 10, 19, 69, 358
amyotrophic lateral sclerosis (ALS)
    208, 209, 273
anger circuit 69
animal cells *see* xenotransplantation/
    xenografting
anorexia nervosa 19
anterior cingulate gyrus 5, 6
anti-substantialism 100
Arendt, Hannah 141–2
Aristotle 146–7, 166, 168
attention-deficit hyperactivity
    disorder (ADHD) 326, 349
automaticity of actions xvi–xvii
autonomy
    abstract concept 134–5
    and freedom 138–40
    and illness 142–4
    and morality 135
    and rational capacity 135
    and the language of the body 141–4
    anthropological focus 135
    connection with embodiment 136–
        44
    effects of degenerative neurological
        disease 141–4

ethical conception 135
freedom of religion and conscience
    134
history of the concept 134–6
legal–political notion 134
modern concept 135–6
neuroethics of pain care 180–1
of sociopolitical entities 134
origins 134
regulation of choice of actions 135
related to emancipation 134, 135
social aspect 134
view within religious thought 135
    see also moral autonomy
autoscopy 16–17
availability heuristic xvii

bed nucleus of the stria terminalis
    (BSTc) 13–15
behavioral genetics
    consequences of scientific
        reductionism 217–22
    epistemological approaches
        217–22
biases xvii–xviii
bioethics xiv, 350
biofeedback, pain control 5
biological clock 3–4, 20, 21, 25
bodily consciousness 138
brain
    central role 2–3
    computer metaphor 3
    constituents of a theory of the brain
        147–8
    energy requirements 3
    functions of neurons 2–5
    metaphors for 3
    structure and functions 2–5
    see also mind–brain relationship
brain cell culture after death 17, 18,
    25

brain–computer interfaces (BCIs)
  connecting minds 271
  EEG-based interfaces 272–5, 277
  enhancement applications 279
  fMRI 276
  history of BCI research 272–4
  imaging technologies 276
  increasing therapeutic options 285
  invasive technologies 275–6
  lie detection 277–8
  neuroprostheses 272, 276–7
  non-invasive technologies 274–5
  potential ethical considerations
    277–9
  range of applications 276–7
  replacing lost functionality 272,
    273–4, 276–7
  threat to privacy of thought 277–9
  types of brain signals used for
    control 272–6
  virtual worlds 271–2
brain development
  changes during 7–15
  early imprinting 7–8, 10–15
  gender identity 7, 8, 10–15
  genetic influences 7, 8
  influence of the environment
    7–15
  interaction with culture 8
  language 7–8
  loss of ability to change 8–9
  plastic and non-plastic aspects 7–9
  prenatal influences 7
  religious convictions 8
  restrictions caused by organization
    8–9
  sexual differentiation 10–15
  sexual orientation 7, 8
brain disorders
  diagnostic and therapeutic
    developments 18–19
  patient-tailored therapy 20–1
  reactivation of atrophic neurons
    23–5
brain function restoration 25–30
  brain–machine interfaces 26
  see also brain–computer interfaces
  bypassing nervous system damage
    26
  gene therapy 28–9
  intervention neurology 27–8
  neural transplantation 26–7
  neuroprosthetics 26
  repair of local lesions 26–7
  spinal cord injury 29–30
  stem cell therapy 29–30
brain–machine interfaces 26
  see also brain–computer interfaces

brain–mind relationship see mind–
    brain relationship
brain prostheses (BPs) 285
brain research, changing focus 1
brain scans
  desire to use predictively 366–7
  diagnostic potential 18–19
  legitimacy conferred by 365–7
  limits of contribution to self-
    understanding 369
  persuasive effects on those viewing
    them 365–7
  separating science from scientism
    355–6
  see also fMRI; neuroimaging
brain stroke, cell therapy 191, 197,
    208

causality, mind–body relationship
    106–14
cell therapy see neurotransplantation
Center for Neurotechnology Studies
    (CNS), workshops on ELSI and
    public policy 305–17
cerebral characterology 260–1
Chalmers, David, hard problem of
    consciousness 66, 72–7
Churchland, Paul 363–4, 368
clinical practice, influence of
    epistemological approach 222–5
cluster headache 21
cochlear implants 272, 285
cognitive neurobiology
  neural-network models of moral
    cognition 148–70
  reciprocal interaction with moral
    theory 147–8
computer metaphor for the brain 3, 78
computers see brain–computer
    interfaces (BCIs)
Comte, Auguste 37
confirmation bias xvii–xviii
congenital adrenal hyperplasia (CAH)
    13
conscience 136
  and embodiment 138
  and moral capacity 138
consciousness
  advent of 114–15
  as a field phenomenon 109
  evolution of 102–3, 110, 112,
    114–15
  mind as 96
  self-organization theory 80–91
  see also hard problem of
    consciousness
consciousness studies
  emergentism 62

historical influences on current
debate 50–60
implications for neuroethics 62–3
influences on postmodern thinking
50–60
insights from the history of ideas
60–3
study of altered states 49–50
use of metaphors from
contemporary technology 61
see also mind, theories of
consent
cell donation from abortion 195
human blastocyst donation 196–7
neurological patients 206–7, 209–10
policy issues in brain interventions
324
consequentialism xx
cranial electrotherapy stimulation
(CES) 284
criminal behavior, and brain disorders
19
critical window concept in
development 1
culture, interaction with brain
development 8
cyberthink 289, 296
``cyborgization´´ (machine interfacing)
of the human body 179
cytoarchitechtonics 261

DARPA, brain–machine interface
program 286
Decade of Pain Control and Research
(2000–2010) xxix
Decade of the Brain (1990–2000) xxv,
xxix
Decade of the Mind project xxix, 306,
319, 345
deep brain stimulation (DBS) 21–2,
284
degenerative neurological disease,
loss of autonomy 141–4
deontology xix, xx
depression
risk factors 20
treatment of 20–1
use of deep brain stimulation 22
depth psychology 97
Descartes, René 2, 97, 100, 101, 106,
109
diagnoscopy 259
Diagnostic and Statistical Manual
(fifth edition) 345
disease, definition 226, 348–9
donor consent
cell donation from abortion 195
human blastocysts 196–7

Dostoevsky, Fyodor 16
drug treatments, causal
interpretations 220–2
dystonia 21

Eccles, John 100
ECoG (electrocorticogram) 275
EEG (electroencephalography) 245,
259–60
EEG-based BCIs 272–5, 277
EEG studies, influence on theories of
consciousness 78
embodiment
and autonomy 136–44
and conscience 138
and personal identity 136–8
language of the body 141–4
embryonic germ cells 192
embryonic stem cells (ESCs) 191, 192–
3
neurotransplantation 29–30, 191,
196–8
emergentism 62, 223
empiricism
controversy with idealism 38, 41–4
debate on limits of 42–4
encapsulated cells, use in
neurotransplantation 193
enhancement
policy issues 326
use of BCIs 279
see also neural engineering;
treatment–enhancement
debate
epilepsy
and religious experiences 15–16
cell therapy 191, 208
epiphenomenalism 107, 112–13, 114
epistemic crisis xxvii–xxviii
epistemological approaches
behavioral genetics 217–22
emergentist framework 223
ethical consequences 222–5
influence on clinical practice 222–5
interpretation of biological
causality 222–3
pharmacogenomics 217–22
scientific reductionism 217–22
epistemological (good, valid) version
of the hard problem 73–7
ethical implications of neuroscience
323
ethical, legal, and social implications
(ELSI) of neurotechnology 303–19
ethics of neurogenetics 225–7
ethics of neuroscience xvi–xxi, 323
ethics of practice 323
eugenics 261

event-related desynchronization BCIs
    273, 274–5
evolution of consciousness 102–3,
    110, 112, 114–15
existential view of human life 141
experimental psychology
    founding of 39–41, 47
    Wundt's restrictions on scope 49–50
experimental spiritism 38
explanation by correlation, avoiding
    68–70, 80
explanatory gap argument 73, 74, 75,
    104
explanatory reduction 364

Fechner, Gustav 40, 43, 44, 45
Flanagan, Owen 166, 169
fMRI (functional magnetic resonance
    imaging)
    BOLD (blood oxygenation level
       dependent) contrast method
       232, 245
    brain scanning 3, 5
    comparison method 231
    data processing 245
    discovery 245
    indirect measurement of neuronal
       activity 231–2
    limitations of functional imaging
       360–2
    non-quantitative nature 231
    raw images produced by scanning
       231–3
    scanning technique 231–3
    spatial resolution of raw data
       232–3
    temporal resolution of raw data
       232–3
    typical experimental method 245–6
fMRI applications
    clinical applications 246–9
    commercial use in lie detection
       237–9
    detection of consciousness in brain
       injury 247, 248–9, 253
    ethical and scientific concerns
       236–41
    ``instant science'' versus
       peer-review 239–40
    lie detection 249–50
    neuromarketing 240–1
    persuasive power of images 230–1
    prediction of political preference
       240–1
    prediction of preferences in
       marketing 239–40
    presentation of results in the media
       230–1, 237–41

presurgical mapping of brain
    function 246, 247–8
fMRI-based BCIs 276
fMRI constraints and limitations 231
    comparison of signals from
       different tasks 235–6
    effects of data processing 233–5
    effects of the experimental design
       237
    factors affecting the BOLD signal
       237
    subtraction method 236, 360–2
    timescale disconnect 362
fMRI data processing 233–6
    data preprocessing 233–4
    generation of pictures showing
       areas of activation 235
    group-based analysis 235
    motion correction (realignment)
       233–4
    multiple comparisons problem
       235
    spatial normalization 234
    statistical analysis 234–5
fMRI interpretation
    deriving meaning from signals
       250–2
    equating structure and function
       252–3
    experimental design and task
       selection 253–4
    neuro-essentialism 256–8
    neuro-policy 257, 260–2
    neuro-realism 257, 258–60
    neuroethical challenge 250–62
    neuroethical responsibilities 262–5
    popular portrayal as mind-reading
       258–62
    scientific interpretation 250–6
    social and cultural interpretations
       256–62
    statistical analysis of fMRI
       data 254–6
fMRI research
    investigation of brain function 246
    social and policy implications 246
fMRI studies
    avoiding explanation by correlation
       68–9
    cortical bias 78–80
    influence on theories of
       consciousness 78–80
    insensitivity to timing 79
Fodor, Jerry 356, 363
freedom
    and autonomy 138–40
    law of 139
    situated freedom 138–40

Freud, Sigmund 15
functionalist versions of physicalism
    104–5

gender identity and brain
    development 7, 8, 10–15
gene therapy, brain function
    restoration 28–9
genethics 338–9
genetic determinism in research
    217–22
genetic factors in susceptibility to
    pain syndromes 174–5
genetic testing
    ethical issues in data interpretation
        222–5
    ethics of pre-symptomatic testing
        224–5
    potential consequences for
        individuals 224–5
genetics
    policy-making 338–9
    use of neurogenetic information
        183
Geschwind syndrome 16
glial celline-derived neurotrophic
    factor (GDNF) treatment 28–9
glial precursor cells,
    neurotransplantation 193
government involvement in
    neuroscience, range of options
        328–30

hard problem of consciousness 66
    avoiding explanation by correlation
        68–70, 80
    epistemological (good, valid)
        version 73–7
    ``explanatory gap´´ argument 73, 74,
        75
    influence of available
        instrumentation 78–80
    ``knowledge argument´´ of
        consciousness 71, 77, 81, 83, 86
    Kuhnian paradigm shifts 78
    mental causation problem 71–2,
        86
    multiple realizability problem 77
    ontological (bad, invalid) version 73,
        74, 75, 76–7
    philosophical paradoxes 70–2
    practical implications 67–70
    search for a general theory of
        consciousness 78–80
    self-organization theory of
        consciousness 80–91
    sources of bias in research 78–80
    two hard problem arguments 72–7

hard problems of neuroscience
    xxvi
health care, ethical use of scientific
    understanding 225–7
heart, and emotions 5–6
Hegel, Georg Wilhelm Friedrich
    139–40
Heidegger, Martin 60
Helmholtz, Hermann von 40, 43–4,
    47, 48
heuristics xvii
higher-level phenomena, explanation
    of 364–5
hippocampus, artificial 285
Hippocrates 2
Hobbes, Thomas 165
homosexuality, and brain
    development 12
human blastocysts, use in
    neurotransplantation 196–8
human condition
    criteria for identifying psychiatric
        disease 348–51
    criteria for normality 348–51
    definition of disease and illness
        348–9
    striving for improvement 343–5
    treatment–enhancement debate
        344–51
Human Genome Project, ELSI
    research 305
human identity see identity; personal
    identity
Huntington´s disease (HD) 27, 191,
    208–9, 210, 211
Huxley, Thomas H. 112
hypothalamic paraventricular
    nucleus 20
hypothalamo-neurohypophysial
    system 20
hypothalamo-pituitary-adrenal (HPA)
    axis 20

``I´´, relationship to the physical brain
    55–60
idealism, controversy with
    empiricism 38, 41–4
identity
    and embodiment 136–8
    and illness 142–4
    see also personal identity
identity theory 102, 105–6, 113
illness, definition 226, 348–9
in vitro fertilization (IVF) treatment,
    donation of surplus blastocysts
    196–8
information-gulping sixth sense 288,
    291–2

informed consent
    cell donation from abortion 195
    human blastocyst donation 196–7
    neurological patients 206–7,
        209–10
    policy issues in brain interventions
        324
interactionism 107, 114
interiority
    and embodiment 136–7
    and personal identity 141
    human capacity for 141, 144
    use of imagination and metaphors
        141–4
international neuroethics policy
    337–8
Internet 271, 278
intervention neurology 27–8

Joan of Arc 16
John Paul II, Pope 139
Johnson, Mark 166
Jonas, Hans 137

Kant, Immanuel xix, 135, 139, 165
Kantian philosophy, influence on
    theories of mind 41–3
``knowledge argument'' of
    consciousness 71, 77, 81, 83, 86
Kuhn, Thomas xxviii
Kuhnian revolutions in the
    philosophy of mind 74, 78

language development 7–8
LBS neurons (Layton BioScience
    neurons) 193
lie detection 327
    and psychological modularity
        358–9, 362
    EDA (electrodermal activity)
        measurement 277–8
    use of neuroimaging 358–9
localization of cognitive processes
    356–60
locked-in syndrome 273, 285

machine interfacing (``cyborgization'')
    of the human body 183
    see also brain–computer interfaces
        (BCIs)
MacIntyre, Alasdair 166–9, 356
maldynia 176–7
McGinn, Colin 55, 56, 58
media portrayal of scientific research
    327
MEG (magnetoencephalography) 245,
    275, 277
Meinhof, Ulrike 9

memory, unreliability of xvii–xviii
mental causation problem 71–2, 86,
    110–14
mental functions
    distributed nature 357–8, 361–2
    gap between the knowable and the
        known 362–4
    limitations of functional imaging
        360–2
    localization thesis 356–60
    modular theory 356–60
    subtraction method of processing
        brain scans 360–2
mental health
    conceptions of 225–7
    ethics of neurogenetics 225–7
metaethics, reciprocal interaction
    with cognitive neurobiology
    147–8
microarray techniques 19
mind
    as product of the brain 3, 5
    taxonomies of 356–60
    versus soul 15–18
mind–body issue
    advent of consciousness 114–15
    anti-substantialism 100
    causal relations 106–14
    causality question 98–9
    consciousness as a field
        phenomenon 109
    epiphenomenalism 107, 112–13,
        114
    evolution of consciousness 102–3,
        110, 112, 114–15
    functionalist versions of
        physicalism 104–5
    identity theory 102, 105–6, 113
    interactionism 107, 114
    interpretation of correlations
        98–9
    mental causation dilemmas
        110–14
    mind as consciousness 96
    nature of the problem 95–9
    non-reductive physicalism 102, 103
    ontological question 97–8, 99
    panpsychism 102
    parallelism 107
    phenomena of depth psychology
        97
    physicalism 103–6, 110–11, 113
    property dualism 101–3, 114
    pros and cons of dualism 99–103
    reductive physicalism 103–4
    soul 97–8, 99–101
    substance dualism (substantialism)
        95, 99–101

supervenience relations 98–9, 113
unconscious or subconscious states
    97
mind–brain relationship
  ethics of neurogenetics 225–7
  limit of contribution from brain
    scans 369
  relevance of ordinary experience
    368–9
mind control 296–7, 325
mind–matter relation, history of
    debate 55–60
mind-merging 289
mind, theories of
  consequences of Kantian
    philosophy 41–3
  controversy between idealism and
    empiricism 38, 41–4
  debate on limits of empiricism
    42–4
  dispute on spiritism (Leipzig 1877)
    44–7
  emergentism 62
  experimental spiritism 38
  historical influences on current
    debate 50–60
  implications for neuroethics
    62–3
  implications of non-Euclidean
    geometry 42–4
  influences on postmodern thinking
    50–60
  insights from the history of ideas
    60–3
  nineteenth century controversies
    41–50
  psychophysical parallelism 50, 55
  psychophysiological theory 38, 40
  rational empiricism 38
  rise of rational and scientific
    concepts 37–8
  separation of psychology and
    philosophy 37–8
  use of metaphors from
    contemporary technology 61
  Wundt´s rejection of spiritism
    46–9
minimally conscious patients, use of
    fMRI 247, 248–9, 253
modular theory of mind 356–62
molecular replacement,
    neurotransplantation 193
molecular treatment,
    neurotransplantation 193
moral ambiguity, neural-network
    model 155
moral argument, neural-network
    model 156

moral autonomy, effects of personal
    maturation 141
  see also autonomy
moral character, neural-network
    model 157–8
moral cognition, developments in
    understanding 146–7
moral cognitive phenomena, neural-
    network models 148–70
moral conflict, neural-network model
    155–6
moral correction, neural-network
    model 160–3
moral deliberation, threats
    from sciences of the mind
    xviii–xxi
moral diversity, neural-network
    model 163
moral knowledge, neural-network
    model 149–53
moral learning, neural-network
    model 153–4
moral pathology, neural-network
    model 158–60
moral perception, neural-network
    model 154–5
moral progress
  comparison with scientific progress
    166–70
  neural-network model 163–5
moral theory, reciprocal interaction
    with cognitive neurobiology
    147–8
moral unity/systematicity, neural-
    network model 165–6
moral virtues, neural-network model
    156–7
MRI scans, diagnostic potential
    18–19
  see also fMRI
multiple realization 106
multiple realizability problem of
    consciousness 77
multiple sclerosis (MS) 21, 29, 191,
    197, 208
multiple systemic atrophy (MSA) 191

NASA, extension of human senses
    program 286
National Nanotechnology Initiative,
    ELSI research 305
National Neurotechnology Initiative
    (NNTI) 319
NBIC (nano-bio-info-cogno)
    convergence 287, 288
near-death experiences 16–18
nerve growth factor (NGF) gene
    therapy 28

neural engineering
    brain–computer interfaces (BCIs)
        285
    brain prostheses (BPs) 285
    converging technologies 287
    cranial electrotherapy stimulation
        (CES) 284
    deep brain stimulation (DBS) 284
    developing field of research 283–4
    enhancing desirable traits 286–7
    increasing therapeutic options 284–
        5
    NBIC (nano-bio-info-cogno)
        convergence 287, 288
    neural prostheses (NPs) 285
    scope of research 283–4
    transcranial magnetic stimulation
        (TMS) 284
neural engineering future prospects
    287–90
    challenge to personal identity 295
    cyberthink 289, 296
    disconnection from real life 297–9
    effects on personal authenticity
        294–5
    ethical challenges of enhancement
        290–9
    improvement of cognitive abilities
        289
    improvement of mood and
        vegetative functions 289–90
    improvement of motor abilities
        288–9
    improvement of sensory abilities
        288
    memory enhancement 289
    mind control potential 296–7
    mind-merging 289
    potential demand for
        enhancements 290
    pressures for limitless
        enhancement 293–4
    privacy of personal information
        295–6
    proportionality between benefits
        and risks 291–2
    shift from therapy to enhancement
        287–8
    social justice and the "neurodivide"
        292–3
    surveillance monopolies 296
    threat to autonomy 297
    transparency in society 295–6
    virtual experience machine 297–9
neural grafting see neurotransplanta-
    tion
neural-network models of cognition
    148–70

moral ambiguity 155
moral argument 156
moral character 157–8
moral conflict 155–6
moral correction 160–3
moral diversity 163
moral knowledge 149–53
moral learning 153–4
moral pathology 158–60
moral perception 154–5
moral progress 163–5
moral unity/systematicity 165–6
moral virtues 156–7
scope of application 149
virtue ethics 166–70
neural prostheses (NPs) 285
neural tissue implantation see neuro-
    transplantation
neural transplantation see neuro-
    transplantation
neuro-essentialism 256–8
neuro-realism 257, 258–60
neuro-talk
    and psychological modularity 358
    separating science from scientism
        355–6
    use of brain scans to support
        355–6
neuroethics
    branches of xiv–xxi
    definition xxvi
    development of the discipline
        xxv–xviii
    drawing together science and
        philosophy xiii
    implications of the debate on
        consciousness 62–3
    links with neuropolicy 323–4
    origin of the term xxvi
    structure and functions xxvi–xxvii
neuroethics agenda see neuropolicy
    making
Neuroethics, Legal, and Social Issues
    (NELSI) initiative 306
neuroethics of pain care 172
    access to new treatments 183–4
    capacities and limitations of
        neuroimaging 182
    caring for vulnerable individuals
        180–1
    consistency with scientific and
        ethical traditions 180
    ethical issues 180–2
    integrative approach 185
    machine interfacing
        ("cyborgization") 183
    nature of "good" pain care 181–2,
        185

neural stem cell research 183
neural transplantation 183
pain in non-human animals
    181
prudent use of scientific knowledge
    184-5
purpose and potential 180-2
questions which it should address
    184-5
respect for autonomy 180-1
threshold for intervention 182
treatment decisions 183-4
use of neurogenetic information
    183
Neuroethics Society 339
neurogenetic data
    ethical issues concerning
        interpretation 222-5
    support for ``disease´´ model of pain
        222-3
neurogenetic testing
    ethical issues in data interpretation
        222-5
    ethics of pre-symptomatic testing
        224-5
    potential consequences for
        individuals 224-5
neurogenetics
    consequences of scientific
        reductionism 217-22
    ethics of neurogenetics 225-7
    explaining phenomenal aspects of
        disease 225-7
    limitations of a reductive approach
        225-7
neuroimaging
    capacities and limitations 182
    desire to use predictively 366-7
    history of development 245
    interpretation of brain images
        356-60
    legitimacy conferred by brain scans
        365-7
    lie detection 358-9
    limits of contribution to self-
        understanding 369
    persuasive effects of brain scans
        365-7
    popular portrayal as mind-reading
        244
    use in psychology 356
    see also brain scans; fMRI; PET;
        SPECT
neuroimaging research
    civic and democratic responsibility
        263-4
    critical and constructive self-
        reflection 265

deriving meaning from signals 250-2
equating structure and function
    252-3
experimental design and task
    selection 253-4
need for responsiveness to inform
    the public 262-3
neuro-essentialism 256-8
neuro-policy 257, 260-2
neuro-realism 257, 258-60
neuroethical challenge of
    interpretation 250-62
neuroethical responsibilities
    262-5
popular portrayal as mind-reading
    258-62
prospective responsibility 264-5
responsibility for prospective uses
    264-5
scientific interpretation 250-6
social and cultural interpretations
    256-62
statistical analysis of data 254-6
neuromarketing 327
neuronal Darwinism 7, 8
neurons
    functions 2-5
    reactivation of atrophic neurons
        23-5
neurophilosophy 368
    of pain 172, 178-80
neuropolicy 257, 260-2
    dimensions 327-30
    government involvement 328-30
    issues of brain intervention 324-7
    links with neuroethics 323-4
neuropolicy making
    agenda-setting stage 330-4
    fragmented nature of the process
        334-5
    international neuroethics policy
        337-8
    lessons from genethics and genetic
        policy 338-9
    role of expert input 335-7
    stages of policy making 330-2
neuroprostheses 26, 272, 276-7
neuropsychological foundation for
    pain 173
neuroscience
    challenges to the sense of self
        125-32
    implications of technologies
        xiv-xvi
    limits to knowing others´ pain
        178-9
    unbalanced view of the human
        condition 140-1

neuroscience of ethics xvi, 323
neuroscience of pain, heuristic value
    174–6
neuroscientific developments
    brain function restoration 25–30
    brain structure and functions 2–5
    central role of the brain 2–3
    changing focus of brain research 1
    computer metaphor for the
        brain 3
    deep brain stimulation 21–2
    development of the brain 7–15
    early imprinting of the brain 7–8,
        10–15
    mechanisms of placebo effects
        22–3
    metaphors for the brain 3
    patient-tailored therapy 20–1
    questions arising from 136
    reactivation of atrophic neurons
        23–5
    restorative neuroscience 25–30
    sexual differentiation of the brain
        10–15
neurotechnology as a public good
    achieving widely supported public
        policy 303–19
    ethical, legal, and social
        implications (ELSI) 303–19
    framework for future studies of
        ELSI 317–19
    mapping the path forward 317–19
    need for evaluation and guidance
        processes 302–3
    workshops on ELSI and public
        policy 305–17
neurotheology 136
neurotherapy, diagnostic and
    therapeutic developments
    18–19
neurotransplantation 26–7, 183
    abortion and the separation
        principle 194–5
    animal cells 193, 198–9
    autologous hESCs 198
    clinical trials in humans 190–1
    consent for cell donation 195
    definition 191
    difficulty of obtaining cells for
        transplantation 192
    donation of in vitro human
        blastocysts 196–8
    embryonic stem cells (ESCs) 191,
        196–8
    encapsulated cells 193
    ethical debate 191
    ethical guidance for retrieval of
        cells 194–9

glial precursor cells 193
    human embryonic or fetal cells
        192–4
    see also stem cells
    molecular replacement 193
    molecular treatment 193
    neural autografts 193
    non-reproductive creation of the
        human blastocyst 197–8
    range of treatment approaches 192
    retrieval of primary cells 194–5
    somatic stem cells (SSCs) 197–8,
        200
    stem cells 191, 192–4, 196–8
    substantia nigra cells 190–1, 192
    types of cell implant 192–4
    viral vector-mediated gene transfer
        198
    xenograft tissue sources 198–9
    xenotransplantation 193
neurotransplantation clinical trials
    202–10
    applicability of animal results to
        humans 202–4
    clinical trial design 204–5
    core assessment protocol (CAP)
        207–9
    defined target for the intervention
        203–4
    ethics of placebo control treatments
        204–7
    informed consent 206–7, 209–10
    irreversible nature of treatment
        202, 204
    justification for human trials
        202–4
    patient expectations 206–7
    role of animal experimentation
        203–4
    sham surgery as control 205–7
    vulnerability of patients 206–7,
        209–10
neurotransplantation risks
    cancer risk 199–200
    genetic quality of implanted cells
        199
    microbiological safety of implanted
        cells 199
    personality effects 200–1
    physiological and behavioral side
        effects 200
    psychic effects 200–1
    surgical risks 199–200
    transfer of psychic elements 202
    weighing against benefits 199–202
    xenografts 202, 211
NIRS (near infrared spectroscopy)
    275

non-reductive physicalism 102, 103
normality, criteria for 348–51

obesity 22
obsessive–compulsive disorder (OCD)
    22
ontological reduction 364
ontological (bad, invalid) version of
    the hard problem 73, 74, 75,
    76–7
out-of-body experiences 16–17

P300 wave-driven BCIs 272–3, 275
pain
    approach to pain research 177–8
    as a spectrum disorder 174, 176
    boundaries of objective information
        179
    classification schemes 174
    cognitive effects of persistent pain
        175
    complex nature of 173–4
    definitions of maldynia 176–7
    effects on the brain and mind 175
    embodiment 173–4
    experiential dimension 173–4
    imperative to evaluate and treat
        179–80
    in non-human organisms 179–80,
        181
    individuality of experience 178–9
    internal and external influences
        177–8
    neuropsychological foundation
        173
    objective explanation 173–4
    relating explanation to experience
        178
    source of the feeling of pain 175–6
    subjective understanding 173–4
    uncertainty of others' subjective
        experience 179
    unique individual experience 175–6
    see also neuroethics of pain care
pain control using biofeedback 5
pain disorders, implications of genetic
    test data 222–5
pain medicine, causal interpretations
    of drug treatments 220–2
pain relief, deep brain stimulation 21
pain research
    consequences of scientific
        reductionism 217–22
    ``disease'' model 222–3
    genetic determinism 217–22
    ``illness'' model 222
    value of integrative pain research
        177–8

pain syndromes, genetic susceptibility
    174–5
pain therapeutics
    approaches to the study of pain
        173–4
    assessment of pain 178–9
    consilience of science and
        philosophy 173
    imperative for right and good care
        172
    imperative to evaluate and treat
        179–80
    limits to knowing others' pain
        178–9
    reciprocity between science and
        philosophy 173
panpsychism 102
parallelism 107
paralysed patients, use of BCIs 273–4,
    276–7, 285
paraventricular nucleus 20
Parkinson's disease (PD)
    clinical trials of neural grafting (cell
        therapy) 190–1, 192
    deep brain stimulation 21
    developments in treatment 19
    GDNF treatment trials 28–9
    gene therapy 28–9
    neurotransplantation interventions
        26–7, 190–1, 194, 197, 201,
        207–9, 211
    placebo effects 22–3
patient-tailored therapy for brain
    disorders 20–1
Paul (apostle) 16
personal identity
    challenges for neuroscience 120–2
    challenges from emerging
        neuroscience 125–32
    definition 122
    importance in the modern age
        119–22
    influence of the modern context
        119–22
    manipulation of 130
    nature of 117–18
    scientific view 120–1
    web of relations 122
PET (positron emission tomography)
    244, 245, 251 see also
    neuroimaging
pharmacogenomics
    consequences of scientific
        reductionism 217–22
    epistemological approaches 217–22
philosophy-science separation xiii
phrenology 260
physicalism 103–6, 110–11, 113

Pinker, Steven 55, 56, 58, 362
placebo effect, neurobiological
    mechanisms 22–3
Plato 95, 97
policy dimensions of neuroscience
    327–30
    ethical, legal, and social
        implications (ELSI) of
        neurotechnology 303–19
    governmental response to
        developments 328–30
    individual use of technologies 328
    neuroethics and public policy
        323–4
    regulatory policy 329–30
    research and development of
        technologies 328
    societal consequences of
        widespread application 328
policy issues of brain intervention
    324–7
    access to services 325–6
    commercial uses of cognitive
        neuroscience 327
    discrimination and stigmatization
        325
    distinction between
        experimentation and therapy
        324–5
    freedom and equality issues 327
    individual responsibility 325
    informed consent 324
    lie detection 327
    media portrayal of scientific
        research 327
    mind control 325
    nature of information to be
        collected 327
    neuromarketing 327
    overall contribution to health
        outcomes 326
    priority in relation to other health
        care areas 326
    risks and uncertainties 324–5
    social advantage from
        enhancement 326
    specific treatment issues 326
    use in non-medical, commercial
        settings 325
    use of information that is collected
        327
    vulnerability of patients 324–5
policy-making process
    agenda-setting stage 330–4
    fragmented nature of the process
        334–5
    international neuroethics policy
        337–8

lessons from genethics and genetic
    policy 338–9
role of expert input 335–7
stages of policy making 330–2
post-traumatic tremor 21
primary cells, retrieval for
    neurotransplantation 194–5
privacy of thought 277–9
property dualism 101–3, 114
proteomics, use in brain disorders 19
psychiatric disease, criteria for
    identifying 348–51
psychiatry, use of deep brain
    stimulation 22
psychology
    explanation of higher-level
        phenomena 364–5
    localization of cognitive processes
        356–60
    modular theory of mind 356–60
    reductive materialism 364–5,
        367–8
    rise of academic psychology 37–8
    separation from philosophy 37–8
    taxonomies of mind 356–60
    use of neuroimaging 356
psychophysical parallelism 50, 55
psychophysiological theory 38, 40
public policy *see* policy

rational empiricism 38
rational enquiry, threat from sciences
    of the mind xvi–xviii
Rawls 165
recovered memories, unreliability
    xvii–xviii
reductionism *see* scientific
    reductionism
reductive materialism in psychology
    364–5, 367–8
reductive physicalism 103–4
reflexivity 136
religion
    and autonomy 134, 135
    contemporary renaissance 58–9
religious convictions, and brain
    development 8
religious experiences, and temporal
    lobe epilepsy 15–16
research bias, sources of 78–80
restorative neuroscience 25–30
retinal implants 272, 285

schizophrenia, causes and treatments
    19
Schrödinger, Erwin 102
science–philosophy separation xiii
scientific reductionism

bias caused by methodology 217–22
brain–mind relationship 225–7
conflation of illness and disease 226
confusing description and explanation 218–22
consequences in behavioral genetics 217–22
consequences in pharmacogenomics 217–22
ethical implications 220–2
scientism, separating science from 355–6
self
    articulacy 123
    challenges for neuroscience 120–2
    challenges from emerging neuroscience 125–32
    commitments which shape personhood 123
    embodiment 122
    features of a plausible view of 122–5
    importance in the modern age 119–22
    influence of the modern context 119–22
    justifiable appropriation claim 122
    manipulation of 130
    multidimensionality 122
    nature of 117–18
    reflective stance 123–4
    reflexivity 123
    relationship to the physical brain 55–60
    scientific view 120–1
    search for 2
    self-distancing relationship 123–4
    sense of see interiority
self-organization theory of consciousness 80–91
self-understanding
    limit of contribution from brain scans 369
    relevance of ordinary experience 368–9
sensory/motor (SMR) and mu-rhythm-driven BCIs 273, 274–5
separation principle
    cell donation from abortion 195
    cell donation from IVF programs 196–7
serotonergic function, interpretation of genetic data 218, 219
sexual differentiation of the brain 10–15

gender identity 7, 8, 10–15
homosexuality 12
influence of testosterone 10–11
sexual orientation 7, 8, 10–15
transsexuality 12–15
sexual orientation, and brain development 7, 8, 10–15
situated freedom 138–40
Slade, Henry 45–7
slow cortical potentials (SCP), use in BCIs 273, 274
somatic cell nuclear transfer (SCNT) 197
somatic stem cells (SSCs) 193, 197–8, 200
soul
    and the mind-body issue 97–8, 99–101
    search for evidence 15–18
SPECT (single photon emission computed tomography) 245, 261, 262
spinal cord injury 277
    cell therapy 191
    experimental repair strategies 29–30
spiritism 44–9
stem cell therapy 29–30
    cancer risk 199–200
stem cells
    cloning in the laboratory 192
    embryonic germ cells 192
    embryonic stem cells (ESCs) 191, 192–3
    genetic quality 199–200
    microbiological safety 199
    neural stem cell research 183
    neurotransplantation 191, 192–4, 196–8
    retrieval for neurotransplantation 196–8
    somatic stem cells (SSCs) 193, 197–8, 200
    sources of 192–3
stroke 27–8, 191, 197, 208
subconscious states 97
substance dualism (substantialism) 95, 99–101
substantia nigra cells, neurotransplantation 190–1, 192
suprachiasmatic nucleus (biological clock) 3–4, 20, 21, 25
synapses in the brain 3

tabula rasa theory of the newborn 8, 11
tardive dyskinesia 21
taxonomies of mind 356–60

technology, metaphors for
  interpreting consciousness 61
testosterone, influence on the
  developing brain 10–11
therapeutic cloning 197
thought, product of the brain 3, 5
Thought-Translation-Device (TTD)
  273, 274
tinnitus in deaf patients 19
Tourette syndrome 21
transcranial magnetic stimulation
  (TMS) 284
transplantation *see*
  neurotransplantation
transsexuality, and brain
  development 12–15
treatment–enhancement debate
  criteria for identifying psychiatric
    disease 348–51
  criteria for normality 348–51
  culture and social conventions 344–8
  definition of disease and illness
    348–9
  human striving for improvement
    343–5
tremor, use of deep brain
  stimulation 21

unconscious states 97
Uttal, William 357–8, 362

Van Gogh, Vincent 16
vegetative state patients, use of fMRI
  247, 248–9, 253
viral vector-mediated gene transfer
  198
virtue ethics 166–70

Wittgenstein, Ludwig 100, 182
Wundt, Wilhelm
  founding of experimental
    psychology 39–41, 47
  psychophysical parallelism 50, 55
  rejection of spiritism 46–9
  restricted scope of experimental
    psychology 49–50
  view on altered states of
    consciousness 49–50

xenotransplantation/xenografting
  193, 202, 211
  guidelines for tissue retrieval 198–9
  tissue sources 198–9

Zöllner, Johann 40, 43, 44, 45–7